ADVANCED MEDICINE RECALL

RECALL SERIES EDITOR

Lorne H. Blackbourne, MD, FACS
Trauma, Burn, and Critical Care Surgeon
San Antonio, Texas

ADVANCED MEDICINE
RECALL

Editor

James D. Bergin, MD
Professor of Medicine
Division of Cardiovascular Medicine
University of Virginia Health System
Charlottesville, Virginia

 Wolters Kluwer | Lippincott Williams & Wilkins
Health

Philadelphia • Baltimore • New York • London
Buenos Aires • Hong Kong • Sydney • Tokyo

Acquisitions Editor: Donna Balado
Managing Editor: Kelley Squazzo
Marketing Manager: Emilie Moyer
Production Editor: Eve Malakoff-Klein
Designer: Teresa Mallon
Compositor: Aptara, Inc.

Library of Congress Cataloging-in-Publication Data

Advanced medicine recall / editor, James D. Bergin.
    p. ; cm.
  Includes index.
  ISBN-13: 978-0-7817-7629-5
  ISBN-10: 0-7817-7629-5
  1. Internal medicine—Examinations, questions, etc.   2. Internal medicine—Outlines, syllabi, etc.   I. Bergin, James D.
  [DNLM: 1. Medicine—Examination Questions. WB 18.2 A2445 2009]
  RC58.A34 2009
  616.0076—dc22

2008003943

DISCLAIMER

Care has been taken to confirm the accuracy of the information present and to describe generally accepted practices. However, the authors, editors, and publisher are not responsible for errors or omissions or for any consequences from application of the information in this book and make no warranty, expressed or implied, with respect to the currency, completeness, or accuracy of the contents of the publication. Application of this information in a particular situation remains the professional responsibility of the practitioner; the clinical treatments described and recommended may not be considered absolute and universal recommendations.

The authors, editors, and publisher have exerted every effort to ensure that drug selection and dosage set forth in this text are in accordance with the current recommendations and practice at the time of publication. However, in view of ongoing research, changes in government regulations, and the constant flow of information relating to drug therapy and drug reactions, the reader is urged to check the package insert for each drug for any change in indications and dosage and for added warnings and precautions. This is particularly important when the recommended agent is a new or infrequently employed drug.

Some drugs and medical devices presented in this publication have Food and Drug Administration (FDA) clearance for limited use in restricted research settings. It is the responsibility of the health care provider to ascertain the FDA status of each drug or device planned for use in their clinical practice.

To purchase additional copies of this book, call our customer service department at **(800) 638-3030** or fax orders to **(301) 223-2320**. International customers should call **(301 223-2300**.

Visit Lippincott Williams & Wilkins on the Internet: http://www.lww.com. Lippincott Williams & Wilkins customer service representatives are available from 8:30 am to 6:00 pm, EST.

Contents

Contributors

EDITOR

James D. Bergin, MD
Professor of Medicine

ASSOCIATE EDITOR

Amy West, MD
Chief Medical Resident

ALLERGY AND IMMUNOLOGY

Jeffrey Culp, MD
Fellow, Division of Allergy
and Immunology

Sean R. Lucas, MD, MPH
Clinical Instructor of Medicine

CARDIOLOGY

Kavita Sharma
Medical student, class of 2007

Matthew Trojan, MD
Clinical Instructor of Medicine

James D. Bergin, MD
Professor of Medicine

ENDOCRINOLOGY

Sacchin Majumdar, MD
Resident, Department of Internal
Medicine

Shetal Padia, MD
Fellow, Division of Endocrinology

Alan Dalkin, MD
Associate Professor of Medicine

GASTROENTEROLOGY

Kavita Sharma
Medical student, class of 2007

Josh Hall, MD
Resident, Department of Medicine

Vanessa Shami, MD
Assistant Professor of Medicine

HEMATOLOGY

Christine Lin, MD
Resident, Department of Medicine

David Mack, MD
Fellow, Division of Hematology

Gail Macik, MD
Associate Professor of Medicine
and Pathology

INFECTIOUS DISEASE

Tedra M. Claytor, MD
Fellow, Division of Infectious
Disease

Brian Wispelwey, MS, MD
Professor of Medicine

NEPHROLOGY

Joshua King, MD
Resident, Department of Medicine

Melisha Bissram, MD
Fellow, Division of Nephrology

Mitch Rosner, MD
Assistant Professor of Medicine

ONCOLOGY

Heather West, MD
Fellow, Division of Hematology
and Oncology

Heidi Gillenwater, MD
Assistant Professor of Medicine

PULMONOLOGY

Brian Hanrahan, MD
Resident, Department of Medicine

Steven Koenig, MD
Professor of Medicine

RHEUMATOLOGY

Ashok Jacob, MD
Fellow, Division of Rheumatology

Wael Jarjour, MD
Associate Professor of Medicine

DERMATOLOGY

Rebecca Rudd Barry, MD
Resident, Department of
Dermatology

R. Carter Grine, MD
Resident, Department of
Dermatology

Barbara Braunstein Wilson, MD
Associate Professor of Dermatology

ENVIRONMENTAL MEDICINE

Barbara Wiggins, PharmD

James D. Bergin, MD
Professor of Medicine

NEUROLOGY

Lee Kubersky, MD
Resident, Department of Neurology

Barnett R. Nathan, MD
Associate Professor of Neurology

Russell H. Swerdlow, MD
Associate Professor of Neurology

Nathan B. Fountain, MD
Associate Professor of Neurology

PHARMACOLOGY

Barbara Wiggins, PharmD

James D. Bergin, MD
Professor of Medicine

PSYCHIATRY

Kurt Miceli, MD
Resident, Department of Psychiatry

Suzanne Holroyd, MD
Professor of Medicine

THE CONSULTANT

James D. Bergin, MD
Professor of Medicine

Acknowledgments

I would like to recognize the hard work of the current authors as well as the contributions from the previous authors whose efforts we have built upon.

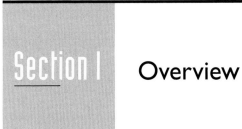

Section I   Overview

Chapter 1

Introduction

A few years ago it was clear that *Medicine Recall* was becoming too large a book to be easily carried around. Feedback from medical students included comments that their coat pockets were being stretched and that they were leaning to one side. We therefore undertook two projects. The first was to shorten *Medicine Recall* to be more concise and pocket friendly, and the second was to write *Advanced Medicine Recall* to target fourth-year students and residents. *Advanced Medicine Recall* is an attempt to focus more on the advanced features of the disease processes. With that in mind, all the sections in *Advanced Medicine Recall* have been reviewed by a Chief or Advanced Medical Resident with the thought that the information presented is something that fourth-year students and interns should be expected to know. There is some (<10%) deliberate repetition between *Medicine Recall* and *Advanced Medicine Recall,* and there are several reasons for this. First, the medical students who reviewed the chapters may have felt that some of the information needed to be there. Second, the Chief Medical Resident and the Attending authors may have felt that some of the information was worthy of repetition or, in some cases, that it made sections flow better. In many instances, when the questions between the two books are similar, answers in *Advanced Medicine Recall* have been adjusted to reflect a higher level of knowledge. Readers are, therefore, referred to *Medical Recall* to review the more basic material for each section.

Like all of the other books in the "Recall" series, this book is organized in a self-study/quiz format with questions on the left and answers on the right. It may be worthwhile for the reader, while reading through the book, to cover the right-hand column with the enclosed bookmark. As in the previous version of *Medicine Recall,* the chapters are organized by systems, with section abbreviations and definitions preceding each discussion. When applicable, a list of appropriate landmark clinical trials completes the chapter.

We hope that you will find this book a helpful addition to your library.

PEARLS

As with *Medicine Recall:*

- Remember to **wash your hands.** Patients really notice this and it is critical. This is one of the few things we can do to prevent the spread of infection. Do it in front of the patient (at the end of the exam or preferably both at the beginning and the end).

- Respect the patient's **modesty.** Always use curtains, gowns, and other appropriate coverings.
- The patient's **confidentiality** should be maintained beyond the patient's room (e.g., the patient's case should not be offhandedly discussed in an elevator, while eating, or while traveling to and from work); the patient's family or friends or others may overhear.
- Remember not to neglect your private life. Relationships require time and effort to build and keep strong. If you are unhappy in your private life you will likely also be unhappy in your professional life.
- In delivering bad news, it is often best to diminish the patient's anxiety by sitting and delivering the information without delay. Because much of the remainder of the conversation will often be forgotten, it is often best to return to the patient later to review important data.
- Depression is common. Approximately 60% of medical patients have depression as an important aspect of their illness.
- Heart disease, smoking-related illness, and cancer are common illnesses. One or more of these should always be considered in the differential diagnosis.
- A common illness presenting in an uncommon fashion is more common than an uncommon illness presenting in a common fashion. (In other words, when you hear hoofbeats, always think of horses, not zebras.) Furthermore, the diagnosis should be in the differential the majority of the time after a careful history and physical. A "shotgun" approach in ordering labs and tests is generally nonproductive and almost always not cost-effective or helpful. This approach can lead to false-positive test results, which can derail a workup.
- Never talk disparagingly about your colleagues. Talking in a disparaging fashion about referring colleagues only undermines the patient's confidence in the referring physician or in you. If the patient has had a long-term relationship with the referring physician, the patient may trust the other physician's word over yours, regardless of who is right. On the attending level, talking negatively about another physician may eventually sever a referral source, and it is just plain wrong to do.
- Before ending an interview or discussion with a patient, always ask whether the patient has questions (and not as you are going to the door).
- Remember to think at least twice before answering emails to make sure that the email conveys what you want it to and nothing more. Emails can easily be copied, sent along, and saved forever. They can come back to haunt you.
- When you write something in the chart, think how it would sound were it to be read aloud in court. If you write your notes that way, you will always be safe.

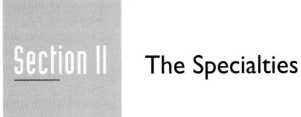

Section II

The Specialties

ABBREVIATIONS

ABPA	Allergic bronchopulmonary aspergillosis
APC	Antigen-presenting cell
AIRE	Autoimmune regulator
APS	Autoimmune polyglandular syndrome
AR	Autosomal recessive
CGD	Chronic granulomatous disease
C_1INH	C_1 esterase inhibitor
CVID	Common variable immunodeficiency
EBV	Epstein-Barr virus
ELISA	Enzyme-linked immunosorbent assay
FESS	Functional endoscopic sinus surgery
HIM	Hyperimmunoglobulin M
HIV	Human immunodeficiency virus
HLA	Human leukocyte antigen
ICF	Immunodeficiency centromeric instability and facial anomalies
ICOS	Inducible T-cell costimulator gene
IFN	Interferon
IL	Interleukin
IVIG	Intravenous immunoglobulin (IgG)
LAD	Leukocyte adhesion deficiency
LPS	Lipopolysaccharide

MCP	Monocyte chemoattractant protein
MHC	Major histocompatibility complex
NARES	Nonallergic rhinitis with eosinophilia syndrome
NK	Natural killer
NSAID	Nonsteroidal anti-inflammatory drug
PAMP	Pathogen-associated molecular patterns
PCP	*Pneumocystis jiroveci* pneumonia
PSS	Progressive systemic sclerosis
RANTES	Regulated on activation, normal T-cell expressed, and secreted chemokine
SADNI	Specific antibody deficiency with normal immunoglobulins
SCID	Severe combined immunodeficiency
TACI	Transmembrane activator, calcium modulator, and cyclophilin ligand interactor
TLR	Toll-like receptor
UP	Urticaria pigmentosa
WHIM	Warts, hypogammaglobulinemia, infection, myelokathexis
XLA	X-linked agammaglobulinemia
XLP	X-linked lymphoproliferative syndrome

DEFINITIONS

Define the following:

Innate immunity	Hard-wired responses encoded by host germ-line genes that recognize patterns on many foreign microbes (nonspecific immunity)
Adaptive immunity	Responses encoded by gene elements that have undergone rearrangement resulting in assembly of antigen-binding structures with high specificity for unique microbial antigens (specific immunity)
Chemokines	Small molecules that induce chemotaxis through G protein–coupled receptors
Antigen	A protein (or carbohydrate) recognized by the immune system
Immunoglobulins	Protein products of mature plasma cells

Antibodies	Immunoglobulins that recognize specific antigens
MHC	The major histocompatibility complex (MHC), or HLA in humans, is the genetic region housing the loci of genes encoded on chromosome 6 (HLA I, II, III). They are responsible for generating cell surface glycoproteins that bind peptides made in cells (MHCI) or ingested by cells and processed (MHCII). These glycoproteins are necessary for the presentation of foreign proteins to T lymphocytes. The absence of MHC may cause a severe immunodeficiency. The presence of different forms (polymorphisms) is associated with the potential for specific disease states (e.g., HLA-B27 and ankylosing spondylitis).

BASIC IMMUNOLOGY

What makes the basic function of the immune system possible?	Recognition of self from nonself by key effector systems
List four nonspecific components of the innate immune system	1. Physical barriers (e.g., skin) 2. Complement 3. Phagocytic cells, many with TLRs that recognize microbial patterns 4. Cytokines
Where do lymphocytes arise?	All lymphocytes arise in bone marrow; 85% are T cells.
Where do lymphocytes undergo maturation?	T cells mature in the thymus and B cells mature in the fetal liver and adult bone marrow.
What is the function of T cells (cell-mediated immunity)?	To facilitate resistance to intracellular microorganisms (e.g., mycobacteria, viruses, fungi, and parasites) and tumors and to regulate specific antibody production by B cells

What is the difference between CD4$^+$ and CD8$^+$ T cells?

Located on the cell surface, CD4 and CD8 receptors are important in determining the recognition of antigen. T cells bearing CD4 can recognize only antigen embedded in MHC class II, which is found only on the surface of a few specialized cells (APCs). T cells bearing CD8 recognize antigen on MHC class I, which is found on all nucleated cells.

What cell markers might be useful clinically?

CD3, a marker used for all T cells.
CD4, a marker for T-helper cells. It generally defines 60% to 70% of T cells in the peripheral blood and lymphoid tissue and is the receptor for HIV.
CD8, a marker for cytotoxic T cells.
CD19 or CD20, B-cell markers.
CD16 and 56, markers for NK cells.

What is the difference between T- and B-cell markers?

T-cell markers (e.g., CD4 and CD8) have functional significance, whereas B-cell markers (e.g., CD19 and CD20) are primarily of maturational significance.

What is the function of B cells (humoral immunity)?

To mature into plasma cells and produce antibody. They can also act as macrophages and APCs.

What are the five major classes (isotypes) of immunoglobulins?

IgA, IgD, IgE, IgG, and IgM

What is the basic structure of immunoglobulins?

A combination of two heavy chains and two light chains

What are the two types of light chains?

Kappa and lambda

What is the role of immunoglobulin?

Recognition and binding of specific extracellular antigens and activation of cells or of the complement-binding system

What are the three phases of the immune response?

Recognition, amplification, and response

Describe each phase of the immune response:
    Recognition

Foreign antigen patterns (e.g., bacterial LPSs) are recognized by the innate immune system.

    Amplification

Signals are generated leading to the release of cytokines that attract other immune components to the site of foreign invasion.

    Response

The stimulating antigen is cleared from the system by effector mechanisms such as inflammation, further innate effector mechanisms (e.g., phagocytosis), and initiation of the adaptive immune response.

What are the basic mast cell products?

Granule-associated mediators (e.g., histamine, tryptase, heparin), lipid derived mediators (e.g., leukotrienes), cytokines/chemokines (e.g., IL-5)

What are the effectors of an IgE-mediated response?

Mast cells, basophils, and eosinophils. Mast cells and basophils are the source of histamine and leukotrienes released in an allergic response. Eosinophils are important in the IgE-mediated killing of helminths. IgE and eosinophils are both produced in response to cytokines expressed by Th2 cells.

What does complement do?

Complement, a component of the innate immune system, lyses pathogens via the membrane activation complex (MAC) in the absence of specific immunity, opsonizes pathogens to target them for destruction, and recruits other cells and proteins to help with target destruction.

IMMUNODEFICIENCY

How are primary immunodeficiencies involving known molecular defects classified?

1. Antibody/B cell deficiencies [Bruton's X-linked agammaglobulinemia, AR agammaglobulinemia, CVID (ICOS and TACI deficiencies), HIM (AR), ICF syndrome]
2. Cellular deficiencies (IFN-γ/IL-12 axis, APS type 1, defective NK function)
3. Combined [SCID, Wiskott-Aldrich, DiGeorge, ataxia telangiectasia, HIM (AR), XLP syndrome, WHIM syndrome, caspase 8 deficiency]
4. Complement
5. Phagocytic (CGD, Chediak-Higashi syndrome, LAD, specific granule deficiency, cyclic neutropenia, X-linked neutropenia)

What are some common primary immunodeficiencies with no known molecular defect?

1. Selective IgA deficiency
2. CVID
3. SADNI
4. Hyper-IgE syndrome
5. Cartilage hair hypoplasia
6. Idiopathic CD4 lymphocytopenia (Nezelof syndrome)

What are common causes of secondary immunodeficiency?

1. Immunosuppression (chemotherapy, steroids, immunomodulators, antilymphocyte antibodies)
2. Infections (HIV, herpes, parasites)
3. Malignancy (Hodgkin's, leukemia, myeloma)
4. Autoimmune disease (diabetes, lupus)
5. Malnutrition
6. Environmental exposure (radiation, chemical)
7. Other (uremia, intestinal lymphangiectasia, pregnancy, aging, stress, hyposplenism)

In general, what does a history of contact dermatitis (e.g., poison ivy) suggest?

Intact cellular immunity

What is a simple test for T-cell function?

The "anergy" panel skin test (e.g., PPD, *Candida, Trichophyton*, tetanus toxoid, saline control) is a measure of delayed-type hypersensitivity; a positive test requires intact T-cell function.

What interferes with an anergy panel?

1. Corticosteroids (topical or higher-dose systemic)
2. Anticoagulants (induration is the result of fibrin deposition)
3. Technique (failure to place antigen intradermally)
4. Infection (HIV, EBV, TB, leprosy)
5. Autoimmune disease (sarcoid, lupus, rheumatoid arthritis)
6. Malnutrition
7. Pregnancy
8. Malignancy (e.g., Hodgkin's lymphoma)

What assays are available to test for T cells?

Flow cytometry for CD3, CD4, CD8, CD45, T-cell receptor

What assays are available to test for B cells?

CD19, CD20, CD21, Ig-associated

What assays are available to test for NK cells?

CD16/CD56

What assays are useful in the evaluation of patients with borderline IgG levels or recurrent sinopulmonary bacterial infections?

Pre- and postimmunization pneumococcal, diphtheria, tetanus titers, isohemagglutinins

What is the treatment for IgA deficiency?

Antibiotics for specific infections and, sometimes, prophylactic antibiotics. IgA-deficient patients who are unable to mount a response to polysaccharide vaccines are occasionally given IVIg.

Are blood transfusions safe in patients with IgA deficiency?

No. Some IgA-deficient patients with anti-IgA antibodies are at increased risk of a severe reaction to trace IgA from IVIg and from blood transfusions (washed packed cells should be given if transfusion is needed).

What constitutes the diagnosis of CVID?

Total serum IgGs are reduced to >2 standard deviations below the age-adjusted mean as well as impaired production of specific antibodies (isohemagglutinins or poor response to vaccines above).

What infections are seen in IgG deficiencies?

Most common, sinopulmonary infections
Common, central nervous system, joint, and gastrointestinal tract infections

What organisms are the most common causes of infection in patients with IgG deficiencies?

Most common, encapsulated bacteria such as *Haemophilus influenzae* or *Streptococcus pneumoniae*
Common, *Staphylococcus aureus,* meningococci, *Pseudomonas, Campylobacter, Ureaplasma,* and *Mycoplasma, Giardia*

Are persons with IgG deficiencies more susceptible to viral infections?

As a rule, no. However, IgG-deficient patients are susceptible to polioviruses (and should not receive live virus vaccine) and to hepatitis B and C. In patients with XLA (but not CVID or HIM), a chronic meningoencephalitis, which is ultimately fatal, can develop with enteroviruses (echovirus or coxsackie) infection.

What are the laboratory and radiographic findings in CVID?

Low IgG, IgA, IgE, variable IgM. B cells (CD19) are present in the peripheral blood and sometimes in exuberant lymphoid tissue. Commonly these patients (25%) have bronchiectasis on high-resolution computed tomography (CT) of the chest.

When are patients with agammaglobulinemia first seen?

Generally, boys with XLA are seen after the first 6 months of life (after maternal antibodies are gone) and within the first 2 years of life.

What are laboratory and radiographic findings in agammaglobulinemia?

XLA patients have essentially no B cells (CD19) in circulation and no discernible lymphoid tissue (a lateral neck view showing no adenoidal tissue is a diagnostic test in children).

What infections are common in patients with agammaglobulinemia?

Sinopulmonary bacterial infections, enterovirus meningoencephalitis

Can a patient have an antibody deficiency with a normal total IgG level?

Yes, there have been reports of patients with B-cell immunodeficiency in spite of a normal total IgG level.

How are patients with B-cell immunodeficiency and normal total IgG level recognized?

Most of these patients have an inability to mount a response to polysaccharide antigens (pneumococcus or unconjugated *Haemophilus*).

How should patients with recurrent pneumonia or other serious bacterial infections be evaluated?

The patient should receive vaccination with unconjugated pneumococcal vaccine and tetanus toxoid; then prevaccination and postvaccination (3 to 4 weeks) titers of antibodies to at least 14 pneumococcal serotypes assayed simultaneously. An adequate response is a fourfold increase in antibody titers between the paired serums. Vaccination with *H. influenzae* (type b) conjugated to a protein may be useful for protecting these patients but is usually not helpful in diagnosis.

What is the treatment for IgG deficiencies?

Monthly infusions of pooled IVIg. The dose is generally begun at 200 to 400 mg/kg and is titrated to maintain an IgG trough level of >400 mg/dL obtained immediately before the next infusion (or sometimes to an adequate clinical response). Despite IgG infusions, many patients with CVID require prophylactic antibiotics.

Name some of the different types of SCID.

ADA deficiency (most common)
PNP deficiency
RAG1, RAG2 (Omenn syndrome)
Defective cytokine signaling
X-linked (common gamma chain)
Autosomal recessive (IL2, IL7 receptor)

For each of the following, list the lymphocyte defect and major abnormalities:

DiGeorge syndrome

T cell; cardiac defects (great vessels) and hypocalcemia (failure of development of the parathyroids), absent thymus, abnormal ears, shortened philtrum, micrognathia, and hypotelorism

Idiopathic CD4 lymphocytopenia (Nezelof syndrome)

T cell; DiGeorge syndrome without the associated congenital anomalies; resembles HIV (failure to thrive, candidiasis, anemia, thrombocytopenia, cancer)

SCID

T and B cell; may be X-linked or autosomal recessive. Affected infants rarely survive the severe immunodeficiency state beyond 1 year. They often present with failure to thrive, diarrhea, respiratory infection, and disseminated infection.

ADA

Most common type of SCID; T and B cells; a form of SCID with deficient purine metabolism (adenosine deaminase)

PNP

Type of SCID; T cells; similar to ADA with deficient purine metabolism leading to toxic intracellular levels of deoxyguanosine triphosphate

Wiskott-Aldrich syndrome

T and B cell; low serum levels of IgM and increased levels of IgE; eczema, thrombocytopenia, repeated infections (encapsulated organisms), lymphoreticular malignancies, and anergy

Ataxia-telangiectasia

T and B cells; cerebellar ataxia and oculocutaneous telangiectasia (butterfly rash over the sclera, face, and ears), truncal ataxia, ovarian agenesis, sinopulmonary infections leading to bronchiectasis and lymphomas, and high levels of α-fetoprotein and carcinoembryonic antigen; highly susceptible to radiation-induced chromosomal injury and subsequent tumors.

Chronic mucocutaneous candidiasis (autoimmune polyglandular syndrome type I)
T cell; superficial candidiasis (not systemic) associated with single or multiple endocrinopathies, iron deficiency, and anergy; molecular defect in AIRE

Hyperimmunoglobulin E
Uncertain, with increased serum levels of IgE (up to 10 times normal); recurrent infections of the skin and sinopulmonary tract with *S. aureus, H. influenzae, and Aspergillus;* coarse facial features; delayed shedding of primary teeth; and chronic eczematous rashes

Do any of the T- and B-cell primary immunodeficiencies discussed occur in adults?
CVID; chronic mucocutaneous candidiasis and hyperimmunoglobulin E are disorders compatible with living to adulthood; the other T-cell or combined immunodeficiencies listed above are severe and generally present early in life; without bone marrow transplantation, they are generally fatal.

In general, how are T-cell and combined immunodeficiencies treated?
Bone marrow, fetal liver, and thymus transplantation may have a role. Gamma globulin infusions ± antibiotics may be given for patients who are IgG deficient or with SADNI. Fresh frozen plasma may be given for other immunoglobulin-deficient states. Good postural drainage helps prevent sinopulmonary infections. Live vaccines, blood transfusions, and x-rays avoided in patients with T-cell deficiencies. Splenectomy, chemotherapy, immunomodulators, antifungals, and antivirals are needed in rare cases.

HIV

See Chapter 7 ("Infectious Disease") and *Medicine Recall*, 3rd ed. for more discussion of HIV.

COMPLEMENT DEFICIENCY

Are complement deficiencies common?

No, they are rare (prevalence = 0.03%).

Name the most common complement deficiencies.

C2, C9, MBL

How are most inherited?

Autosomal recessive

What diseases are seen in patients with complement deficiency?

1. Autoimmune disease
2. Recurrent infections

What is a common complement deficiency?

C2 deficiency is seen in approximately 1 in 25,000 Caucasians, in whom there is an increased tendency for autoimmune disease.

What immune issues do patients with complement deficiency have troubles with?

Persons are rarely clinically affected by a decreased ability to opsonize pyogenic bacteria.

In what ethnic groups are terminal complement deficiencies seen?

These deficiencies are probably more common in ethnic groups other than Caucasians.

What infections are most common with this problem?

People with terminal complement component deficiencies (C5 to C9) are predisposed to *Neisseria* infections.

What complement deficiency is associated with recurrent episodes of angioedema?

Deficiency of C_1INH

What types of processes cause complement consumption?

1. Autoimmune disease (lupus, rheumatoid arthritis, vasculitis)
2. Infections
3. Serum sickness

AUTOIMMUNITY

See *Medicine Recall*, 3rd ed.

ANAPHYLAXIS

What is the acute treatment for anaphylaxis?

Stop the causative agent (e.g., penicillin infusion), provide basic life support, and:

1. Epinephrine, intramuscular injections of 0.3 to 0.5 mL of 1:1000 every 5 minutes as necessary to control symptoms.
2. IV fluids for hypotension.
3. H_1 blockers (diphenhydramine, >50 mg up to 300 mg/day) and H_2 blockers (cimetidine, 4 mg/kg) intravenously.
4. Glucagon, atropine, dopamine if patient is on beta blockers or refractory to epinephrine.

Why should patients who have had an anaphylactic reaction be monitored after successful therapy?

Episodes can recur for up to several hours after the event.

What are some of the drug and food causes of anaphylaxis?

Drugs: antibiotics (particularly beta lactams), protamine, insulin, muscle relaxants, general anesthetics, and vaccines

Food: peanuts, tree nuts, fish, shellfish, milk, and eggs (including vaccines made from egg products, such as the influenza vaccine)

What are other common causes and causative agents of anaphylaxis?

Antitoxins, insect venom, latex, exercise, exercise within 4 to 6 hours of ingesting certain foods (e.g., wheat, celery), systemic mastocytosis, malignancy, semen, and unknown or idiopathic causes

How is the correct diagnosis of anaphylaxis made?

History is the major diagnostic modality (most cases present with urticaria and decreased blood pressure, increased heart rate). Specific IgE testing [either by skin testing or by IgE immunoassays (ELISA), formerly done with radiation and known as radioallergosorbent tests or RASTs] may be helpful when IgE is suspected.

Skin testing should be performed more than 6 weeks after the event or else false-negative tests will be more common due to the anergic state of mast cells after anaphylaxis.

What blood test can be evaluated to confirm anaphylaxis?

Serum tryptase (within 3 to 4 hours of the event)

What is an anaphylactoid reaction and what agents usually cause them?

It is clinically similar to anaphylaxis but is not IgE-mediated. Agents such as radiocontrast media, NSAIDs, muscle relaxants, and paclitaxel cause direct stimulation of mast cells and basophils. Anaphylactoid reactions can often be prevented with glucocorticoids and antihistamines.

Can people with fish allergy tolerate IV contrast media?

Yes, there is no relationship between fish allergy and adverse reactions to contrast media.

URTICARIA AND ANGIOEDEMA

What are the causes of physical urticaria/angioedema?

Dermographism, cold, heat, sun, cholinergic stimulation, vibration, exercise

What are the complement-mediated causes of urticaria (and angioedema)?

Hereditary and acquired angioedema, necrotizing vasculitis, serum sickness, reactions to blood products, viral infections including hepatitis B and EBV, and pregnancy

What are the nonimmunologic (non–IgE mediated) causes of urticaria (and angioedema)?

Opiates (direct histamine release from mast cell), vancomycin, dextran, radiocontrast, acetylsalicylic acid, NSAID, azo dyes, and benzoates

What is the most common cause of chronic urticaria?

After excluding acute and physical urticarias, etiologies of chronic urticaria may be found in <2% of cases.

What factors should be considered in the evaluation of the patient with chronic urticaria?

Thyroid disease, physical urticarias, food sensitivity, drug reaction, chronic infections (sinus, dental, and genitourinary), systemic disease (vasculitides), and malignancy

What tests/labs should one evaluate for chronic urticaria?

CBC with differential, sedimentation rate, thyroid antibodies, thyroid function, liver function; consider autologous serum skin testing to demonstrate autoantibodies to Fc receptor; urinalysis if symptoms of UTI or history of recurrent UTI, skin biopsy for atypical urticaria (painful, residual bruising, if lesions last more than 24 to 48 hours, or other systemic complaints) to rule out vasculitis

What organs other than skin are affected in angioedema?

There is submucosal edema of the gastrointestinal system (lips, esophagus, gastrointestinal tract), nasopharynx, larynx, trachea, or urogenital system.

Is the differential diagnosis different for angioedema than for urticaria?

Yes; isolated angioedema is much less common than chronic urticaria with or without angioedema. Isolated angioedema suggests drug allergy; C_1INH deficiencies, either hereditary or acquired; and vasculitis.

What are the causes of angioedema?

Same as urticaria with the addition of ACE inhibitors

What is the time course of ACE inhibitor–related angioedema?

This side effect is most commonly seen in the first week of treatment but may occur any time, affecting at least 3 in 1000 patients.

If a patient has a history of angioedema, must the ACE inhibitor be discontinued?

If the patient is taking an ACE inhibitor, it should be stopped, because the side effect of angioedema is life-threatening. Most patients with ACE inhibitor–related angioedema can tolerate angiotensin-receptor blockers (ARBs).

How is the cause of angioedema established?

If the C4 level is normal during an episode of angioedema, there is no problem with C_1INH because C4 is used up in this process. If the C4 level is low or if a person is seen in an asymptomatic period, C_1INH level and functional activity should be measured (to determine if it is HAE I or II), as should the C1q level. C1q levels are normal in hereditary angioedema and decreased in acquired C_1INH deficiency. C2 is reduced during acute episodes. Acquired C_1INH is associated with malignancy, particularly B-cell lymphomas.

What is the first-line therapy for urticaria and angioedema not related to C_1INH deficiency?

H_1 antihistamines (preferably long-acting; e.g., cetirizine, fexofenadine). If control is not achieved, H_2 antihistamines (e.g., ranitidine) can be added or doxepin can be used, which has both H_1 and H_2 antihistaminic activity.

Where do steroids fit in the treatment of urticaria and angioedema not related to C_1INH deficiency?

Daily steroids are to be avoided as they provide only short-term relief.

What other agents can also be used for the treatment of urticaria and angioedema not related to C_1INH deficiency?

Leukotriene modifiers (montelukast, zileuton) can also be used. A short course of cyclosporine for those with autoimmune urticaria that is refractory to their medications may be beneficial. Epinephrine 1:1,000 IM is used if angioedema is threatening the airway.

What is the treatment for urticaria and angioedema secondary to C_1INH deficiency?

C_1INH deficiency is treated with attenuated androgenic steroids, which increase the production of C_1INH. This is effective in patients with deficient production, deficient activity, and increased catabolism of C_1INH. Epinephrine may not work in a crisis, and a tracheostomy is indicated for laryngeal edema. Antifibrinolytics (epsilon-aminocaproic acid or tranexamic acid) may be helpful.

MASTOCYTOSIS

What is mastocytosis?	Mastocytosis is a disease of excess mast cells; it can be localized to the skin or may occur in systemic form.
How common is mastocytosis?	Approximately 1 in 5000 patients seen in dermatology clinics has mastocytosis. It is slightly more common in men than in women (1.5:1).
What is the most common lesion found on skin examination in mastocytosis?	Urticaria pigmentosa (UP)
What are symptoms and signs of mastocytosis?	Symptoms: pruritus, flushing, abdominal pain, fatigue, musculoskeletal pain, recurrent anaphylaxis Signs: skin lesions (UP), hepatosplenomegaly, ascites, bone lesions
What are the features of the seven categories of mastocytosis?	1. Cutaneous: includes UP, nodular or telangiectasia macularis, eruptive persistent, diffuse cutaneous 2. Indolent systemic mastocytosis: involving skin and bone marrow only (UP and diffuse cutaneous) and systemic (marrow, gastrointestinal, and UP) 3. Systemic: associated with a hematologic non–mast cell disorder (dysmyelopoietic syndrome, acute nonlymphocytic leukemia, myeloproliferative disorders, malignant lymphoma, chronic neutropenia) 4. Aggressive systemic: lymphadenopathy and eosinophilia 5. Mast cell leukemia 6. Mast cell sarcoma 7. Extracutaneous mastocytoma
How is the diagnosis of mastocytosis made?	One major diagnostic criterion + one minor criterion or three minor criteria

Major criteria:
> Bone marrow biopsy and aspirate with dense infiltrates of mast cells

Minor criteria:
1. Spindle-shaped mast cells
2. Detection of 816 *c-kit* mutation
3. Flow cytometry with CD2, CD25, and CD117 expression
4. Serum tryptase >20 μg/mL

What is the treatment for mastocytosis?

H_1 antihistamines for pruritus, flushing, and tachycardia.
H_2 antihistamines for gastric hypersecretion.
Epinephrine.
Cromolyn (200 mg before meals and at bedtime) may help with gastrointestinal symptoms.
Tricyclic antidepressants for headaches.
Avoidance of ethanol, NSAIDs, opiates, friction, and physical exertion.

What is the prognosis for mastocytosis?

Those with the cutaneous form usually have high rates of spontaneous remission. The indolent form is usually associated with a normal life expectancy. The prognosis of patients with systemic disease and an associated hematologic non–mast cell disorder is determined by the hematologic abnormality. Aggressive systemic disease is the rarest and has the most fulminant course. Mast cell leukemia is rapidly progressive over 1 to 2 years.

What are the poor prognostic indicators for mastocytosis?

Constitutional symptoms, anemia, thrombocytopenia, abnormal liver function tests, lobulated mast cell nucleus, low percentage of fat cells in the marrow, associated hematologic disorder, absence of UP, male gender, absence of skin and bone symptoms, hepatosplenomegaly, and normal bone films

What therapies are available for more severe forms of systemic mastocytosis?

IFN-α (controversial), hydroxyurea (may reduce mast cell progenitors in type III disease), and other chemotherapy for leukemic forms (types II and IV)

DRUG ALLERGIES

How common are immune-mediated drug-induced allergic reactions?

Allergies account for 6% to 10% of all adverse drug reactions. The rest are commonly known, predictable pharmacologic actions of the drug.

Is skin testing helpful for patients with a history of hives to antibiotics?

Penicillin skin testing with penicillin major and minor is reliable for the diagnosis of immediate hypersensitivity. A negative test has a 99% negative predictive value, whereas a positive skin test indicates a high risk for immediate hypersensitivity reactions.

How common is antibiotic cross-reactivity in penicillin-sensitive patients?

The history of a reaction to penicillin carries a 5% to 15% risk of immediate hypersensitivity to first-generation cephalosporins (4% to second and 1% to 3% to third and fourth) and increases the risk of an adverse response to other, unrelated drugs eightfold. A positive penicillin skin test increases the risk of a reaction to cephalosporins (and probably imipenem).

What drugs interfere with immediate skin tests?

Most antihistamines if used within 3 days of the test (astemizole, 6 weeks) and tricyclic antidepressants

Are there skin tests for other antibiotics?

Clinically proven skin tests have not been developed for other pharmacologic agents. Testing is sometimes performed for other drugs, but a negative test must be interpreted with caution (poor negative predictive value). Nonirritating doses are available for testing which, if positive, suggest IgE-mediated sensitization. There are no prospective challenges published other than for beta lactams.

What if there is no alternative agent than the drug allergen?

Desensitization protocols decrease the risk of uncontrolled anaphylaxis. Once therapy is initiated, it cannot be interrupted without resuming the risk of anaphylaxis.

How does desensitization work?

It is not known for certain, but there may be a gradual cross linking of IgE by antigen, causing a controlled anaphylaxis.

Are drug rashes possible with a negative penicillin skin test?

Penicillin skin testing predicts only immediate IgE-mediated hypersensitivity. With a negative penicillin skin test, it is still possible for a non–IgE-mediated drug rash, serum sickness, mucocutaneous syndrome, or other adverse side effects to develop.

Which reactions are contraindications to drug use?

A history of serum sickness, Stevens-Johnson syndrome/toxic epidermal necrolysis, erythroderma, hemolytic anemia, interstitial nephritis, or exfoliative dermatitis

ATOPIC DERMATITIS (SEE CHAPTER 12, "DERMATOLOGY")

CONTACT HYPERSENSITIVITY (SEE CHAPTER 12, "DERMATOLOGY")

RHINITIS AND SINUSITIS

What is the differential diagnosis of chronic rhinitis?

1. Allergic
2. Nonallergic
   A. Inflammatory [infectious, NARES, nasal polyps (NSAID allergy), atrophic rhinitis]
   B. Noninflammatory
      1. Vasomotor
      2. Systemic disease (hypothyroidism, diabetes)
      3. Rhinitis medicamentosa (oral contraceptives, topical decongestants, cocaine, ACE inhibitors)
      4. Chronic sinusitis
      5. Structural defects (trauma/cerebrospinal fluid rhinorrhea, tumor, foreign body)
      6. Pregnancy

What is chronic sinusitis?

Symptoms ≥12 weeks
Requires two or more of the following:
1. Anterior or posterior mucopurulent drainage
2. Congestion
3. Facial pain/pressure
4. Decreased sense of smell
5. Objective documentation:
   Rhinoscopy
   X-ray (sinus CT preferred)

How is the diagnosis of chronic sinusitis made?

Radiographically by sinus CT scan (plain films not very sensitive)

What is the treatment for acute sinusitis?

Antibiotics that cover beta lactamase–positive organisms for 10 to 21 days
Promotion of nasal drainage
Topical nasal decongestants for 3 to 5 days

What is the treatment for chronic sinusitis?

Nasal steroids
Short course of oral steroids
FESS (in certain patients—i.e., nasal polyps)

What are potential adverse effects of antihistamines?

Somnolence and a theoretical thickening of mucus, therefore possibly reducing clearance

ASTHMA (SEE ALSO CHAPTER 10, "PULMONOLOGY")

What is the differential diagnosis for wheezing?

1. Asthma
2. Pulmonary edema
3. Airway obstruction (laryngospasm, tracheomalacia, vocal cord dysfunction, tracheal web, foreign body)
4. Chronic obstructive pulmonary disease (COPD)
5. Congestive heart failure
6. Pulmonary embolus
7. Primary eosinophilic lung disease (hypereosinophilic syndrome, eosinophilic pneumonia, Churg-Strauss syndrome)

8. Secondary eosinophilic lung disease [allergic bronchopulmonary aspergillosis (ABPA), hypersensitivity pneumonitis, drugs, malignancy, collagen vascular disease, sarcoid]
9. Bronchiolitis obliterans
10. Interstitial lung disease

GASTROENTEROLOGY

What is eosinophilic esophagitis/gastroenteritis?

An eosinophilic infiltrate of the bowel potentially involving all layers of the gut; symptoms include nausea, vomiting, diarrhea, malabsorption, weight loss, and dysphagia

How is the diagnosis of eosinophilic esophagitis/ gastroenteritis made?

Biopsy shows >15 to 20 eosinophils per high-power field. Involvement is sporadic, so multiple biopsy samples may be required. Usually, about half of patients have a peripheral eosinophilia and some have high levels of IgE. IgE testing (skin test may be more sensitive than serum immunoassays) to foods should be performed. Patch testing is still experimental.

What is the treatment for eosinophilic esophagitis/ gastroenteritis?

Treatment of coexisting acid reflux may relieve symptoms. Swallowed metered-dose-inhaler steroids; a trial of strict avoidance of any identified offending foods in esophagitis; an elemental diet in gastroenteritis or severe esophagitis; oral glucocorticoids in very severe cases.

TRANSPLANTATION IMMUNOLOGY

Are all grafts matched?

Although matching for intrafamilial transplants of all types is performed, nonfamilial cardiac, lung, and liver grafts are not MHC-matched because other factors such as size, location, and availability limit the transplants much more. Kidney transplantation, for which there is the potential for living related and unrelated donors, allows for matching. Bone marrow transplants must be matched, whereas matching in liver transplants may actually decrease survival.

What is hyperacute rejection?

Rejection mediated by preformed complement-fixing antibodies. It occurs in <24 hours and is irreversible.

What is accelerated rejection?

Rejection mediated by preformed but not complement-fixing antibodies. Onset is 3 to 5 days.

How is accelerated rejection treated?

Treatment is with antithymocyte or antilymphocyte globulin or newer anti–monoclonal antibodies against T-cell surface antigens (e.g., CD3). Treatment is successful in approximately 60% of cases.

What is acute rejection?

Rejection mediated by recipient T cells and antibodies as a primary response. It occurs 6 to 90 days after transplantation and is thought to be directed at passenger APCs. There is prominent infiltration of CD8 cells and polymorphonuclear neutrophils.

How is acute rejection treated?

Immunosuppression with pulse steroids and agents used in accelerated rejection is successful 80% to 90% of the time.

What is chronic rejection?

Mostly antibody deposition leading to hyperplasia and endothelial necrosis >60 days posttransplant. It is slowly progressive and does not respond well to treatment.

What is graft-versus-host disease?

Graft-versus-host disease is an immune response of the donor T cells against the recipient usually 6 or more days after transplant. It is a problem only when transplanting hematopoietic tissue (bone marrow, nonirradiated blood transfusions).

Why not purge the T cells from marrow before transplantation?

Sometimes the donor marrow is purged of T cells before transplant, but without T cells, engraftment is less often successful and the incidence of leukemia increases.

What immunosuppressive drugs specifically target T cells?

1. Antithymocyte globulin, antilymphocyte globulin, and anti–monoclonal antibody to T-cell antigens (CD3, OKT3), which, in part, bind with the activation sites of T cells via foreign proteins (horse, rabbit, or mouse) and are then selectively cleared by the host's immune system
2. Calcineurin inhibitors (cyclosporine, tacrolimus) and anti–IL-2 receptor antibodies, which decrease IL-2 and interfere with growth and function

Should blood transfusion be avoided?

Yes, for persons likely to need a bone marrow transplant; however, it may enhance renal and cardiac allograft survival by selecting for patients who are hyporesponsive for antibody production. Transfusions with irradiated or filtered blood are usually safe, however.

TUMOR IMMUNOLOGY

What are common alterations that lead to cancer?

1. Increased activity of proto-oncogenes
2. Decreased activity of suppressor genes
3. Alterations in genes that regulate apoptosis
4. Defect in genes that regulate DNA repair

What are causes of antigenic differences between normal and tumor cells?

1. Chemical carcinogens and ionizing radiation may alter protein synthesis.
2. Viruses may introduce new DNA or RNA into cells.
3. Malignant cells may revert to synthesis of fetal markers such as alpha fetoprotein, carcinoembryonic antigen, or other fetal proteins.
4. Genetic mutation may lead to expression of inappropriate antigens such as ABO.

Why are antigenic differences potentially important?

If differences between normal cells and malignant cells can be found, immunotherapy may be effective in curing patients.

What immunotherapeutic agents are currently under investigation?

Interleukins and interferons, monoclonal antibodies, and antitumor vaccines

What are potential uses for monoclonal antibodies?

1. To direct action against tumors through antibody- or complement-dependent cytotoxicity
2. To carry cytotoxic substances such as radiolabeled compounds, chemotherapeutic agents (e.g., methotrexate or doxorubicin), naturally existing toxins, or immunoconjugates (e.g., ricin)

Chapter 3 — Cardiology

ABBREVIATIONS

A2	Second heart sound, aortic valve component
AAA	Abdominal aortic aneurysm
ABI	Ankle brachial index
ACE	Angiotensin-converting enzyme
ACE-I	Angiotensin-converting enzyme inhibitor
ACS	Acute coronary syndrome
ADP	Adenosine diphosphate
AF	Atrial fibrillation
AI	Aortic insufficiency
AIVR	Accelerated idioventricular rhythm
ALCAPA	Anomolosis left coronary artery originating from the pulmonary artery
AMI	Acute myocardial infarction or anterior myocardial infarction
APB	Atrial premature beat
aPTT	Activated partial thromboplastin time
ARB	Angiotensin-receptor blocker
AS	Aortic stenosis
ASA	Acetylsalicylic acid
ASD	Atrial septal defect
AST	Aminotransferase
AV	Atrioventricular
AVNRT	AV node reciprocating tachycardia
AVRT	AV reciprocating tachycardia
BBB	Bundle branch block
BCLS	Basic cardiac life support
bNP	b-type natriuretic peptide
BP	Blood pressure
BiVD	Biventricular ICD
BiVP	Biventricular pacemaker
BSA	Body surface area
CABG	Coronary artery bypass grafting
CAD	Coronary artery disease
CCU	Cardiac care unit
CEA	Carotid endarterectomy
CHB	Complete heart block
CHD	Congenital heart disease
CHF	Congestive heart failure
CI	Cardiac index
CK	Creatine kinase
CKMB	Creatine kinase, MB isoform
CO	Cardiac output
COPD	Chronic obstructive pulmonary disease

CMRI	Cardiac magnetic resonance imaging
CTA	CT angiogram
cTn	Cardiac troponin (either cTnI or cTnT)
CVA	Cerebrovascular accident
CVP	Central venous pressure (also RA pressure)
DCA	Directional coronary atherectomy
DCM	Dilated cardiomyopathy
DM	Diabetes mellitus
DORV	Double-outlet right ventricle
DP	Dipyridamole
EBCT	Electron beam CT
ECG	Electrocardiogram
EECP	External enhanced counterpulsation
EF	Ejection fraction
EP	Electrophysiology
ESR	Erythrocyte sedimentation rate
GPIIb/IIIa	Glycoprotein IIb/IIIa
GXT	Graded exercise test
HF	Heart failure
HDL	High-density lipoprotein
HIT (or HITT)	Heparin-induced thrombocytopenia (with thrombosis)
HMG-CoA	3-Hydroxy-3-methylglutaryl coenzyme A
HOCM	Hypertrophic obstructive cardiomyopathy (also IHSS)
HR	Heart rate
hsCRP	Highly sensitive C-reactive protein
HTN	Hypertension
IABP	Intra-aortic balloon pump
ICD	Implantable cardioverter-defibrillator
ICU	Intensive care unit
IE	Infective endocarditis
IHD	Ischemic heart disease
IHSS	Idiopathic hypertrophic subaortic stenosis (also HOCM)
IMA	Internal mammary artery
IMI	Inferior myocardial infarction
INR	International normalized ratio
IVC	Inferior vena cava
IVNC	Isolated ventricular noncompaction
IVUS	Intravascular ultrasound
JVD	Jugular venous distension (also JVP)
JVP	Jugular venous pressure (also JVD)
LA	Left atrium
LAD	Left anterior descending artery or left axis deviation

LAFB	Left anterior fascicular block
LBBB	Left bundle branch block
LCx	Left circumflex artery
LDH	Lactate dehydrogenase
LDL	Low-density lipoprotein
LIMA	Left internal mammary artery (also abbreviated **LITA** for left internal thoracic artery)
LMCA	Left main coronary artery
LMWH	Low molecular weight heparin
LPFB	Left posterior fascicular block
LV	Left ventricle
LVED	Left ventricular end-diastolic
LVEDP	Left ventricular end-diastolic pressure
LVEF	Left ventricular ejection fraction
LVES	Left ventricular end-systolic
LVH	Left ventricular hypertrophy
LVOT	Left ventricular outflow tract
MAP	Mean arterial pressure
MAT	Multifocal atrial tachycardia
MET	Metabolic equivalent
MI	Myocardial infarction
MIBI	Methoxyisobutyl isonitrile
MR	Mitral regurgitation
MRI/A	Magnetic resonance imaging/angiography
MS	Mitral stenosis
MUGA	Multigated acquisition
MVP	Mitral valve prolapse
NCEP	National Cholesterol Education Program
NSTEMI	Non-ST-elevation MI
NSVT	Nonsustained ventricular tachycardia
NTprobNP	N terminal pro-b-type natriuretic peptide
NYHA	New York Heart Association
P2	Second heart sound, pulmonic valve component
PA	Posteroanterior or pulmonary artery
PAD	Peripheral arterial disease
PAF	Paroxysmal atrial fibrillation
PAOD	Peripheral arterial occlusive disease
PAOP	Pulmonary artery occlusion pressure
PCI	Percutaneous coronary intervention
PCWP	Pulmonary capillary wedge pressure (also PAOP)
PDA	Posterior descending artery or patent ductus arteriosus
PE	Pulmonary embolism
PEA	Pulseless electrical activity

PI	Pulmonic insufficiency
PMI	Posterior myocardial infarction or point of maximal impulse
PND	Paroxysmal nocturnal dyspnea
PS	Pulmonic stenosis
PTCA	Percutaneous transluminal coronary angioplasty
PTCI	Percutaneous transluminal coronary intervention
PVC	Premature ventricular contraction
PVD	Peripheral vascular disease
PVE	Prosthetic valve endocarditis
PVR	Pulmonary vascular resistance
PVRI	Pulmonary vascular resistance index
RA	Right atrium
RAD	Right axis deviation
RBBB	Right bundle branch block
RCA	Right coronary artery
RV	Right ventricle
RVEF	Right ventricular ejection fraction
RVH	Right ventricular hypertrophy
RVR	Rapid ventricular response
saECG	Signal-averaged ECG
SR	Sinus rhythm
STEMI	ST-elevation MI
SK	Streptokinase
SVR	Systemic vascular resistance
SVRI	Systemic vascular resistance index
SVT	Supraventricular tachycardia
TAA	Thoracic aortic aneurysm
TEE	Transesophageal echocardiogram
TG	Triglycerides
TGA	Transposition of the great arteries
TIA	Transient ischemic attack
TIMI	Thrombolysis in Myocardial Infarction
TNK-tPA	Tenecteplase-tPA
tPA	Tissue plasminogen activator
TR	Tricuspid regurgitation
TS	Tricuspid stenosis
TTE	Transthoracic echocardiogram
UFH	Unfractionated heparin
UA or USA	Unstable angina
VF	Ventricular fibrillation
VLDL	Very low density lipoprotein
$\dot{V}o_2$	Oxygen consumption
VPB	Ventricular premature beat (also PVC, VPC)

VPC	Ventricular premature contraction
VSD	Ventricular septal defect
WPW	Wolff-Parkinson-White

ICU

What are the potential complications of placing a pulmonary artery (PA) catheter?	Bleeding, infection, pneumo- or hemothorax, arrhythmias, death
What arrhythmias occur during placement of PA catheters?	VT and heart block
What group of patients are prone to developing heart block?	Those with a LBBB
When do the arrhythmias usually occur?	When the catheter passes through the RV
What are the normal filling pressures?	
RA pressure or CVP	0 to 8 mm Hg (mean)
RV pressure	15 to 30/0 to 8 mm Hg (systolic/diastolic)
PA pressure	15 to 30/3 to 12 mm Hg (systolic/diastolic)
PCWP	3 to 12 mm Hg (mean)
What is the PCWP?	Approximation of the LA and LV pressure during ventricular filling (LVEDP)
What is the danger of overinflating the balloon while measuring the PCWP?	PA rupture, which can be fatal

What are three sources of error encountered when measuring pressures with a fluid-filled catheter (e.g., arterial line, Swan-Ganz catheter)?

1. Zeroing error
2. Deterioration in frequency response—check for air in the catheter or transducer
3. Catheter impact—catheter impact is caused by a valve or other structure hitting the catheter
4. Catheter whip—as the catheter is hit by the pulse wave and motion is generated, increasing systolic pressures and lowering diastolic pressures (i.e., the mean pressure is unaltered)

How can you test for catheter whip?

In arterial lines, by inflating a BP cuff proximal to the line; as the cuff is deflated, the pressure that corresponds to the first pressure wave recorded on the arterial line is the true systolic pressure.

What is the normal CO?

5 ± 1 L/min

What is the normal CI?

3 ± 0.5 L/min/m^2

How is SVR calculated?

SVR = {[systemic BP (mean) – RA (mean)]/CO} × 80 dyne · cm · sec^{-5}

What is the normal SVR?

1200 ± 300 dyne · cm · sec^{-5}

How is the SVRI calculated?

SVRI = SVR × BSA

What is the normal SVRI?

2100 ± 500 dyne · cm · sec^{-5} × m^2

How is the PVR calculated?

PVR = [(PA mean – PC mean)/CO] × 80 dyne · cm · sec^{-5}

What is the normal PVR?

100 ± 50 dyne · cm · sec^{-5}

How is the PVRI calculated?

PVR × BSA

What is the normal PVRI?

170 ± 70 dyne · cm · sec^{-5} × m^2

How are Wood units calculated?

PVR = [PA (mean) – PCWP (mean)]/CO

What is the appropriate value for PVR in Wood units?

<4

DETERMINATION OF CARDIAC OUTPUT

Name five pitfalls of the thermodilution method.

1. Low outputs (outputs <2.5 L/min average a 35% overestimation)
2. Tricuspid regurgitation
3. Improper technique (i.e., slow injection, incorrect volume)
4. Intracardiac shunts (VSD)
5. Extracardiac shunts (AV fistula)
6. Cold patients
7. Distal tip of the catheter in the main PA
8. Changes in blood viscosity (anemia or polycythemia)
9. Invasive insertion

What is the Fick equation?

$CO = [\text{oxygen consumption} \times 10]/[(AoO_2 \text{ sat} - PAO_2 \text{ sat}) \times (Hgb \times 1.36)]$

What is the estimated value for oxygen consumption?

110–150 mL/kg/min (110 for stable patients; 150 for ICU patients)

Name at least three pitfalls of the Fick equation.

1. Intracardiac shunts
2. Difficult measurement of oxygen consumption (generally estimated)
3. Incorrect data
4. Invasive insertion
5. PA sample drawn too quickly, which pulls pulmonary capillary (oxygenated) blood into the sample, thus overestimating the PA saturation

In general, what PA saturation levels would be in a normal range?

A PAO_2 saturation of >65% and <80% is consistent with a normal CO. A PAO_2 saturation >80% is consistent with some types of left-to-right shunting, and <65% is consistent with a reduced cardiac output.

How can errors in CO determination affect SVR?

The SVR, PVR, and so on are calculated numbers, and errors in pressure or CO measurements affect these numbers. For example, a patient with a normal CO of 6.0 L/min and significant tricuspid regurgitation may have a measured CO of 3.0 L/min. This would double the calculated SVRI and may result in inappropriate treatment.

HISTORY AND PHYSICAL EXAMINATION

HISTORY

What seven historical features of chest pain must be identified to differentiate cardiac pain from noncardiac pain?	Think **PQRST: P**recipitating factors, **Q**uality, **R**adiation and location, **R**elief, **R**isk factor, **S**ymptoms, and **T**ime and duration

PHYSICAL EXAMINATION

What causes an S_1?	Closure of the mitral and tricuspid valves
What causes a loud S_1?	Sometimes with MVP, sometimes MS and ASD
What causes a soft S_1?	MR (rheumatic or calcific), severe acute AI (valve closes prematurely)
What causes a widely split S_1?	TS, Ebstein's anomaly, VT, RBBB, LV pacing
What causes an S_2?	Closure of the aortic and pulmonic valves
What is the first sound of a split S_2?	Aortic valve closure
What is on the differential of paradoxical splitting?	Pulmonary hypertension, LBBB, aortic stenosis, HOCM, patent ductus arteriosus (left-to-right shunt), TR
What causes a single S_2?	Either absence of A_2 or P_2 (i.e., single ventricle, pulmonary atresia), or very soft P_2 (Tetralogy of Fallot), or fusion in VSD or PA HTN
What causes a loud A_2?	Thin chest wall, systemic HTN, aortic coarctation, and corrected TGA
What causes a soft A_2?	Either AS (decreased mobility) or AI (fails to coapt)
What causes a loud P_2?	PA HTN
What causes a soft P_2?	Valvular or infundibular PS

What is in the differential when an S_4 is noted?

LVH (HTN, AS, HOCM), RVH, IHD, hyperdynamic circulation, acute valvular regurgitation, and restrictive cardiomyopathy

When is the click heard in MVP?

Usually midway through systole

What maneuvers can affect the click?

Things that shrink the ventricle push the click closer to S_2 (sitting up, part of Valsalva).

What is an ejection click?

A click usually heard during systole due to a congenitally abnormal aortic or pulmonic valve

What is an opening snap?

An early diastolic sound associated with abnormal mitral or tricuspid valve opening. Heard with MS or TS.

When does cyanosis occur?

When the concentration of deoxyhemoglobin in the blood is >5 mg/dL

What are the two main categories of cyanosis?

Central and peripheral

What are the general causes of central cyanosis?

Decreased arterial oxygen saturation caused by right-to-left shunting, impaired ability of hemoglobin to bind oxygen (e.g., in methemoglobinemia or abnormal hemoglobin variants), or impaired pulmonary function

What causes peripheral cyanosis?

Cutaneous vasoconstriction due to low CO or exposure to cold

What are the causes of peripheral edema?

Chronic venous insufficiency

Venous obstruction

Lymphatic obstruction

Thrombosis

Heart failure (high- and low-output)

Constrictive pericarditis

Nephrotic syndrome

Hepatic cirrhosis

Angioneurotic edema

Myxedema

What is the formula for converting cm H$_2$O to mm Hg?

cm H$_2$O × 0.75 = mm Hg

In the jugular venous tracing below,* identify the various numbered waveforms.

1. a wave
2. c wave
3. v wave
4. x descent
5. y descent

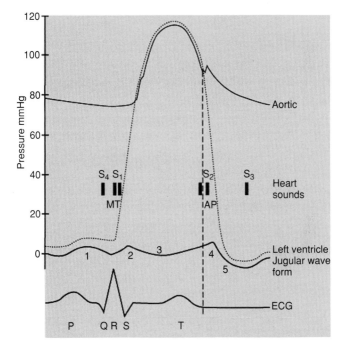

Passive ventricular filling

What is the abdominal–jugular (also called hepatojugular) reflux?

An increase in JVP of >3 cm H$_2$O with 10 to 30 seconds of periumbilical pressure

---

*Modified from Fuster et al: Hurst's *The Heart*, 10th ed. New York: McGraw-Hill, 2001:64.

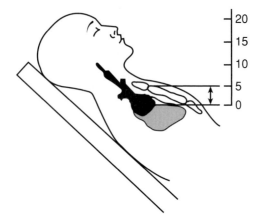

When does abdominal–jugular reflux occur?	It is associated with RV or LV failure, TR, or any cause of elevated CVP or PCWP.
How high is the JVP if the earlobes have a bobbing motion while the patient is sitting?	>15 cm H_2O
What is the differential diagnosis of Kussmaul's sign?	Constrictive pericarditis, restrictive cardiomyopathy, RV infarction or failure
What is the differential diagnosis of pulsus paradoxus?	Pericardial tamponade, constrictive pericarditis, restrictive cardiomyopathy, COPD (exacerbation), asthma (exacerbation), superior vena cava obstruction, pulmonary embolus, hypovolemic shock, pregnancy, and obesity
What is the differential diagnosis of pulsus alternans?	Severe HF, anything causing rapid respiratory rates, pericardial tamponade
What is a bisferiens pulse?	A pulse waveform with two upstrokes
List five causes of a bisferiens pulse.	AI, HOCM, exercise, fever, PDA

With what are the following findings associated?

Pulsus tardus	Obstruction to LV outflow (valvular AS or nonvalvular AS)
Pulsus parvus	Reduced LV stroke volume
Pulsus parvus et tardus	Severe AS
Bisferiens pulse (both peaks in systole)	Conditions in which a large stroke volume is ejected rapidly from the LV (aortic regurgitation, combined AS and AI), hypertrophic cardiomyopathy, hyperkinetic circulation, normal variant
Dicrotic pulse (first peak in systole, second peak in diastole—based on the relation to S$_2$)	Hypotension, fever with decreased SVR, tamponade, severe heart failure, hypovolemic shock
Pulsus alternans	Severe LV dysfunction and a regular rhythm
What is the pulse pressure?	The systolic BP minus the diastolic BP; index = (systolic BP – diastolic BP)/(systolic BP)
What are causes of a wide pulse pressure?	Aortic regurgitation, PDA, truncus arteriosus, CHB, sinus bradycardia, fever, anemia, strenuous exercise, thyrotoxicosis, AV fistulas, and hot weather

CARDIOVASCULAR PROCEDURES

CHEST RADIOGRAPHY

See *Medicine Recall*, **3rd ed.**

ELECTROCARDIOGRAM

What is the normal size of the P wave measured in II?	≤120 ms (3 boxes)—if longer, consider LA enlargement
	≤0.25 mV (2.5 boxes)—if taller, consider RA enlargement

Table 3–1.   Calculating the Heart Rate on the ECG

Number of Large Boxes	Time	Rate (bpm)
1	200 ms	300
2	400 ms	150
3	600 ms	100
4	800 ms	>75
5	1 s	60
6	1.2 s	50

What is the 300, 150, 100 rule?

The 300, 150, 100 rule is used to quickly calculate the rate on the ECG. The HR = 150/(number of small boxes between R waves) or 300/(number of large boxes between R waves)

What is the normal range for the PR interval?

120 to 200 ms (3 to 5 boxes)

List three causes of a short PR interval.

1. Accelerated AV conduction
2. Tachycardia
3. Accessory AV pathway (e.g., WPW syndrome)

List five causes of a long PR interval.

1. High vagal tone
2. AV conduction system degenerative disease
3. IHD
4. Drugs that impair AV conduction (e.g., beta-adrenergic blockers and digoxin)
5. Dual AV node physiology using the slow pathway

What is the normal range for the QRS interval?

60 to 119 ms (1.5 to 3 boxes). A conduction delay is present if the QRS is ≥110 ms, and a BBB is present if the QRS is ≥120 ms.

What is the QTc?

The corrected QT interval (corrects for the HR)

Why is it important to measure intervals?	The measurement allows determination of blocks (e.g., first-degree or RBBB).
What prolongs the PR interval?	AV blocks
What prolongs the QRS interval?	BBBs Premature ventricular beats LVH Preexcitation syndromes (e.g., WPW syndrome) Electrolyte abnormalities (e.g., hyperkalemia) Paced beats Medications (e.g., amiodarone, procainamide, tricyclic antidepressants)
What prolongs the QT interval?	Medications [tricyclic antidepressants, antiarrhythmics (e.g., quinidine, procainamide, amiodarone, sotalol, dofetilide), methadone, antipsychotics, terfenadine plus macrolide antibiotics (e.g., erythromycin)] Electrolyte deficiencies (e.g., potassium, magnesium, calcium) Congenital long QT IHD Hypothermia MVP Intracranial events (e.g., subarachnoid hemorrhage)
What is the I, aVF rule?	From the previous example, if leads I and aVF are both more positive than negative, the axis is normal.
What is a significant Q wave?	40 ms or one third the height of the QRS
What does the Q wave represent?	A previous MI

Does the absence of a Q wave mean that no infarction has occurred?

Some infarctions tend to lose Q waves over time: inferior infarctions lose Q waves 50% of the time; anterior infarctions lose Q waves <10% of the time.

Describe the QRS complex in the following:

RBBB

QRS ≥120 ms

rSR′ pattern in V_1

Deep slurred S wave in V_6, I

LBBB

QRS ≥120 ms

All negative in V_1

All positive in V_6, I

LAFB

QRS <120 ms (unless associated with an RBBB)

LAD (>−30 degrees)

Small Q waves in I, aVL

R waves in II, III, aVF (i.e., no IMI)

LPFB

QRS <120 ms (unless associated with an RBBB)

RAD (>120 degrees)

Small Q waves in II, III, aVF

R waves in I, aVL (i.e., no lateral MI)

If an RBBB pattern is observed with paced beats (transvenous), what should be considered?

Septal perforation by the wire, a high RV septal location (the impulse crosses to the LV side) and biventricular pacing

Name the causes of ST elevation.

AMI, ventricular aneurysm, pericarditis, Prinzmetal's angina, myocardial contusion, hypothermia (Osborne or J wave), hyperkalemia, early repolarization, and artifact. ST elevation is also occasionally seen with LBBB, LVH, myocardial neoplasms, hypertrophic cardiomyopathies, and after VT.

Name the causes of ST depression.	Acute posterior MI, ischemia, digitalis, LVH, and BBB
What does the $S_1S_2S_3$ pattern (i.e., S waves in leads I, II, and III) or the $S_1Q_3T_3$ pattern (i.e., S wave in lead I and Q wave and inverted T wave in lead III) suggest?	Acute pulmonary embolus causing acute RV strain
How frequently is this ECG abnormality seen?	In 10% of cases
What is electrical alternans?	Alternating ECG voltage beat by beat

ECG CASE STUDIES

The following ECGs, on pages 47 through 49, are those of a 74-year-old man with chest pain. He was admitted to the CCU.

> **What is the rate, rhythm, and axis of the ECG below?**

Rate = 80 bpm; rhythm = sinus; axis = (–)10

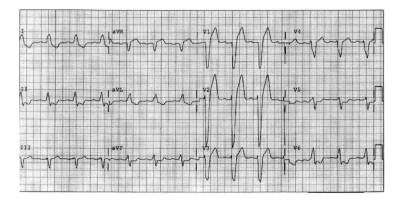

What is the other important finding?	A LBBB
With the chest pain and a new LBBB, what therapy should be considered?	Emergent PCI or thrombolysis
You are then called for tachycardia and hypotension. What is the rate, rhythm, and axis on the ECG below?	Rate = 120 bpm; rhythm = atrial fibrillation; axis = 0

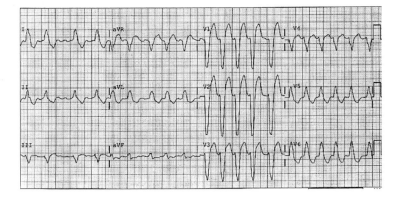

What else is demonstrated on the ECG?	The same LBBB
What is the clue that this rhythm isn't VT?	The rhythm is irregularly irregular.
You treat the rhythm with a beta blocker and the patient's symptoms resolve. You are then called a few hours later for bradycardia and dizziness. What is the rate, rhythm, and axis of the ECG on page 49?	Rate = 33 bpm; rhythm = complete heart block (3rd degree AV block) axis = (–)80

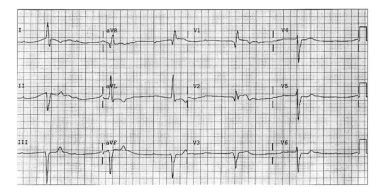

**What are the other
findings on the ECG?**

An atypical RBBB, RVH, and LVH. There
is likely a recent anterior infarction (Q
waves in V_1 through V_3 with ST
elevation), although that can sometimes
be related to LVH.

**Is it odd that the patient
does not have the same
LBBB?**

Yes, and very concerning. He now shows
severe conduction system disease with an
alternating BBB.

**What therapy should be
considered for this man?**

An emergent temporary pacemaker.

**The ECG on below is that of
a 42-year-old man who has
been referred for the
evaluation of heart failure.**

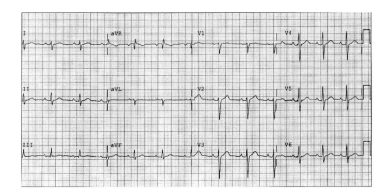

What is the rate, rhythm, and axis?	Rate = 76 bpm; rhythm = sinus; axis = (+)120
What is the conduction abnormality?	He has an isolated LPFB.
What are the features of this conduction abnormality?	The right axis, lack of evidence of a lateral MI (no Q waves noted in I or aVL), and the small Q waves in leads II, III, and aVF

The ECG below is that of a 47-year-old man involved in a head-on crash. The car did not have airbags and he was not wearing a seat belt.

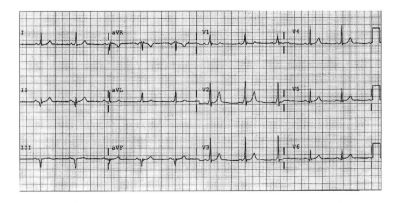

What is the rate, rhythm, and axis?	Rate = 64 bpm; rhythm = sinus; axis = (−)45
He complains of chest pain. Did he have an MI?	There are Q waves in II, III, and aVF, consistent with an IMI; however, an MI is unlikely owing to other findings.
What other findings are there?	The PR interval is short (100 ms). Delta waves are present in all leads but best seen in V1 through V3, also I and aVL. The delta waves are also noted in II, III, and aVF, explaining the IMI pattern.

What is the cause of the ECG findings?

WPW syndrome—an abnormal connection between the atrium and ventricle, allowing conduction to pass to the ventricle outside the AV node

The ECG below is that of a 60-year-old man in the CCU.

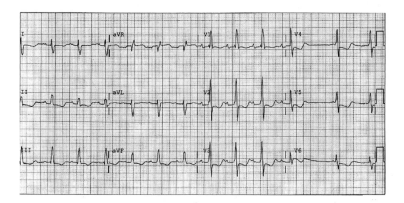

What is the rate, rhythm, and axis?

Rate = 79 bpm; rhythm = Wenckebach; axis = (+)130. The PR interval is shortest at the start and end of the tracing with the longest PR right at the transition to leads V_4 through V_6 with the dropped beat at V_4 through V_6.

What else is demonstrated on this ECG?

There is a RBBB. Possibly LA enlargement and diffuse STT changes suggesting ischemia.

What do the T waves in the chest leads suggest?

The T inversions in those leads could be consistent with ischemia or an evolving MI (now age-indeterminate). Usually, age-indeterminate MIs do not have as deep a T-wave inversion.

**The ECG below is that of a
75-year-old woman.**

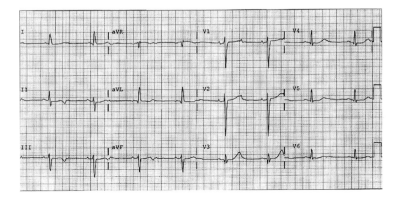

**What is the rate, rhythm,
and axis?**

Rate = 49 bpm; rhythm = 2:1 AV block;
axis = (–)45. The extra P waves are best
noted in leads V_1 and V_2.

**How is it possible to
tell whether this is
Wenckebach or Mobitz 2?**

It isn't absolutely possible. The PR
interval on the conducted beats does not
change consistent with the 2:1 cycle. If
the patient has other cycles, like a 3:1 or
4:1 with a constant PR, this would likely
be Mobitz 2. An exercise test can be
helpful in that patients with Wenckebach
tend to improve their conduction (or at
least not worsen).

**What else is noted on this
ECG?**

An LAFB and inferior T changes that may
represent ischemia. The anterior T waves
are also quite broad, suggesting
hypokalemia, hypomagnesemia, or
hypocalcemia.

**The ECG on page 53 is that
of a 74-year-old man who
presents to your clinic
complaining of palpitations.**

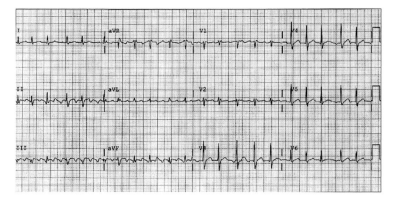

What is the rate, rhythm, and axis?

Rate = 130 bpm; rhythm = atrial flutter with predominant 2:1 conduction; axis = (–)43. This has a fairly typical sawtooth appearance, although the rate is a little slower than the usual 150 bpm.

The ECG below is that of a 70-year-old man complaining of dyspnea.

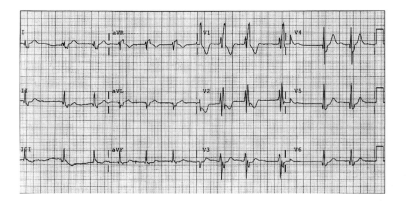

What is the rate, rhythm, and axis?

Rate = 75 bpm, rhythm = atrial fibrillation, axis = (+)165

What is the major finding?	The RBBB and the left posterior fascicular block
Is there anything of concern about the RBBB configuration?	The voltage is quite high, suggesting pulmonary hypertension.
Of interest, the image below shows the ECG of the same man 2 years earlier. What is the rate, rhythm, and axis?	Rate = 80 bpm; rhythm = atrial fibrillation; axis = (+)100

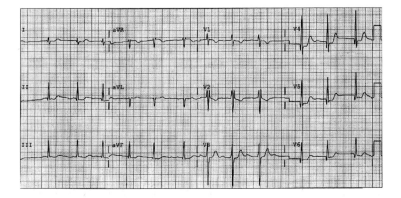

What does the axis and taller R wave suggest?	RVH

The ECG below is that of a 70-year-old man with a dilated cardiomyopathy. He is admitted to Neurology owing to a change in mental status and you are called to assess VT.

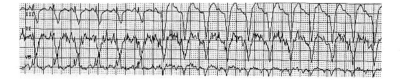

What is the rate, rhythm, and axis?

Rate = 130 bpm at the beginning and 140 bpm from the middle of the strip onward. The rhythm begins as paced. The VT is actually sinus rhythm with his baseline LBBB as P waves seen on the shoulder of the T wave. The axis cannot be determined as it is just a single lead.

The ECG below is that of a 65-year-old man with chest pain.

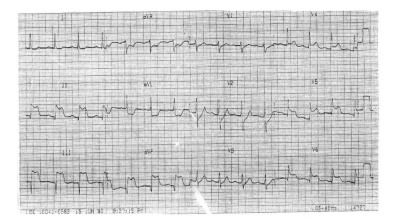

What is the rate, rhythm, and axis?

Rate = 84 bpm; rhythm = sinus; axis = (−)40

What is the reason for the chest pain?

This is a classic inferior posterior lateral MI, given the anterior ST depression with the inferior and lateral ST elevation.

What noninvasive test should be considered next?

There are a couple options, but an ECG with right-sided chest leads would give prognostic information (looking for RV infarction). An echocardiogram could help to look at RV and LV function but would take longer to obtain.

This patient is given aspirin and nitroglycerin and nitropaste is applied. The patient then becomes hypotensive. What should be considered?

This would be a typical scenario for an RV infarction with hypotension secondary to the nitropaste. If the paste is removed and some volume given, the hypotension is likely to resolve.

The ECG below is that of a 61-year-old man with chest pain.

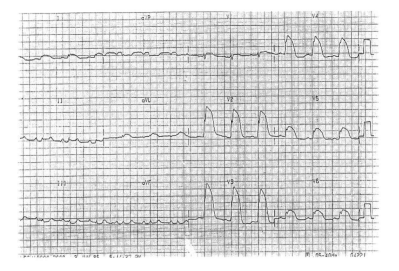

What is the rate, rhythm, and axis?

Rate = 75 bpm; rhythm = sinus rhythm; axis = (+)30

If this patient presented 30 minutes into chest pain, what therapy should be considered?

Thrombolysis for the very large anterolateral MI

If this patient presented 2 hours into pain and did not have contraindications, what could be considered?

Direct PCI

SIGNAL-AVERAGED ELECTROCARDIOGRAPHY

What is signal-averaged ECG (saECG)?

An ECG technique used to look for late depolarizations from the ventricle (small depolarizations that occur after the QRS complex)

What are late depolarizations called?

Late ventricular afterdepolarizations

What is the significance of late afterdepolarizations?

They can be a substrate responsible for some VTs.

When is saECG helpful?

When you suspect that a patient's symptoms are caused by VT and you want to risk-stratify that patient for risk of VT and sudden death. A patient with a low LVEF and an abnormal saECG has a higher risk of VT and sudden death (approximately 30% at 1 year of follow-up).

HOLTER MONITORING, LONG-TERM EVENT RECORDERS

What is the advantage of a Holter monitor?

Allows the evaluation for symptomatic and asymptomatic rhythm disturbances (such as silent PAF). Allows the evaluation for cardiac and noncardiac causes of palpitations.

What is the disadvantage of a Holter monitor?

It can be cumbersome to wear and can be used for only 24 to 48 hours.

What are two types of recording modes for an event recorder?

Continuous looping and noncontinuous recording

What is the advantage of a nonlooping device?

It does not have to be worn continuously. It is placed in contact with the skin only during symptoms.

What are the disadvantages of a nonlooping device?

It is not helpful for patients with syncope or brief symptoms.

What is the advantage of a looping device?	When the event is tagged by the patient, the ECG recording immediately prior to the event is saved, allowing the triggering event to be studied.
What is another type of long-term ECG recorder?	An implantable device.
How is this device placed?	Much like a single-lead pacemaker. The device is implanted under the skin (usually the left shoulder) and a lead is placed into the ventricle.
How are data from the device obtained?	Much like the interrogation of a pacemaker.
How long can these devices be used?	Usually over a year.

TILT TABLE

What is the tilt table test used for?	To look for vasovagal syncope
How is a tilt table test performed?	The patient is strapped to a table, and the table is tilted to 70 degrees from horizontal for 45 minutes with continuous ECG and arterial BP monitoring.
What medication can be added to tilt table testing to bring out autonomic instability?	Isoproterenol.

ECHOCARDIOGRAPHY

What Doppler findings correspond to significant aortic valve stenosis?	Peak instantaneous gradients >50 mm Hg
What equation is used during the Doppler exam to calculate the aortic valve area?	The continuity equation

What Doppler findings correspond to significant mitral valve stenosis?

Gradients >10 to 15 mm Hg

What equation is used during the Doppler exam to calculate the mitral valve area?

The pressure half-time formula

What Doppler technique is used to estimate the PA pressure?

A simplified Bernoulli equation: $4v^2 + RA$ pressure. If the Doppler velocity is 3 m^2 and you estimate the RA pressure at 10 mm Hg, then the PA pressure (assuming no PS) is $4 \times (3)^2 + 10 = 46$ mm Hg.

How is the RA pressure estimated?

By evaluating the size and dispensability of the IVC.

How are shunts detected?

Color-flow and pulsed Doppler sonography can identify abnormal flows (e.g., ASD and VSD). Agitated saline or Albunex, a contrast agent, can be rapidly injected into a peripheral vein while the heart is imaged.

What are the echo findings when there is a shunt at the atrial level?

If there is an ASD, contrast can be seen flowing from the RA to the LA. Often, shunts are bidirectional and flow into the RA of noncontrasted blood, which creates a contrast-negative jet.

STRESS TESTING

What are some contraindications to exercise stress testing (i.e., a GXT)?

Uncontrolled HTN

Decompensated CHF

AMI or unstable angina

Critical AS

Severe idiopathic subaortic stenosis

Known severe LMCA disease

Uncontrolled arrhythmia or heart block

Inability to walk on treadmill because of neurologic or musculoskeletal abnormalities or vascular disease

Acute myocarditis or pericarditis

Acute systemic illness

What are contraindications to DP testing?

Significant asthma or COPD (due to stimulation of adenosine a2b receptors, causing bronchospasm), and recent CVA. Caffeine and theophylline compounds must be withheld before testing.

What are contraindications to dobutamine testing?

Significant HTN, known catechol-induced arrhythmias, and a large AAA (i.e., ≥6 cm)

What variables indicate a high-risk GXT?

Inability to exercise or poor exercise performance (<5 METs) because of a cardiac reason

Significant ECG changes within the first 3 to 6 minutes

Extensive ischemic changes (>2-mm ST depression, many leads involved)

Decrease in BP or flat BP response to exercise

Significant arrhythmias

What ECG findings are noted during a positive but not a high-risk test?

ST depression (usually the lateral leads)

ST elevation (usually the anterior leads when it occurs)

Heart block or VT

How much should the HR increase during a GXT?

10 bpm/stage

When is a delay in HR acceleration commonly noted?

May be noted in athletes and patients taking beta-adrenergic blockers

How much should the BP increase during a GXT?

10 mm Hg/stage (a delay may be noted in athletes and fit individuals)

What is the sensitivity and specificity of GXT for detecting CAD?

65% and 65%

| List the causes of false-positive GXT results. | Female gender, hyperventilation, MVP, LVH, digitalis |
| What is the mortality rate for a stress test? | 1:10,000 |

CARDIOPULMONARY EXERCISE TESTING

What is cardiopulmonary exercise testing?	Measurement of the body's oxygen consumption during peak exercise.
How is cardiopulmonary testing performed?	During a standard treadmill or bicycle stress test, snorkel-like equipment or a mask is attached to the patient so that all the inspired O_2 and expired CO_2 can be measured by the machine.
In general terms, what affects the peak $\dot{V}o_2$ a patient can achieve?	Age, gender, and size all affect the peak $\dot{V}o_2$. Severe lung disease, anemia, beta blockers, and deconditioning will also affect the results.
In general, when is cardiopulmonary testing used?	To determine the prognosis in patients who have LV dysfunction
What peak $\dot{V}o_2$ level is associated with a poor long-term prognosis?	A peak $\dot{V}o_2$ <14 mL/kg/min or <50% of the predicted value for a given patient is associated with poor long-term survival. A peak $\dot{V}o_2$ <10 mL/kg/min or <35% predicted carries an abysmal 1-year survival rate.
What peak $\dot{V}o_2$ level is associated with a good long-term prognosis?	$\dot{V}o_2$ >20 mL/kg/min

STRESS ECHOCARDIOGRAPHY

| What is the stress-echocardiographic appearance of ischemia? | Normal wall motion at rest that becomes abnormal (asynergic) during stress |

What is the stress-echocardiographic appearance of infarcted myocardium?	Generally asynergic segments of myocardium that are thinned
What is the stress-echocardiographic appearance of hibernating myocardium?	Asynergic regions that improve with stress (treadmill or dobutamine)

RADIONUCLIDE IMAGING

Why does thallium provide useful information?	It behaves like potassium; that is, it is taken up by viable cells, and thallium uptake is directly proportional to coronary blood flow.
How does MIBI work?	MIBI is a lipophilic compound that diffuses across intact cell membranes (cells with working mitochondria).
Why is it important to determine viability?	Hibernating myocardium improves function after revascularization.
What are indications for radionuclide ventriculography (MUGA)?	A rest study is used to assess LVEF with or without RVEF.
How does a MUGA scan work?	Red blood cells are removed from the body and labeled with pyrophosphate. The labeled cells are then returned to the patient and technetium is injected into the patient. The technetium binds to the pyrophosphate-labeled cells. The gamma rays are then tracked. LVEF = (LVED counts – LVES counts)/LVED counts. This provides an accurate means of monitoring the LVEF.

POSITRON EMISSION TOMOGRAPHY

What is PET imaging?	Imaging with the use of positrons.
What is the advantage of PET over other imaging techniques?	Less tissue attenuation (better imaging of all body types) Can be used to study metabolism (e.g., fatty acid, glucose)

What are the disadvantages of PET?	Requires a linear accelerator to manufacture the positrons. The equipment is expensive.

ELECTROPHYSIOLOGIC PROCEDURES

What general rhythm disturbances can be treated by catheter ablation?	SA node modification for inappropriate sinus tachycardia Atrial flutter Pulmonary vein modification for atrial fibrillation Ablation of preexcitation pathways Ablation of ventricular tachycardia
How do the EP physicians gain access to the left side of the heart for evaluation?	Either through the coronary sinus, through a transseptal approach (right atrium into the left atrium), or retrograde across the aortic valve

PACEMAKERS AND INTERNAL DEFIBRILLATORS

What do the letters in a three-letter pacemaker code represent?	The first letter is the chamber or chambers paced (i.e., A, V, or D). The second letter is the chamber or chambers sensed (i.e., A, V, or D). The third letter is the mode of response to a sensed event (i.e., T, I, or D). The fourth letter refers to the rate response or not (i.e., R or blank)
In a rate-responsive pacemaker (R), what are the triggering modes?	Changes in respiratory rate, CO_2 level/minute ventilation, or motion
How is the LV paced with a biventricular pacemaker?	By threading a pacemaker lead through the coronary sinus up to the great cardiac vein (drains the LAD territory) or down a lateral wall vein. Can also be implanted on the LV directly with surgery.
What are the indications for biventricular pacing?	Patients with NYHA class II to III/IV heart failure despite medical therapy with EF <35% who are in sinus rhythm and have evidence of LV dyssynchrony with a QRS >130 msec

What are the capabilities of a three-zone ICD?	Antitachycardia pacing, defibrillation, and single- or dual-chamber pacing
What is antitachycardia pacing?	Termination of VT by pacing the ventricle at a rate 10% or so faster than the tachycardia, which results in shifting the tachycardia circuit to a new location. When the pacing is terminated, the tachycardia is also terminated.
What is a potential complication of antitachycardia pacing?	The tachycardia speeds up to the paced rate and does not terminate.
What is the advantage of antitachycardia pacing?	Painless termination of the VT

CARDIAC CATHETERIZATION

What is the ramus intermedius?	A branch from the LMCA (in between the LAD and circumflex)
How common is right dominance?	This occurs in 90% of cases. The other 10% of the time, the PDA comes from the LCx (left dominant).
Which artery supplies the SA node?	The RCA in 55%, the LCx in 45%
Which artery supplies the AV node?	The RCA if dominant (85% to 90%); the LCx otherwise.
What are the important complications of cardiac catheterization?	Allergic contrast reaction, bleeding, infection, renal failure, 1/1000 incidence of stroke, MI, arrhythmias, cardiac perforation, and death
What are the benefits of cardiac catheterization?	It provides a map of all vessel stenoses, distal vessels, collaterals, and LV function. It also provides information as to the severity of valvular regurgitation, allows calculation of stenotic valve areas, and directly measures intracardiac pressures.

What are the coronary flow findings for TIMI 0 flow?

Absence of any antegrade coronary blood flow

What are the coronary flow findings for TIMI 1 flow?

Faint filling beyond the coronary stenosis but not to the distal portion of the artery

What are the coronary flow findings for TIMI 2 flow?

Complete filling of the artery with delayed or sluggish flow

What are the coronary flow findings for TIMI 3 flow?

Normal coronary blood flow

How can restenosis be treated?

Redilatation, stenting, brachytherapy, atherectomy, and CABG

What common drugs are used in the drug-eluting stents?

Sirolimus and paclitaxel

What factors of a stent are associated with a higher restenosis rate?

A smaller stent diameter and a longer stent length

What is subacute stent thrombosis?

A platelet-mediated phenomenon that occurs before reendothelialization of the stent

When does subacute stent thrombosis occur?

Typically early after intracoronary stent implantation, usually within the first 30 days. However, this can also occur late out.

How does subacute thrombosis present?

Patients present with chest pain and ST elevation.

How is subacute stent thrombosis prevented?

Cotreatment with ASA (325 mg for the first month; 81 mg thereafter) and clopidogrel (75 mg every day) has been shown to limit its occurrence to about 2%.

What are the options for bifurcation lesions?

Usually crushed or kissing stents.

What is brachytherapy?

Intracoronary radiation (beta or gamma).

What is the downside of brachytherapy?

"Candy wrapper" restenosis. Stenosis that occurs at the proximal and distal margins of the brachytherapy field.

What are the indications for aortic valvuloplasty?

A bridge for patients with AS who require noncardiac surgery. May be helpful to determine if the AS is the cause of LV dysfunction prior to valve replacement in very ill patients. Can be a lasting therapy for patients with congenital noncalcific AS.

How do you time an IABP?

The device inflates during diastole (the dicrotic notch), augmenting coronary blood flow, and deflates during systole (just prior to the aortic pressure upstroke), causing a reduction in afterload. This can be timed off the aortic pulsation or the ECG tracing.

What are three contraindications to an IABP?

1. Significant aortic regurgitation
2. Aortic dissection
3. Severe peripheral vascular disease

CORONARY ARTERY BYPASS GRAFTING

What are the mechanisms of chest pain reduction after CABG?

Restoration of blood flow to the myocardium, MI during surgery, placebo effect, and denervation.

What is an OPCAB?

Off-pump coronary bypass

What is an advantage of an OPCAB?

Since it is done off "pump," there is the theoretical advantage of less neurologic complications due to the bypass machine and less manipulation of the aorta.

What is a disadvantage of an OPCAB?

It can be difficult to revascularize all areas of the heart.

What is robotic surgery?

Using human-controlled robotic "hands" to perform heart surgery

What is a potential advantage of the robotic surgery?

It can be done remotely. For example, a technician could place the cannulae and the surgeon could operate from thousands of miles distant.

What is hybrid surgery?

Using a combination of percutaneous (i.e., stents) and operative procedures.

CORONARY ARTERY DISEASE

What is the incidence of CAD?

On an annual basis in the United States, 5.4 million people are diagnosed with CAD, and CAD is responsible for in excess of 500,000 deaths per year.

What is the coronary perfusion pressure?

Mean arterial pressure − LVEDP

What factors can lower perfusion pressure?

Coronary perfusion pressure—hypotension, coronary stenosis

High LVEDP—hypertrophy (HTN <AS), HF, MR, and AR

How is coronary flow determined?

Coronary flow = (perfusion pressure)/(vascular resistance)

How are the different types of hyperlipoproteinemia classified (Fredrickson and Lee)?

Type I: increased chylomicrons, normal cholesterol, increased triglycerides

Type IIA: increased LDL and cholesterol; may have increased triglycerides; normal VLDL

Type IIB: increased LDL, VLDL, and triglycerides

Type III: floating beta lipoprotein; increased cholesterol and triglycerides

Type IV: increased VLDL and triglycerides; normal to increased cholesterol

Type V: increased chylomicrons, VLDL, and cholesterol; greatly increased triglycerides; reduced LDL and HDL

What LDL should be the goal (based on NCEP III guidelines) in patients with known CAD or CAD equivalent (i.e., DM)?

<100 mg/dL, consider <70 mg/dL in high-risk patients

How much cardiovascular mortality benefit do you get for lowering the LDL by 40 mg/dL?

About 20%

How much fat is in the average American diet?

35% to 40% of all calories ingested

How much can dietary modification lower LDL cholesterol?

Reducing ingested fat to 20% to 25% of the total calories taken in can lead to a 15% reduction in LDL cholesterol.

What HMG-CoA reductase inhibitors are available for the treatment of hyperlipidemia?

Fluvastatin, lovastatin, pravastatin, simvastatin, atorvastatin, and rosuvastatin

What bile-acid sequestrants are available for the treatment of hyperlipidemia?

Cholestyramine [Questran], colestipol [Colestid], and colesevelam [Welchol]

What fibric acid derivatives are available for the treatment of hyperlipidemia?

Gemfibrozil [Lopid] and fenofibrate [Tricor]

What cholesterol absorption inhibitors are available for the treatment of hyperlipidemia?

Ezetimibe [Zetia], Benecol, Take Control, and B-sitosterol

What else is available for the treatment of hyperlipidemia?

Nicotinic acid and fish oil. Garlic may also have a mild benefit.

Besides CAD, what is a potential complication of elevated TG?

Pancreatitis

What are the side effects of:

HMG-CoA reductase inhibitors?

Constipation, rhabdomyositis (<1%; more frequent with drug combinations such as gemfibrozil and cyclosporine and potentiated by large quantities of grapefruit juice), hepatitis (<3%), myopathy, and transaminitis

Bile-acid resins?

Gastrointestinal complaints (e.g., constipation, bloating)

Niacin?

Flushing, pruritus, hepatitis, hyperglycemia, hyperuricemia, gout

Fibric acid derivatives?

Gastrointestinal complaints, hepatitis, and myopathy/myositis

What is LP(a)?

A derivative of LDL that is substantially more atherogenic than LDL alone

What are the features of the "metabolic syndrome"?

Waist >40 inches [men], >35 inches [women], fasting glucose >110 mg/dL, BP ≥130/85 mm Hg, HDL <40 mg/dL, TG ≥150 mg/dL

BIOMARKERS IN ACUTE CORONARY SYNDROMES

Name seven causes of CK elevation.

AMI, myocarditis, rhabdomyolysis (trauma, status epilepticus, surgery, severe prolonged exercise), polymyositis or muscular dystrophy, devastating brain injury, familial elevation, renal injury

Name four causes of CK-MB elevation.

Acute MI, cardiac surgery, muscular dystrophy, and myocarditis

Name four causes of CK-BB elevation.

Brain injury or Reye's syndrome, uremia, malignant hyperthermia, and small intestine necrosis

Name six causes of LDH elevation.

Acute MI, hemolytic anemia, pernicious anemia or sickle cell crisis, large pulmonary embolus, renal infarction, prosthetic heart valves, hepatic injury, and myoglobin

What are the circumstances where troponin I and T may remain elevated for prolonged periods?

Some patients with heart failure may "leak" troponin at all times. Patients with renal failure may have prolonged elevations due to decreased clearance.

What else causes a rise in AST?

Hepatic congestion/ischemia, skeletal muscle injury (including IM injections), PE, and during shock

When does the LDH elevate, peak, and resolve in AMI?

Elevation at 24 to 48 hours, peak at 3 to 6 days, and resolution at 8 to 14 days

What else causes LDH to elevate?

Hemolysis, megaloblastic anemia, leukemia, liver disease, hepatic congestion/ischemia, renal disease, some neoplasms, PE, myocarditis, skeletal muscle disease, and shock

In the figure below, label the curves for the appropriate enzyme:

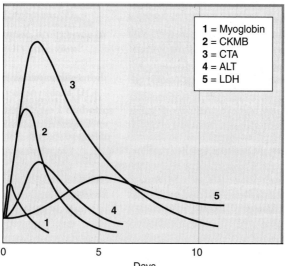

1 = Myoglobin
2 = CKMB
3 = CTA
4 = ALT
5 = LDH

Days

Troponin

CK

LDH

What is hsCRP?	A biomarker of inflammation
What is b-type natriuretic peptide?	A peptide released by the myocardium in response to stretch
What are the two commonly used b-type natriuretic peptides?	bNP and NTproBNP
What conditions elevate b-type natriuretic peptide levels?	Congestive heart failure, acute MI, PE

ACUTE CORONARY SYNDROMES—GENERAL CONSIDERATIONS

What is the incidence of AMI?	1.5 million people per year; accountable for 25% of all deaths in the United States

TREATMENT OF ACUTE CORONARY SYNDROMES

If argatroban and warfarin are used in patients with HITT, when is the argatroban discontinued?	Patients are usually treated to an INR of 6 and then the argatroban is withdrawn. If the INR falls below 2, the argatroban is restarted.
Which of the GPIIb/IIIa inhibitors has the shortest half-life?	Abciximab (30 minutes versus 120 to 150 minutes for the other two)
What is the onset of action of	
Abciximab	120 minutes
Tirofiban	5 minutes
Eptifibatide	60 minutes

What is the duration of action of the GPIIb/IIIa inhibitors on the platelet function?

    Abciximab?   48 hours

    Tirofiban?   4 to 6 hours

    Eptifibatide?   4 to 6 hours

Are any of the GPIIb/IIIa inhibitors reversible?
Yes, tirofiban and eptifibatide (theoretically abciximab is also if you give enough platelets)

Name the direct thrombin inhibitors.
Lepirudin, bivalirudin, argatroban

What are the disadvantages of drug-coated stents compared with bare metal stents?
Cost and late subacute thrombosis

How is subacute thrombosis prevented?
Full deployment of the stent and at least a year of thienopyridine use following placement of a drug-eluting stent

List five of the seven risk factors in the TIMI risk score for patients with UA or NSTEMI.
Age >65 years, >3 CAD risk factors, known prior CAD, ASA use last 7 days, >2 anginal events in <24 hours, ST deviation, and elevated troponin or CK

How is the risk score used?
If the TIMI score is ≥3, the outcome is worse, suggesting a more aggressive approach (GPIIb/IIIa inhibitors and early catheterization) in these patients.

What are the indications for thrombolysis?
ST elevation in two contiguous ECG leads in patients with pain onset within 6 hours who have been refractory to sublingual nitroglycerin (with or without heparin), who cannot have primary PCI within 90 minutes of first medical contact, and who have no contraindications; therapy may also be beneficial in patients

presenting at 6 to 12 hours and perhaps at 12 to 24 hours. Also, new LBBB with typical pain.

When is thrombolysis generally preferred over PCI?

When the patient presents early after symptom onset

When PCI is not an option

When there would be a prolonged transport time

When the door to balloon time would exceed 1 hour

What are seven absolute contraindications to thrombolysis?

1. Any prior intracranial hemorrhage
2. Known structural cerebral vascular lesion (e.g., AVM)
3. Significant closed head or facial trauma within 3 months
4. Ischemic CVA in the past 3 months (excludes an ischemic CVA in the past 3 hours)
5. Malignant intracranial neoplasm (primary or metastatic)
6. Known bleeding disorder or active bleeding not including menses
7. Suspected aortic dissection

What are nine relative contraindications to thrombolysis?

1. Active peptic ulcer disease or internal bleeding within the last 2 to 4 weeks
2. A history of uncontrolled or poorly controlled HTN
3. Severe uncontrolled HTN on presentation: systolic pressure >180 mm Hg, diastolic pressure >110 mm Hg
4. Traumatic CPR or CPR >10 minutes
5. Ischemic or embolic CVA more than 3 months ago, dementia or other known intracranial process
6. Use of warfarin or other anticoagulants
7. Significant trauma or major surgery <3 weeks
8. Pregnancy
9. Noncompressible vascular punctures

When is primary PCI generally preferred over thrombolysis?

When an invasive lab is available

When the expected door to balloon time is <90 minutes

When the (door to balloon) – (door to needle) <1 hour

For high-risk patients (shock and heart failure)

When there are contraindications to lysis

When patients present late out from the event

When the diagnosis of STEMI is in question

What is rescue PCI?

Patients who fail thrombolysis at 90 minutes are taken urgently to PCI.

What is facilitated PCI?

Patients who receive thrombolysis are then brought to the catheterization laboratory for immediate PCI. This is generally not pursued owing to higher complication rates.

What are the four hemodynamic classes (Forrester) for post-MI patients?

Warm and dry (good CO and low PC)

Warm and wet (good CO and high PC)

Cold and dry (poor CO and low PC)

Cold and wet (poor CO and high PC)

MECHANICAL COMPLICATIONS OF MYOCARDIAL INFARCTION

List six mechanical complications that may follow an AMI.

Left ventricular aneurysm or rupture, papillary muscle rupture or dysfunction, thromboembolism, reinfarction or extension, pericardial effusion or tamponade, and heart failure

What is the incidence of ruptured papillary muscle in patients who die after AMI?

1% to 5% in patients who die of AMI

When does a ruptured papillary muscle typically occur?

2 to 10 days after the MI. Primarily, the posterior papillary muscle is involved.

When does a VSD typically occur?

9 to 10 days after MI, although it may occur earlier after revascularization

What is the incidence of left ventricular rupture after AMI?

More common than VSD or papillary muscle rupture; accountable for up to 25% of fatal AMIs

When does left ventricular rupture typically occur?

50% of cases within 5 days of AMI; 90% within 2 weeks

What is the mortality rate for left ventricular rupture?

>95%

What are the risk factors for LV rupture?

Female gender, hypertensive patients, usually larger infarct size (at least 20% of the free wall), treatment with lytic therapy.

How can acute MR caused by papillary muscle rupture be differentiated from an acute VSD?

    By history?

Patients with VSDs have little or no orthopnea early after the event, whereas patients with acute MR often have severe orthopnea.

    By auscultation?

The VSD murmur is heard best over the sternum. The MR murmur can be heard at the apex but frequently radiates superiorly in posterior leaflet papillary muscle ruptures and posteriorly in anterior leaflet papillary muscle ruptures.

    Echocardiogram and Doppler?

Probably the best way—allows direct visualization of the defect or flow.

Right heart catheterization with measurement of the oxygen saturation?

An increase in oxygen saturation by more than 5% between chambers is consistent with a shunt (i.e., VSD). For example, RAo_2 saturation, 61%; RVo_2 saturation, 75%; PAo_2 saturation, 78%; arterial O_2 saturation, 95%.

How is an LV aneurysm recognized on imaging procedures?

By a resting dyskinetic region

What is a pseudoaneurysm?

A ventricular free wall rupture contained by a section of pericardium (commonly a scarred section that prevents tamponade)

How is a pseudoaneurysm recognized on imaging?

A narrow neck feeding into a nontrabeculated sac

What is ventricular remodeling?

Abnormal reshaping of the ventricle at sites not involved in the initial injury owing to abnormal loading conditions

OTHER CARE AFTER MYOCARDIAL INFARCTION

How are high-embolic-risk LV thrombi recognized?

Highest risk is seen with thrombi that project into the LV cavity—i.e., that are not layered.

What is the prognostic significance of VF early after an AMI (within 48 hours)?

None

What is the prognostic significance of VF late after an AMI (longer than 48 hours)?

The mortality rate significantly increases owing to recurrent VF, which requires evaluation and long-term treatment.

Are ICDs indicated early after MI associated with LV dysfunction (LVEF <35%)?

No. A study (Defibrillator After Acute Myocardial Infarction Trial—DINAMIT) has suggested a higher death rate within the first 40 days.

When are ICDs indicated post-MI?	In patients with sustained or symptomatic VT, otherwise in those >40 days post MI with LV dysfunction and mild to moderate symptoms of heart failure. One study [Multicenter Automatic Defibrillator Implantation Trial (MADIT) II] also suggested a benefit in patients post-MI with LVEF <30% and no symptoms.
Besides VT/VF, what rhythm is seen after some IMIs?	First-, second- and then third-degree heart block

ARRHYTHMIAS

COMMON ARRHYTHMIAS

List the common SVTs	Sinus tachycardia, AV node reentry, atrial tachycardia, AV reciprocating tachycardia (accessory pathway), atrial flutter with rapid ventricular response, AF, and MAT
How is sinus tachycardia treated?	Always search for the underlying cause and treat that.
How is atrial tachycardia treated?	
With evidence of block?	Digitalis intoxication should be high on the list of causes and treated appropriately (Digibind if needed).
Without evidence of block?	AV node–blocking agents like diltiazem, beta blockers, and digoxin.
What is inappropriate sinus tachycardia?	A rhythm from the region around the sinus node that inappropriately accelerates periodically. It is an atrial tachycardia.
What are the ECG indicators to look for to determine if a patient is in VT?	P waves not connected to the QRS (AV dissociation), fusion beats, complexes >140 ms, and common-looking BBB complexes.

What is a fusion beat?

A combination of a normal QRS and a VT beat, so it is more narrow than the VT beats.

What is the name of the wide complex rhythm at 100 to 120 bpm seen in patients with MI undergoing treatment?

AIVR (accelerated idioventricular rhythm)—often associated with reperfusion

What is the best question to ask to determine whether a patient has an SVT with aberrancy or VT?

"Have you had a heart attack?" If the answer is yes, the rhythm is most likely VT; if the answer is no, consider SVT.

What is torsades de pointes?

A polymorphic VT where the axis shifts up and down as if it were turning about a point.

ATRIAL FIBRILLATION

What is the yearly risk for CVA for the average patient in AF on ASA?

5%, depending on the risk group

What is the yearly risk for CVA for the average patient in AF on warfarin?

About 1%

Considering *all* patients with AF, what factors place patients at:
  High risk for CVA?

Prior CVA/TIA, mitral stenosis, prosthetic valves (metal)

  Intermediate risk for CVA?

Age >75 years, hypertension, heart failure, LVEF ≤35%, diabetes mellitus

  Low risk for CVA?

Female gender, age 65 to 74 years, CAD, and thyrotoxicosis

What are the factors that place a patient at high risk for CVA with *nonvalvular* AF?	Prior CVA/TIA Age >75 years Hypertension Diabetes Heart failure
Do all patients with AF require anticoagulation with warfarin?	No. Those with minimal risk or none of the risk factors above may just require ASA.
In patients who are on warfarin for atrial fibrillation, what is the goal INR?	1.8 to 2.5
What else can be done for patients with AF and symptoms?	Ablation of the regions around the pulmonary veins

ANTIARRHYTHMIC MEDICATIONS

Name the antiarrhythmics according to the Vaughan Williams classification.	Class Ia (quinidine, procainamide, disopyramide) Class Ib (lidocaine, mexiletine) Class Ic (flecainide, propafenone) Class II (beta-adrenergic blockers) Class III (amiodarone, bretylium, sotalol (also a beta-adrenergic blocker), propafenone, dofetilide, and ibutilide) Class IV (nondihydropyridine calcium channel blockers)
What causes quinidine syncope?	Torsades de pointes
What is a cause of arthritis in patients taking procainamide?	Drug-induced lupus reaction

EMERGENT TREATMENT—PROTOCOLS

What is the presumptive diagnosis in a patient with a wide-complex, regular tachycardia, and no pulse?	VT
What is your first intervention?	Cardioversion
What is the diagnosis in a patient with a wide-complex, regular tachycardia who is comfortable, awake, and has a pulse?	VT or SVT with a BBB
What is your first intervention?	Intravenous amiodarone, lidocaine, beta blockers, or possibly procainamide
If the monitor shows sinus rhythm but the patient is unresponsive and has no pulse, what is the diagnosis?	Pulseless electrical activity [formerly known as electromechanical dissociation (EMD)]
In a patient with no blood pressure, what agents should be used?	Epinephrine (1 mg) and vasopressin (40 IU)
What are the reversible causes of PEA	Hypoxemia, hypovolemia, hypothermia, pneumothorax, pulmonary embolism, acidosis, coronary thrombosis, and cardiac tamponade
In patients with torsades de pointes, what therapies should be considered?	Cardioversion, treatment of electrolyte disarray, Magnesium 1 to 2 g IV, isoproterenol, pacing
What are some of the common medication causes of torsades?	Disopyramide, procainamide, quinidine, dofetilide, ibutilide, and sotalol
What antibiotics can cause torsades?	Clarithromycin, erythromycin, and the fluoroquinolones

SYNCOPE

What percentage of syncope cases are:	
Cardiovascular?	10% to 25% (mortality rate at 12 months = 30%)
Noncardiovascular?	40% to 60% (mortality rate at 12 months = 12%)
Unknown?	50% to 70% (mortality rate at 12 months = 6%)
List 10 noncardiac causes of syncope.	Vasovagal, orthostatic, hypovolemic (includes bleeding), CVA/TIA (rare), seizure, psychogenic, hypoglycemic, hyperventilation, pulmonary embolus
List six cardiovascular causes of syncope.	AS, CAD catastrophic event (e.g., ventricular free wall rupture or acute VSD), dissecting aortic aneurysm, congenital lesions, dysrhythmias (including long QT and heart block), neurocardiogenic

VALVULAR HEART DISEASE

What are the *common* systolic murmurs?	AS, MR, and VSD
What are the *uncommon* systolic murmurs?	HOCM, MVP, supravalvular aortic stenosis, RV outflow obstruction, pulmonic stenosis, tricuspid regurgitation
What are the *common* diastolic murmurs?	Aortic regurgitation and MS
What are the *uncommon* diastolic murmurs?	Tricuspid stenosis, left atrial myxoma, left-to-right shunts, Austin Flint murmur, pulmonic regurgitation
What are the *common* continuous murmurs?	PDA and the combination of AS and AI
What are the *uncommon* continuous murmurs?	Surgically created systemic-to-pulmonary shunts, venous hums

What are the Jones criteria? Screening criteria for the diagnosis of acute rheumatic fever. Patients with two major or one major and two minor criteria have a high probability of acute rheumatic fever.

What are the major Jones criteria? Carditis, erythema marginatum, chorea (St. Vitus' dance), polyarthritis, subcutaneous nodules

What are the minor Jones criteria? Fever, arthralgia, elevated ESR or positive C-reactive protein, previous rheumatic fever or rheumatic heart disease, and prolonged PR interval. There is also supporting evidence for a preceding streptococcal infection—that is, history of recent scarlet fever, positive throat culture for group A streptococcus, or increased ASO titers or titers for other streptococcal antibodies.

VALVULAR SURGERY

Name some of the sources of bioprosthetic valves. Porcine, bovine, pericardial, and human (cadaveric)

What are the common names of the bioprosthetic valves? Hancock, Carpentier, and homograft (human valve tissue)

Why is immunosuppression not required for tissue valves? The valves are fixed in glutaraldehyde; there is no active surface protein.

How long do tissue valves last? There is a 30% failure rate at 15 years.

Which are the two groups at higher risk of tissue valve failure? Younger patients and those with chronic kidney disease.

Name some of the mechanical valves available. St. Jude's, Medtronic-Hall, Star-Edwards, Lillehei-Kaster. Bjork-Shiley valves are uncommon.

What medication is required after placement of a metal valve?

Warfarin with or without aspirin

In whom should anticoagulation be avoided?

Young children, older persons (especially those prone to falling), young women who desire to bear children, and patients with a history of peptic ulcer disease or bleeding diathesis (in whom a tissue valve would be required)

In patients undergoing mitral valve surgery, why is it important to maintain the subvalvular apparatus?

It helps maintain normal ventricular geometry.

AORTIC STENOSIS

What is the normal aortic valve area?

2 to 3 cm^2

What valve area is considered to be critically narrowed?

<0.7 cm^2 (<0.5 cm^2/m^2)

What are the nonauscultatory findings of severe AS?

Sustained apical impulse

Low pulse pressure

Delayed pulse peak and low amplitude (pulsus parvus et tardus; best appreciated at the brachial artery)

What are the auscultatory findings of severe AS?

Diamond-shaped systolic murmur (the later the peak, the tighter the valve) heard at the base with radiation to the carotids

S_4; S_3 if in CHF

Ejection click

Reduced (or absent) A_2

Delayed A_2 closure (or paradoxic splitting of A_2P_2)

Mild AI (severe AS and severe AI cannot occur together)

What is an easy formula to calculate the aortic valve area?	Aortic valve area $= \dfrac{CO}{\sqrt{\text{Peak LV systolic Pressure} - \text{peak Ao systolic pressure}}}$
Why isn't percutaneous aortic balloon valvuloplasty the standard of care for severe AS?	The average patient obtains only 6 months of relief prior to restenosis of the valve.

AORTIC REGURGITATION

What connective tissue and arthritic syndromes are associated with AI?	Marfan's syndrome, Ehlers-Danlos syndrome, Reiter's, rheumatoid arthritis, systemic lupus erythematosus, Takayasu's aortitis
Why is *acute* AI difficult to diagnose?	The murmur is soft because of the rapid equalization of the aortic diastolic pressure and the LVEDP.
What are the common nonauscultatory physical findings of *chronic* severe AI?	Wide pulse pressure (If pulse pressure is <50 mm Hg or aortic diastolic pressure is >70 mm Hg, the AI is probably not severe.)
What is the description of the murmur in AI?	Midfrequency decrescendo diastolic murmur
Name the common signs associated with AI.	Corrigan's pulse (rapid increase and decrease) DeMusset's sign (head bob with pulsations) Pistol-shot pulses Duroziez's murmur (femoral artery systolic and diastolic murmur) Mueller's sign (uvular bobs) Quincke's sign (nail-bed pulsation) Hill's sign (augmented femoral artery systolic and diastolic pressure)
What is the Austin-Flint murmur?	It occurs in severe AI. The regurgitant jet strikes the anterior leaflet of the mitral valve, causing it to move into the mitral inflow and resulting in relative MS.

When is surgery needed for patients with AI?	Some studies have shown improved survival when the LV is >70 mm at end diastole or >50 mm at end systole.

MITRAL STENOSIS

What is the normal mitral valve area?	4 to 6 cm^2
At what valve area and valve gradient do symptoms commonly begin?	Mitral valve area <2 cm^2 and gradients >20 mm Hg
What are some nonvalvular causes of LV inflow obstruction?	Atrial myxoma, LA thrombus, and cor triatriatum
What is cor triatriatum?	A congenital abnormality where the left atrium remains a septated chamber
What are the common nonauscultatory physical findings of MS?	Malar flush. Peripheral cyanosis. Elevated JVD (when right heart failure occurs). Augmented v wave on jugular inspection. All signs increase with exercise and pregnancy.
What is the description of the murmur in MS?	A diastolic rumble that increases with exercise and is heard best in the left lateral decubitus position
What are the other auscultatory findings in patients with MS?	Increased S_1 Opening snap—the closer the A_2 opening snap interval, the tighter the valve Presystolic augmentation of the rumble
When patients present with symptoms of MS, what is the usual ECG finding?	Atrial fibrillation
Why does atrial fibrillation cause symptoms in patients with MS?	Loss of the atrial kick to fill the ventricle

| What features of the valve determine whether the valve can be repaired? | If the valve is not heavily calcified or the submitral apparatus is not too severely thickened, the valve can be repaired. |

MITRAL REGURGITATION

How does LV cavity dilatation cause MR?	It results in a stretch of the mitral annulus and consequent leaflet noncoaptation. Enlargement of the ventricle also causes malposition of the papillary muscle structure and leaflet malcoaptation.
How does CAD cause MR?	Recurrent MIs lead to LV dilatation.
	MIs involving the inferior or inferoposterior walls can tether the leaflet and prevent full closure.
	Papillary muscle infarction causes papillary muscle dysfunction or disruption, leading to leaflet malcoaptation.
What connective tissue diseases cause MR?	Marfan's syndrome, Ehlers-Danlos syndrome, osteogenesis imperfecta, and systemic lupus erythematosus
How does HOCM cause MR?	As the column of blood accelerates across the obstruction in the LVOT, the anterior mitral leaflet is pulled into the LV cavity (SAM: systolic anterior movement of the mitral valve).
What are some examples of congenital heart diseases with MR?	Corrected transposition, endocardial fibroelastosis, partial AV canal, and cleft leaflet
What populations are most commonly affected by mitral annular calcification?	Older women and patients with renal failure
Where does the murmur of *acute* MR radiate if the anterior papillary muscle or leaflet is injured?	The regurgitant jet (and murmur) is reflected to the back below the scapula.

Where does the murmur of *acute* MR radiate if the posterior papillary muscle or leaflet is injured?

The regurgitant jet (and murmur) is reflected superiorly to the clavicular region.

What is the common auscultatory finding of *chronic* MR?

Holosystolic murmur radiating to the apex

What are the common physical examination findings of *chronic* severe MR?

Loud holosystolic murmur, S_3 gallop, rales, JVD, liver distension, and edema

What maneuvers cause the click and murmur of MVP to move early into the systolic cycle?

Any maneuver that shrinks the LV cavity—that is, decreases the preload or afterload (e.g., by sitting or standing up)—causes the click and murmur to occur earlier.

What maneuvers cause the click and murmur of MVP to move late into the systolic cycle?

Any maneuver that increases the cavity size—that is, increases preload or afterload (e.g., by raising the legs up or gripping the hands)—causes the click and murmur to occur later.

What is the typical body habitus for patients with MVP?

Pectus excavatum, asthenic features, and straight back

INFECTIVE ENDOCARDITIS

What organisms are frequently seen in patients with acute endocarditis?

It is caused by more virulent organisms, such as *Staphylococcus aureus*, *Streptococcus pneumoniae*, and *Streptococcus pyogenes*.

What historical feature is more common in patients presenting with subacute endocarditis?

It is more common in patients with prior valvular disease.

What congenital heart defects are risk factors for IE?

Patent ductus, VSD, coarctation of the aorta, bicuspid aortic valve, tetralogy of Fallot, and pulmonary stenosis

What are some of the other risk factors for IE?	Rheumatic heart disease
	Degenerative cardiac lesions (aortic sclerosis and mitral calcification)
	Some MVP with regurgitation
	Intracardiac pacemakers or intracardiac prostheses
	Intravascular access procedures in ill, hospitalized patients
	Intravenous drug use
What are the symptoms and signs of IE?	Almost any organ can be involved. Symptoms and signs include fever, constitutional symptoms, heart murmur, peripheral manifestations (see below), musculoskeletal symptoms, HF, emboli, and neurologic symptoms.
How often is a heart murmur heard in IE?	In >85% of cases
How often is a new or a changing murmur heard with IE?	In <10% of cases
How often are peripheral findings of IE seen?	In <50% of cases
What are the signs and symptoms of IE due to?	Infectious process on the valve
	Bland or septic embolization
	Sustained bacteremia
	Circulating immune complexes
What are the peripheral manifestations of IE?	Splinter hemorrhages, Roth's spots, petechiae, Osler's nodes, and Janeway lesions
What else causes splinter hemorrhages and how are IE splinters differentiated from them?	They may also occur with trauma and are more suggestive of IE if they are close to the nail matrix.
How often is the ESR elevated?	90% to 100% of cases

What are the typical findings on urinalysis with IE?	Proteinuria, hematuria, and red blood cell casts
How should blood cultures be drawn in patients with suspected IE, and how many should be drawn?	Three sets of specimens should be drawn within 24 hours, but no more than two vials should be drawn from one site at one time. Cultures should be held for 21 days (for fastidious organisms).
In patients with culture-positive IE, how commonly are all the blood cultures positive?	In two thirds of patients, all blood cultures are positive.
How often are the first two blood cultures positive in culture-positive IE?	If the patient has not been exposed to antibiotics, the first two blood cultures yield a pathogen more than 90% of the time.
What findings are seen on TTE in patients with IE?	A vegetation, valvular dysfunction, or the presence of an abscess.
How much more sensitive is TEE than TTE for the evaluation of IE?	TEE is more sensitive (95%) than TTE (65%). Consider TEE when TTE is negative and there is suspicion of IE.
How often are strep and staph species the cause in IE?	Streptococci and staphylococci cause approximately 90% of all cases of IE.
What are the pathogens involved in IE?	Streptococci (*viridans, mutans,* or *bovis* and enterococci, among others)
	Staphylococci (*S. aureus;* coagulase-negative)
	Gram-negative bacilli (uncommon, high mortality rate)
	Fungi
	Miscellaneous bacteria
	Culture-negative causes [including the HACEK organisms: ***H****aemophilus* species *(H. parainfluenzae, H. aphrophilus,* and *H. paraphrophilus),* ***A****ctinobacillus actinomycetemcomitans,* ***C****ardiobacterium hominis,* ***E****ikenella corrodens,* and ***K****ingella* species]

How likely is endocarditis if a blood culture is positive for the following:

    Streptococcus mutans? — 15 cases of IE for every one case of bacteremia without valvular involvement

    Streptococcus sanguis? — Three cases of IE for every one case of bacteremia without valvular involvement

    Enterococci? — Equal likelihood of IE or bacteremia without valvular involvement

    Group A streptococcus? — Only one case of IE for every seven cases of bacteremia without valvular involvement

Why does culture-negative endocarditis occur?

Possible explanations include subacute right-sided endocarditis, mural endocarditis, timing [cultures drawn at the end of a chronic course (>3 months)], prior antibiotic use, slow-growing fastidious organisms (HACEK, nutritionally variant streptococci), fungal infection, obligate intracellular pathogens, noninfectious endocarditis, or the wrong diagnosis.

What are the *major* Duke criteria to define IE?

Positive blood cultures (typical microorganisms and persistently positive cultures)

Evidence of endocardial involvement (mass, abscess, valve dehiscence, worsening murmur)

What are the *minor* Duke criteria to define IE?

Predisposing heart condition or IV drug use

Fever ($\geq 38.0°C$)

Vascular phenomenon (arterial embolism, septic pulmonary infarcts, mycotic aneurysms, intracranial hemorrhage, Janeway lesions)

Immunologic phenomenon (Roth spots, Osler's nodes, glomerulonephritis)

Microbiologic (positive cultures not meeting the major criteria)

Using the Duke criteria, what is:

Definite evidence of IE?

Two major criteria

One major and three minor criteria

Five minor criteria

Possible evidence of IE?

Evidence short of definite but not rejected

One major and one minor criterion

Three minor criteria

Evidence of IE rejected?

Firm alternative diagnosis

Resolution of IE syndrome with ≤4 days of antibiotic therapy

No pathologic evidence of IE at surgery or autopsy with antibiotic therapy ≤4 days

What is the general principle of the antibiotic treatment?

Parenteral antibiotics with sustained bactericidal activity, shown on susceptibility testing, should be selected and used for a prolonged course (6 to 8 weeks).

Why should the patients with suspected IE have continuous monitoring?

To watch for heart block due to a ring abscess.

Why are repeat blood cultures drawn after starting therapy?

To document clearing, therefore response to treatment.

Should these patients be anticoagulated?

Anticoagulation is associated with bleeding complications and should be avoided.

What are the indications for surgery in a patient with IE?

Refractory CHF, uncontrolled infection, significant valvular dysfunction, repeated systemic embolization, large vegetation size (>1 to 2 cm), ineffective antimicrobial therapy (against, e.g., fungi), mycotic aneurysm, most cases of prosthetic valve endocarditis and local (cardiac) suppurative complications with conduction abnormalities

PROSTHETIC VALVE ENDOCARDITIS

Are mechanical or bioprosthetic valves more prone to develop PVE ?	Probably about the same
Are prosthetic aortic and mitral valves similar in rates of PVE?	Aortic valves are about twice as likely to develop PVE.

ANTIBIOTIC PROPHYLAXIS

Is transient bacteremia common with dental manipulation?	Extremely. With tooth extraction, this occurs 10% to 100% of the time. In periodontal surgery, it occurs 40% to 90% of the time, and with teeth cleaning up to 40%.
Does bacteremia occur during common tasks?	Yes. With tooth brushing and flossing, up to 70% of the time; with toothpicks, up to 40% of the time; and with water irrigation devices, up to 50% of the time. Chewing food causes bacteremia up to 50% of the time.
How high is the risk of endocarditis with dental procedures?	The estimation is 1 case of IE per 14 million dental visits.
Is the risk of IE higher in patients with valvular heart disease?	Yes. The estimate is 1 case of IE per 1.1 million dental visits in patients with MVP; 1 per 475,000 dental visits in patients with congenital heart disease; 1 per 140,000 in patients with rheumatic heart disease; 1 per 115,000 visits in patients with prosthetic valves; and 1 per 95,000 visits in patients with previous IE.
How common are fatal anaphylactic reactions in patients receiving penicillin?	Estimated at 15 to 25 individuals per 1 million patients

Based on the 2007 guidelines, which of the patient groups below should receive endocarditis prophylaxis?

Patients with prosthetic heart valves?	Yes
Patients with a history of IE?	Yes
Patients with unrepaired congenital heart disease?	Yes
Patients with completely repaired congenital defects with prosthetic material or devices?	Yes for the first 6 months
Patients with repaired congenital disease but residual defects?	Yes
Patients who have had a heart transplant and some valvulopathy?	Yes
An isolated ASD (secundum) or patients >6 months out from a repair of an ASD, VSD, or PDA (surgical or percutaneous)	No
Innocent or functional murmur or echo evidence of MR but a normal valve	No
Aortic valve sclerosis with a mild gradient (<2 m/s) and good leaflet motion	No
Physiologic TR or PI with normal valves	No

Give examples of procedures that do or do not require antibiotic prophylaxis in selected patients:

Skin and musculoskeletal tissue

Do—any procedure where the skin or musculoskeletal tissue is infected

Respiratory

Do—any procedure with an incision or biopsy of mucosal tissue

Do not—ET intubation, flexible bronchoscopy without biopsy

Gastrointestinal

Do—Esophageal dilatation or sclerosing therapies, any procedure of the biliary tree, any operation involving the intestinal mucosa

Do not—TEE and endoscopic procedures

Genitourinary

Do—urethral, prostate, or cystoscopic procedures only if the GU tract is infected

Do not—cesarean and vaginal deliveries, vaginal hysterectomy, and procedures on uninfected uterine tissues

Dental

Do—any procedure involving the manipulation of gingival tissue or the periapical tooth region or breaking of the mucosal barrier in the selected patient groups above

Do not—restorations, orthodontic adjustments, fluoride treatments, and loss of primary teeth

In patients with the appropriate indications who *are able* to take oral medications, what antibiotics are indicated as prophylaxis against bacterial endocarditis (non-GI/GU procedures)?

Amoxicillin: adults, 2.0 g (children, 50 mg/kg) given by mouth 1 hour before the procedure

Penicillin allergic—clindamycin: adults, 600 mg (children, 20 mg/kg) given by mouth 1 hour before the procedure OR

Cephalexin or cefadroxil: adults, 2.0 g (children, 50 mg/kg) by mouth 1 hour before procedure OR

Azithromycin or clarithromycin: adults, 500 mg (children, 15 mg/kg) by mouth 1 hour before the procedure

Antistaphylococcal coverage should be added if indicated.

In patients with the appropriate indication who are *unable* to take oral medications, what antibiotics are indicated as prophylaxis against bacterial endocarditis (non-GI/GU procedures)?

Ampicillin: adults, 2.0 g (children, 50 mg/kg) given IM or IV within 30 minutes before procedure)

Penicillin allergic—clindamycin: adults, 600 mg (children, 20 mg/kg) given IV 30 minutes before procedure OR

Cefazolin or ceftriaxone: adults, 1.0 g (children, 25 mg/kg) IM or IV 30 minutes before procedure

Antistaphylococcal coverage should be added if indicated.

In patients with the appropriate indication, what antibiotics are indicated as prophylaxis for GU and GI procedures?

Amoxicillin 2.0 g orally (adults) or 50 mg/kg orally (children) 1 hour before procedure or ampicillin 2 g IM or IV (adults) or 50 mg/kg (children) IM or IV 30 minutes before procedure

Or vancomycin 1 g IV (adults) or 20 mg/kg (children) IV 1 to 2 hours before procedure in penicillin-allergic patients

ATHLETES AND CARDIOVASCULAR DISEASE

What are the common ECG findings in athletes?

Owing to the high vagal tone: sinus bradycardia, junctional rhythms, first-degree AV block, and Wenckebach (Mobitz 1)

What are the three most common cardiovascular causes of sudden death in young athletes?

Hypertrophic cardiomyopathy, commotio cordis, and coronary artery anomalies

What is commotio cordis?

VT/VF following a blow to the chest

Why does commotio cordis occur?	The blow hits at the time of the T-wave vulnerable period, causing and R-on-T initiation of VT/VF.
What is the survival rate for victims of commotio cordis?	About 15%
For all athletes, what four sports are associated with the highest number of sudden deaths?	Football, soccer, basketball, running/orienteering

CARDIOMYOPATHIES

GENERAL CARDIOMYOPATHIES

What are the three classic types of cardiomyopathy?	Dilated, hypertrophic, and restrictive
What is an ischemic cardiomyopathy?	Recurrent MIs cause abnormal loading conditions and consequent ventricular remodeling.
Do all patients with heart failure have poor systolic function?	No. There is a large group, perhaps 40% of the heart failure population, with normal ejection fractions.
Do all patients with heart failure and normal ejection fractions have diastolic dysfunction?	No. Patients with volume overload due to renal failure and those with pericardial constriction are examples of patients with heart failure and normal diastolic function.
Compared to NYHA class assignment, what is a more accurate way to determine prognosis in patients with advanced heart failure?	Metabolic exercise testing (determination of oxygen consumption)
What are the four stages of heart failure?	Stage A—high risk for developing heart failure
	Stage B—asymptomatic heart failure
	Stage C—symptomatic heart failure
	Stage D—refractory end-stage heart failure

What are the classic *cardiovascular* physical signs of heart failure?

Distended neck veins, lateral PMI, S_3 and/or S_4 gallop, murmurs of mitral or tricuspid regurgitation, and a narrow pulse pressure

What is the significance of a narrow pulse pressure in a patient with cardiomyopathy?

A pulse pressure index of <25% is associated with a CI of <2 L/min/m^2.

List the common chest radiograph features of heart failure.

Cardiomegaly, Kerley B lines, venous congestion or cephalization, and pulmonary edema

From the above list, what is the most common chest radiograph finding in patients with HF?

Cardiomegaly

List some of the potentially reversible causes of a dilated cardiomyopathy.

Alcoholic cardiomyopathy, hypocalcemia, hypokalemia, hypophosphatemia, hemochromatosis (also casuses restrictive), pheochromocytoma, myocarditis, sarcoid heart disease, lead poisoning, selenium deficiency, uremic cardiomyopathy, and ischemic cardiomyopathy

What are some of the viruses that can cause myocarditis?

Coxsackie A and B, influenza B and A, echovirus, hepatitis, and HIV, among others.

What is the most common cause of myocarditis and the most common cause of HF worldwide?

Chagas' disease [a parasitic infection caused by a trypanosomal infection after the bite of a reduviid bug (bedbug)]

What are some classic medication-induced forms of myocarditis?

Adriamycin (doxorubicin) and cyclophosphamide cardiotoxicity

What other drugs can cause myocarditis?

Cocaine, methamphetamine, alcohol, and arsenic.

What are some of the causes of myocarditis that occur secondary to things in the environment?

Wasp, bee, and scorpion stings. Snake and spider bites.

Why is the muscle injured in myocarditis?

It is uncertain, and likely heterogenous, but there may be a close HLA match between viral proteins and the myocardium, or autoimmune, or direct induction of apoptosis.

How common is myocarditis?

It shows up on 0.5% of all autopsies.

What elements predict recovery in virally induced myocarditis?

Short time interval between disease onset and presentation as well as fairly low filling pressures (e.g., PCWP <20 mm Hg)

Do steroids help in the treatment of virally induced myocarditis?

There are no good studies to answer this question.

How often does LV function improve in patients with viral myocarditis, alcohol-induced myocarditis, or peripartum myopathies?

Improvement in LV function occurs about 50% of the time.

What are the restrictive cardiomyopathies?

Impairment of myocardial relaxation (i.e., diastolic dysfunction)

What are some examples of restrictive cardiomyopathies?

Amyloidosis, eosinophilic infiltration, and hemochromatosis

What is a hypertrophic cardiomyopathy?

Impaired relaxation due to disordered hypertrophy of the myocardium

Do all hypertrophic cardiomyopathies have impairment to LV outflow?

The classic is HOCM, but there are variations, including progressive apical thickening and generalized myocardial thickening.

What is IVNC?

An ill-defined cardiomyopathy thought to result from an arrest in the normal compaction of the loose myocardial meshwork during fetal development

What are the characteristic findings of IVNC on echocardiography?

Isolated regions of thickened myocardium with deep myocardial trabeculations

What is Takotsubo's cardiomyopathy?

An apical ballooning syndrome (also called "broken heart")

What group of people are more prone to this cardiomyopathy?

It usually occurs in women under stressful situations.

What is the natural history of this cardiomyopathy?

90% or more of affected individuals recover over time.

What is the standard therapy for patients with systolic dysfunction?

ACE-I plus a beta-adrenergic blocker.

What are some potential side effects of ACE-Is?

Hypotension, renal failure (in patients with bilateral renal artery stenosis), hyperkalemia, allergic reactions (the most serious of which is angioedema), and cough

Are ARBs as good as ACE-Is in reducing mortality in patients with LV systolic dysfunction?

Probably. They can also be used as add-on therapy to ACE-Is.

If ACE-Is and ARBs are used together, what are the potential complications?

Hyperkalemia, hypotension, and renal failure

If ACE-Is or ARBs are not tolerated, what drug combination is generally used?

Hydralazine and isosorbide

Is there a specific group of patients to whom hydralazine and isosorbide may offer a mortality benefit in addition to ACE-I and beta-adrenergic blockers?

African Americans

If an aldosterone inhibitor is added onto a regimen of a beta-adrenergic blocker and ACE-I, what must be followed?	The potassium level. It is suggested that labs should be drawn at 1 week, 1 month, and then every 3 months.
What are potential cardiovascular side effects of inotropic medications?	Arrhythmias (e.g., sinus tachycardia, VT, VF), hypotension (all vasodilate), and tolerance secondary to beta-adrenergic receptor downregulation
What is the cardiorenal syndrome?	Worsening renal function noted in patients with heart failure.
How is this diagnosed?	A ≥ 0.3 mg/dL rise in serum creatinine
Why is the cardiorenal syndrome an issue?	It is associated with a longer stay in the hospital, more days in the ICU, more rapid readmission rates, and worse in- and out-of-hospital prognosis.

TRANSPLANT

What medications lower cyclosporine or tacrolimus levels?	Dilantin, phenobarbital, rifampin, and isoniazid
What medications increase cyclosporine or tacrolimus levels?	Macrolides (e.g., erythromycin), ketoconazole, itraconazole, diltiazem, and amiodarone
What medications may potentiate renal dysfunction when used with cyclosporine or tacrolimus?	Aminoglycosides, amphotericin, nonsteroidal anti-inflammatory agents
Besides cyclosporine and tacrolimus, what is a third IL-2 inhibitor approved for use?	Sirolimus
What are some of the side effects of mycophenolate mofetil?	Marrow suppression, lymphoma, nonlymphoma malignancies, diarrhea, and hyperlipidemia

Name six side effects of steroids.	Glucose intolerance, adrenal insufficiency if acutely withdrawn, cataracts, osteoporosis, cushingoid appearance, and skin fragility
What medications should not be used to treat SVT after heart transplantation?	Adenosine and digoxin. A transplanted heart is more sensitive to adenosine and adenosine may cause prolonged and/or fatal asystole. Digoxin is ineffective due to lack of vagal innervation.
Does reinnervation of the transplanted heart ever occur?	Yes; 75% of heart recipients show some sympathetic reinnervation after 1 year. A smaller number show parasympathetic innervation.
Does reinnervation have any practical implication?	Yes; patients with reinnervation have improved exercise performance (faster HR response), and some recipients in whom CAD develops complain of chest pain.
What noninfectious process can masquerade with fever and an infiltrate after organ transplantation?	Transplant-associated B-cell lymphoma, which occurs in 1% to 5% of patients over time (frequency depends on the organ transplanted).

ASSIST DEVICES

What is the most common assist device used in treatment of HF?	IABP
What are the disadvantages of balloon pumps?	Limb ischemia of the leg where they are inserted. Limited mobility due to insertion in the femoral artery and infection. The level of support is only moderate.
What two types of flow patterns are associated with LV assist devices?	Continuous and pulsatile
What is the advantage of pulsatile flow?	It closely mimics the natural pumping of the human heart.

What are the disadvantages of pulsatile flow?

The devices tend to be more complex to insert, must be larger than the continuous-flow devices because of the obligatory size of the pumping chamber, and must vent to the outside or into some other chamber because of the displaced air.

PERICARDIAL DISEASE

ACUTE AND CHRONIC PERICARDITIS

What are some of the autoimmune causes of pericarditis?

The common ones are systemic lupus, rheumatoid arthritis, and scleroderma. Others include Sjögren's syndrome, dermatomyositis, ankylosing spondylitis, Reiter's syndrome, Wegener's granulomatosis, Felty's syndrome, and serum sickness.

What other autoimmune-type illnesses can have associated pericarditis?

Temporal arteritis, inflammatory bowel disease, Kawasaki's disease, Familial Mediterranean fever, Whipple's and Behçet's diseases.

What are infectious causes of pericardial disease?

Viral (Coxsackie B, echovirus, influenza, herpes simplex virus)

Bacterial (*S. aureus, S. pneumoniae,* and *Histoplasma capsulatum*), commonly from a pleuropulmonary focus from trauma, surgery, or local spread of an abscess. Also Acute rheumatic fever

Fungal or other infections, such as toxoplasmosis and Lyme disease

What are some of the inflammatory disease causes of pericarditis?

Sarcoidosis and amyloidosis

What are some of the common medications that can cause acute pericarditis?

Hydralazine and procainamide. Odd causes include penicillin, cromolyn sodium, minoxidil, dantrolene sodium, and methylsergide.

What is the most important physical finding of pericarditis?

Pericardial friction rub, which is heard best at the apex with the patient leaning forward

When does each occur in the cardiac cycle?

During ventricular systole, ventricular diastole, and atrial systole. Commonly at least two components are heard.

What does the ECG show in patients with acute pericarditis?

There is diffuse ST elevation and PR depression

What else causes PR depression?

Atrial infarction, which is uncommon

How is chronic pericarditis recognized?

There is chronic and generally relapsing pain after a bout of acute pericarditis

What are the symptoms and signs of chronic pericarditis?

Pleuritic chest pain and often a rub

What is the treatment for chronic pericarditis?

Search for an underlying cause (e.g., infection). NSAIDs and colchicines are the mainstays of treatment. Steroid use should be avoided if possible. Other agents, such as azathioprine, and other immunosuppressants may be helpful. Pericardial resection has also been reported.

EFFUSIONS AND TAMPONADE

What is a pulsus paradoxus?

A drop of ≥ 12 mm Hg in the systolic blood pressure during inspiration.

How is a pulsus paradoxus exam performed?

The BP cuff is inflated and lowered to the first Korotkoff sound (which is audible initially only during expiration). The cuff is then slowly deflated until the first Korotkoff sound is heard throughout the entire respiratory cycle. The difference in systolic pressure between the first Korotkoff sound occurring in expiration and then the Korotkoff sounds occurring throughout the respiratory cycle is the pulsus paradoxus.

What else is found on physical examination of pericardial tamponade?

Beck's triad: Decreased systolic BP, distended neck veins (with rapid x descent and attenuated y descent), and "distant" heart sounds. Sinus tachycardia is seen in most patients.

CONSTRICTIVE PERICARDITIS

What are the physical examination signs of constrictive pericarditis?

Clear lungs (usually)

Kussmaul's sign (elevation of JVP with inspiration)

Rapid y descent on jugular venous pulsations

Hepatic congestion

What procedures are helpful in making a diagnosis of constrictive pericarditis?

MRI, CT, echocardiogram, and cardiac catheterization

What is seen on MRI in pericardial constriction?

Demonstrates pericardial thickening and adhesion to the epicardium

What is seen on the echocardiogram in pericardial constriction?

Can sometimes demonstrate pericardial adhesions, stranding, or thickening. The atria are commonly enlarged with normal-sized ventricles.

What is seen on CT in pericardial constriction?

The same as the echocardiogram. Sometimes the pericardial thickness can be exaggerated by tangential cuts.

What is seen on the hemodynamic portion of a cardiac catheterization in constrictive pericarditis?

Elevation of all the diastolic filling pressures, similar to tamponade. In contrast to tamponade, however, there is an exaggerated y descent and the PA systolic pressure is almost never >50 mm Hg.

CENTRAL AND PERIPHERAL VASCULAR DISEASE

What is the definition of an aneurysm?

Dilatation to >50% of the normal vessel size

What is the diameter of a normal *ascending* aorta?

3 cm

Where are most thoracic aortic aneurysms found?

50% ascending, 10% arch and 40% descending

When should you consider operating on a patient with Marfan's syndrome who has an aortic aneurysm?

When it is around 4.5 cm

When should you consider operating on a patient with a bicuspid aortic valve?

4.5 to 5 cm

What is Takayasu's disease?

Also called pulseless disease, Takayasu's disease is inflammation and then scarring of the aorta, major branches, and pulmonary arteries, leading to occlusion (hence pulselessness) or pulmonary HTN if the pulmonary arteries are involved.

What is the cause of Takayasu's disease?

Thought to be secondary to an autoimmune process. It affects women 9:1 over men.

What are the causes of aortic dissections?

Marfan's syndrome and other connective tissue abnormalities (Ehlers-Danlos)

Cystic medial necrosis (without overt Marfan's syndrome)

Bicuspid aortic valves and aortic coarctation (predisposing factors to dissection)

Pregnancy (with 50% of dissections occurring in women younger than 40 years of age during the last trimester of pregnancy; often associated with coronary dissection)

Trauma, possibly causing a tear in the aorta at the isthmus

What are the common physical examination features of a dissecting aorta?

Shock, although, initially 50% of patients are hypertensive

Pulse deficits (right-to-left difference; occurs in 50% of proximal dissections and may occur in distal dissection secondary to compression of the subclavian artery)

Aortic regurgitation (50% of patients with proximal events; may cause severe, rapid-onset CHF)

Neurologic deficits

What are the causes of hypotension during an aortic dissection?

Cardiac tamponade

Intrapleural or intraperitoneal rupture

Pseudohypotension (impingement on the brachiocephalic vessels by the dissecting hematoma interfering with BP measurement)

RV failure (IMI)

Bradycardia (IMI rhythms)

What is the mortality rate for medical treatment in patients with type A dissections in the first 48 hours?

50%; roughly 1% mortality/hour

What are the indications to operate on a type B dissection?

Evidence of continued dissection (pain) or organ or limb ischemia.

What is the surgical mortality rate for a type B dissection?

10% to 20% if uncomplicated and up to 60% if complicated

What is the diameter of a normal *descending* aorta (at the level of the renal arteries)?

<2 cm

What percentage of the general population has an AAA?

1% to 4%

What percentage of abdominal aneurysms larger than 6 cm will rupture by 1 year?

50% (the larger the aneurysm, the greater the percentage); 80% if symptomatic

How is an aortic rupture recognized?

Patients complain of severe back and abdominal pain and present with hypotension or the appearance of frank hemorrhagic shock. Most patients have a palpable pulsatile abdominal aorta.

What is the mortality rate for a recognized rupture of an AAA?

50% to 80%

How common is peripheral vascular disease?

Symptomatic in 2% of adults and asymptomatic in 10%

How common are amputations in patients with PAD?

25% of patients with PAD require an amputation at 1 year and only 50% are alive with two legs at 5 years

In patients with PAD, where are the stenoses located?

20% iliac arteries, 40% femoral arteries, 20% lower limb arteries, and 20% diffusely

What are the six "Ps" of acute arterial occlusion?

Pain, paresthesias, paralysis, pallor, pulselessness, poikilothermy

What should you think of in a patient who complains of claudication symptoms but has good distal pulses or good ABIs?

Small vessel disease (DM) and spinal stenosis

Where are the common arterial entrapment sites?

Superficial femoral artery, popliteal artery, and thoracic outlet

How is the diagnosis of thoracic outlet syndrome made?

When the arm is abducted to 90 degrees and externally rotated, paresthesias and numbness occur, a bruit is heard over the supraclavicular fossa, and symptoms resolve when the arm is returned to baseline position.

What dermatologic clues suggest venous rather than arterial disease?

Patients with venous disease usually have thick, scaly skin; those with arterial disease usually have thin, shiny skin.

Where are venous ulcers usually seen, and what is their usual course?

The medial malleolar area; these ulcers usually resolve and recur.

CONGENITAL HEART DISEASE

What are the causes of CHD with each of the following:

    Left-to-right shunts with cyanosis?

ASD (secundum type)

Atrioventricular septal defects (primum type)

Complete AV canal defect

VSD

Patent ductus arteriosus (PDA)

Truncus arteriosus

Tricuspid atresia with a VSD

    Right-to-left shunts (cyanosis)?

Tetralogy of Fallot

Ebstein's anomaly

Tricuspid atresia

PA atresia with intact ventricular septum

Transposition of the great arteries

Total anomalous pulmonary venous return

Double-outlet right ventricle with pulmonary stenosis or atresia (DORV will have a VSD)

    Obstructive valvular or vascular lesions (with or without cyanosis)?

Hypoplastic left heart syndrome

Congenital valvular AS or AI, MS or MR

Pulmonary vein atresia

Cor triatriatum (the left atrium fails to become a common chamber)

Peripheral pulmonary artery stenosis (with or with a VSD)

Tetralogy of Fallot

Transpositions?	Transposition of the great arteries
	Congenitally corrected transposition of the great arteries (the aorta and pulmonary arteries are transposed, but the RV and LV are also transposed leading to a functionally "normal" circulation)
What are some of the other congenital heart defects?	The left coronary artery originating from the PA (ALCAPA)
	Atrial septal and sinus of Valsalva aneurysms
	AV fistula
	Double-outlet right ventricle without pulmonary stenosis
	Congenital heart block
What is Eisenmenger's syndrome?	Any CHD with consequent pulmonary HTN and reversal of flow to right to left (e.g., ASD, VSD, patent ductus, and AP window)
What is a Blalock-Taussig shunt?	A connection created between the systemic circulation and the PA (e.g., the subclavian artery and PA)
Why is this performed?	To establish or improve blood flow to the lung (and hence oxygenation)
What is a Fontan procedure?	Anastomosis of the IVC or right atrium to the pulmonary artery. A bidirectional Glenn adds the SVC to PA anastomosis.
What are the acyanotic forms of CHD seen in adults?	Bicuspid aortic valve, supra-aortic or sub-aortic valvular stenosis, aortic coarctation, valvular PS, ASD, patent ductus unless associated with Eisenmenger's syndrome, and corrected TGA
What are the cyanotic forms of CHD seen in adults?	Tetralogy of Fallot; VSD, some ASDs, and some PDAs when associated with Eisenmenger's syndrome; atrioventricular septal defect (formerly AV canal defect); pulmonary atresia with a VSD, and Ebstein's anomaly

What are the complications seen in adult patients who have had a TOF repair?	VT, atrial fibrillation, RV failure due to obstruction, and pulmonary hypertension
For the long-term care of patients with CHD, what else is important to remember prior to procedures?	Endocarditis prophylaxis

NEOPLASMS

What is the location of most myxomas?	LA (75%). Myxomas in children are found in increased frequency in the ventricle.
What is the classic examination feature of a myxoma?	A tumor plop (occurs when the patient shifts position)
What percentage of metastatic tumors affect the myocardium?	5%
What percentage of metastatic tumors affect the pericardium?	10%
What metastatic tumors most frequently involve the heart (endocardium, myocardium, and pericardium)?	Bronchogenic carcinoma, breast cancer, leukemias, and lymphomas

MAJOR TRIALS IN CARDIOLOGY

The following is a list of the pivotal trials in cardiology, with references.

PRIMARY PREVENTION STUDIES

WOSCOPS: Pravastatin versus placebo was studied in 6595 men with hyperlipidemia (average cholesterol 272 mg/dL, average LDL 192 mg/dL) followed for a mean of 4.9 years; 31% relative risk (RR) reduction in MI or death (1.6% versus 2.3%, $P < 0.001$), similar reduction in nonfatal MI (31%) and cardiovascular death (28%) with pravastatin. *N Engl J Med* 1995;333:1301–1307.

SECONDARY PREVENTION

CAPRIE: Clopidogrel versus ASA was studied in 19,185 patients with known atherosclerotic disease (CVA/MI/PVD) followed for a mean of 2 years; 9.4% RR reduction in death/MI/CVA (5.32% versus 5.83%, $P = 0.043$) in the clopidogrel group. *Lancet* 1996;348:1329–1339.

PROVE IT-TIMI 22: High-dose atorvastatin (80 mg) versus standard therapy (pravastatin 40 mg) was compared in 4162 patients with ACS with a mean follow-up of 24 months. The composite triple endpoint of death, myocardial infarction, and rehospitalization for recurrent ACS was assessed at 30 days (3.0% of atorvastatin patients versus 4.2% of pravastatin patients, $P < 0.046$) and demonstrated a hazard reduction of 24% after the mean of 24 months (15.7% versus 20.05%, $P = 0.0002$). There was also a highly significant difference in LDL between the atorvastatin and pravastatin groups (60 mg/dL versus 88 mg/dL). *J Am Coll Cardiol.* 2005;46:1405–1410.

ASYMPTOMATIC CAD

ASTEROID Trial: A total of 507 patients with coronary artery disease were treated with rosuvastatin 40 mg after a baseline IVUS study and followed up at 24 months with a repeat IVUS. There was a 53% reduction in LDL (130.4 mg/dL to 60.8 mg/dL, $P < 0.001$). The mean reduction in atheroma volume for the group was 0.98% for the entire vessel; for the most diseased 10 mm, there was a 6.8% median reduction ($P < 0.001$ compared to baseline). 1.2% of patients had a CK elevation of >5 times the upper limit of normal, but only 0.2% had elevation on two sequential visits. There were no occurrences of rhabdomyolysis. Likewise, 1.8% of patients had an elevation in ALT >3 times the upper limit of normal, with 0.2% having an elevation on two sequential visits. *JAMA* 2006;295:1556–1565.

COURAGE Trial: Optimal medical treatment was compared with PCI in 2287 patients with stable angina. All patients were treated to an LDL of 60 to 85 mg/dL; 95% of patients had ischemia and 69% of those with multivessel disease. At 5 years, the primary endpoint of death occurred in 18.5% of the medical treatment patients and 19.0% of the PCI group ($P = 0.62$). No difference was noted for the secondary endpoint of death, MI or stroke. At 3 years, the PCI group averaged $5295 higher than the medical treatment group ($P < 0.0001$).

STENTS

RAVEL: A total of 238 patients with primary native single coronary lesions were randomized to sirolimus coated (2.5 to 3.5 mm and <18 mm length) or bare metal stents. At 6 months, late lumen loss was significantly less in the sirolimus group compared with the bare metal stent group (–0.01 mm versus 0.9 mm, $P < 0.001$). Stent restenosis was 26.6% in the bare metal group versus 0% in the sirolimus group at 6 months ($P < 0.001$). *N Engl J Med* 2002;346:1773–1780.

TAXUS I NIRx: A total of 61 patients with de novo or restenotic lesions with vessel diameter 3.0 to 3.5 mm and <15 mm in length were randomized to paclitaxel versus bare metal stents. Major adverse events had occurred in 3% of the paclitaxel group and 10% of the control group at 12 months. Minimal lumen diameter, diameter stenosis, and late lumen loss were all significantly less in the paclitaxel group ($P < 0.01$ for all three categories). *Circulation* 2003;107:38–42.

REPLACE-2: A total of 6010 patients undergoing urgent or elective PCI were randomized to IV bivalirudin (0.75 mg/kg bolus + 1.75 mg/kg/hr during the PCI) $\pm$ IIb/IIIa versus heparin $\pm$ IIb/IIIa inhibitor. Patients were followed for 30 days for the primary endpoint of death, MI, urgent repeat revascularization, or in-hospital bleeding and the secondary endpoint of death, MI, or urgent repeat revascularization. The primary endpoint occurred in 9.2% of those receiving bivalirudin and 10.0% of the heparin group ($P = 0.32$). The secondary endpoint occurred in 7.6% of the bivalirudin group and 7.1% of the heparin patients. In-hospital bleeding occurred less often in the bivalirudin group (2.4% versus 4.1%; $P < 0.001$). *JAMA* 2003;289:853–863.

USA/NSTEMI

ESSENCE: Enoxaparin versus heparin was studied in 3171 patients with USA/NSTEMI followed for 30 days; the result was 16% and 15% RR reduction in death/MI/recurrent ischemia at 14 days (16.6% versus 19.8%, $P = 0.019$) and 30 days (19.8% versus 23.3%, $P = 0.016$) in the enoxaparin-treated patients *N Engl J Med* 1997;337:447–452.

TIMI 18 (TACTICS): In a comparison of early invasive versus early conservative strategy, 2220 patients with NSTEMI were treated with ASA/heparin/tirofiban and randomized to catheterization within 4 to 48 hours versus early conservative strategy and followed out to 6 months; the result was a 22% RR reduction in death/MI/rehospitalization in the early invasive strategy (15.9% versus 19.4%, $P = 0.025$) at 30 days and a 26% RR reduction in death/MI at 6 months (7.3% versus 9.5%, $P < 0.05$) *N Engl J Med* 2001;344:1879–1887.

PURSUIT: Eptifibatide/heparin versus ASA/heparin was studied in 10,948 patients with USA/NSTEMI followed for 30 days; the result was an 11% RR reduction in death/MI (14.2% versus 15.7%, $P = 0.04$) for the eptifibatide group. *N Engl J Med* 1998;339:436–443.

SYNERGY: This was a safety and efficacy trial of enoxaparin compared with UFH in high-risk ACS patients treated with an early invasive strategy. The primary endpoint of death or nonfatal MI at 30 days occurred in 14% (enoxaparin) versus 14.5% (UFH) and met the noninferiority criteria.

However, in the patients not pretreated with antithrombotic therapy or those who were pretreated but continued on the same therapy postrandomization, there was a lower rate of death or MI with enoxaparin. *JAMA* 2004;292:45–54.

ACUITY: A total of 9207 patients with moderate- to high-risk ACS undergoing an invasive strategy were randomized to IIb/IIIa use as an initial strategy (upstream use) versus deferred/selective use in the catheterization lab. At 30 days, death, MI, or unplanned revascularization for ischemia occurred in 7.1% of patients in the upstream use group versus 7.9% of patients in the selective use group ($P = 0.044$ for noninferiority). Selective/deferred use was associated with less major bleeding (4.9% versus 6.1%, $P < 0.001$ for noninferiority and $P = 0.009$ for superiority) *JAMA* 2007;297:591–602.

STEMI

ExTRACT-TIMI 25: Fibrinolysis followed by randomization to UFH or enoxaparin was studied in 20,506 patients. Patients were given 7 days of SQ enoxaparin versus at least 48 hours of UFH. At 30 days, death or nonfatal recurrent MI outcome was significantly less frequent in the enoxaparin group (9.9% versus 12%; $P < 0.001$). At 30 days, major bleeding was slightly more frequent in the enoxaparin group (2.1% versus 1.4%, $P < 0.001$). All 4676 patients in the cohort were treated with PCI with similar results (death + nonfatal MI; 10.7% with enoxaparin versus 13.8% with UFH, $P = 0.001$) with no difference in major bleeding (1.4% enoxaparin versus 1.6% UFH, $P = 0.56$). *N Engl J Med* 2006;354: 1477–1488.

OASIS-5: A total of 20,078 patients with acute coronary syndromes received either fondaparinux (2.5 mg daily) or enoxaparin (1 mg/kg/bid) for a mean of 6 days. At 9 days, 579 patients treated with fondaparinux and 573 patients treated with enoxaparin experienced the primary endpoint of death, MI, or refractory ischemia ($P = NS$). At 30 days, there was a trend favoring the fondaparinux group (805 patients versus 864 patients; $P = 0.13$), and also at 6 months (1222 patients versus 1308 patients; $P = 0.06$). Major bleeding occurred less often in the fondaparinux group at all time points (9 days: F 217, E 412; 30 days: F 313, E 494; 180 days: F 417, E 569; $p = NS$). *N Engl J Med* 2006;354:1464–1476.

SHOCK trial (follow-up): A total of 302 patients who presented with STEMI and cardiogenic shock within 36 hours of admission were randomized to early invasive therapy versus initial medial stabilization. Among patients randomized to early revascularization, there was no difference between CABG and PCI. At 1, 3, and 6 years there was a 13% to 13.2% absolute reduction in mortality in the early invasive group ($P < 0.05$ at all three time points). *JAMA* 2001;285:190–192; *JAMA* 2006; 295:2511–2515.

HEART FAILURE

MERIT-HF: Metoprolol CR/XL versus placebo was studied in 3991 patients (on ACE-I) with class II to IV CHF followed for an average of 1 year; the study was terminated early because of a 34% RR reduction in mortality (7.2% versus 11.0%, $P < 0.0062$) in the metoprolol group. *Lancet* 1999;353:2001–2007.

REMATCH: A total of 129 patients with severe heart failure not eligible for cardiac transplantation were randomized to device therapy with the HeartMate LVAD versus optimal medical therapy (OMT); 68 patients received LVAD and 61 OMT. At 1 year, survival was 52% in the LVAD patients and 25% in the OMT group ($P = 0.002$). At 2 years, survival was 23% in the LVAD group and 8% in the OMT group ($P = 0.09$). A serious adverse event (infection, bleeding, or device malfunction) was 2.35 times more likely to occur in LVAD-treated patients. *N Engl J Med* 2001;345: 1435–1443.

COMET: Carvedilol versus immediate release metoprolol was studied in 3029 patients with primarily class II to III CHF with an average daily dose of 42 mg carvedilol and 85 mg metoprolol. Patients were followed for a mean of 58 ± 6 (SD) months. The primary endpoint of all-cause mortality was improved in the carvedilol group (33.9% versus 39.5% in the metoprolol group, $P = 0.0017$). The coprimary endpoint of all-cause mortality or all-cause hospitalization did not have statistical significance. *Lancet* 2003;362:7–13.

CARE-HF: A total of 813 patients were followed for 29.4 months and randomized to biventricular pacing or medical therapy. The primary endpoint of death from any cause or cardiovascular hospitalization occurred in 39% of the biV group (159 patients) and 55% of the medical therapy group (224 patients; $P < 0.001$). Other findings included reduction in LV end-systolic volume, MR jet, ejection fraction, and quality of life ($P < 0.01$). *N Engl J Med* 2005;352:1539–1549.

ATRIAL FIBRILLATION/SUDDEN DEATH TRIALS

AFFIRM: A total of 4060 patients with atrial fibrillation were randomized to rate versus rhythm control and followed for a mean of 3.5 years; 26% had a reduced ejection fraction, 39% were women, 70.8% had hypertension, and 38.2% had CAD. In the rate-control group, 21.3% of patients died; 23.8% died in the rhythm-control group ($P = 0.08$). In addition, 77 patients experienced strokes in the rate-control and 80 in the rhythm-control group. Most patients experienced strokes when warfarin was discontinued or when the warfarin was subtherapeutic. More patients in the rhythm-control group were hospitalized with drug-related side effects. *N Engl J Med* 2002;347:1825–1833.

MADIT-II: ICD versus conventional therapy was studied in 1232 patients with CAD and LVEF <30% who had had a least one MI. The study was stopped early owing to a 31% RR reduction in mortality in the ICD arm ($P = 0.016$) when followed for an average of 2 years. The survival benefit was seen after 9 months. *N Engl J Med* 2002:346:877–883.

SCD-HeFT: ICD versus amiodarone or placebo when added to standard medical therapy was studied in 2521 patients with class II to III CHF due to ischemic and nonischemic causes and LVEF <35%. After a median follow-up of 45 months, ICD patients had a reduction in all-cause mortality of 23% when compared with placebo (17.1% versus 22.3%, $P = 0.007$). *N Engl J Med* 2005;352:225–237.

POSTINFARCTION

AIRE: Ramipril versus placebo was studied in 2006 patients with therapy initiated on day 3 to 10 after STEMI with clinical evidence of CHF at any time after the MI and followed for an average of 15 months; a 27% RR reduction in all-cause mortality was found in the ramipril-treated patients (17% versus 23%, $P = 0.002$). *Lancet* 1993;342:821–827.

TOAT: A total of 223 patients approximately 1 month following a LAD-related STEMI with no evidence of ischemia were randomized to elective PCI versus medical therapy. The PCI group had an increase in LV volume (systolic:diastolic; 106.6 $\pm$ 37.5/162.0 $\pm$ 51.4) compared to the medical treatment group (79.7 $\pm$ 34.4/130.1 $\pm$ 46.1), $P < 0.01$ for both. The PCI group did show an increase in exercise time compared with the medical treatment group ($P = 0.05$). Quality of life (impact on lifestyle) was reduced in the medical treatment arm and remained stable in the PCI group ($P = 0.025$). *J Am Coll Cardiol* 2002;40:869–876.

ABBREVIATIONS

ACTH	Adrenocorticotropic hormone
ADH	Antidiuretic hormone
AI	Adrenal insufficiency
BMD	Bone mineral density
BUN	Blood urea nitrogen
CRH	Corticotropin-releasing hormone
CT	Computed tomography
DCCT	Diabetes Control and Complications Trial
ddAVP	1-desamino-8-d-arginine vasopressin
DHEA-S	Dehydroepiandrosterone-sulfate
DI	Diabetes insipidus
DKA	Diabetic ketoacidosis
DTR	Deep tendon reflex
FSH	Follicle-stimulating hormone
GFR	Glomerular filtration rate

GH	Growth hormone
GLP	Glucagon-like peptide
GnRH	Gonadotropin-releasing hormone
GHRH	Growth hormone–releasing hormone
hCG	Human chorionic gonadotropin
HHS	Hyperglycemic hyperosmolar states
IDDM	Insulin-dependent diabetes mellitus
IGF	Insulin-like growth factor
ITT	Insulin tolerance test
IVF	Intravenous fluids
LH	Luteinizing hormone
MEN	Multiple endocrine neoplasia
MRI	Magnetic resonance imaging
MSH	Melanocyte-stimulating hormone
NIDDM	Non–insulin-dependent diabetes mellitus
NPH	Neutral protamine Hagedorn
PCOS	Polycystic ovary syndrome
PO	By mouth
PPI	Protein pump inhibitor
PRL	Prolactin
PTH	Parathyroid hormone
PTHrP	Parathyroid hormone related protein
PTU	Propylthiouracil
RAI	Radioactive iodine
SERM	Selective estrogen receptor modulators
SIADH	Syndrome of inappropriate ADH
T_3	Triiodothyronine
T_3RU	T_3 resin uptake
T_4	Thyroxine
TB	Tuberculosis
TBG	Thyroxine-binding globulin
TPO	Thyroid peroxidase antibody
TRH	Thyrotropin-releasing hormone
TSH	Thyroid-stimulating hormone (thyrotropin)
TSS	Transsphenoidal surgery
UKPDS	United Kingdom Prospective Diabetes Study
UTI	Urinary tract infection
VIPoma	Vasoactive intestinal peptide (oma)

ENDOCRINE EMERGENCIES

Name five endocrine emergencies.

1. Pituitary apoplexy or sudden loss of pituitary function
2. Thyrotoxic crisis (thyroid storm)
3. Myxedema coma

4. Addisonian crisis/acute adrenal insufficiency
5. Hyperglycemic crises—DKA and HHS

PITUITARY EMERGENCIES

What is pituitary apoplexy?

The clinical syndrome that occurs after a sudden infarction or hemorrhage into the pituitary gland

What are some causes of pituitary apoplexy?

Hemorrhagic infarction of a pituitary tumor—often an adenoma, which is a neurosurgical emergency

Head trauma, skull base fractures, stalk compression. Hypertension, sickle cell, diabetes, and acute hypovolemic shock/hypoperfusion can precipitate this as well.

What are the most common presenting features of pituitary apoplexy?

Sudden onset severe headache (frontal or retro-orbital) and visual field defects

What are some additional presenting features of pituitary apoplexy?

Neck stiffness, nausea, vomiting, progressive cranial nerve dysfunction

Hypotension, visual disturbances, hypoglycemia, fever, and altered consciousness; even coma can occur

How is it diagnosed?

CT—favored in acute setting (MRI in the subacute setting) with evidence of bleed, mass, pituitary trauma

How is pituitary apoplexy managed?

Urgent neurosurgical consultation for possible transsphenoidal surgery. Indicated for failure of optic tract pressure to resolve or progressive pituitary compression.

Stress-dose corticosteroids (100 mg hydrocortisone IV q8h or 4 mg dexamethasone IV q8h) until stability is achieved.

Most patients will require long-term cortisol, thyroid, and gonadal steroid replacement.

What features suggest posterior pituitary trauma or loss of function?

Hypernatremia, polyuria, and polydipsia—from central diabetes insipidus (loss of vasopressin secretion)—occur in ~4% of cases of pituitary apoplexy.

THYROID EMERGENCIES

What is thyroid storm?

Clinically severe or accelerated thyrotoxicosis that results in multiorgan and multisystem dysfunction

What are some characteristic features of thyroid storm?

High fever and profuse sweating

Altered mental status—delirium, psychosis, seizures; if untreated, coma can develop

Hyperreflexia, hyperkinesis

Tachycardia or arrhythmia, systolic hypertension, wide pulse pressure

High-output heart failure and pulmonary edema

Gastrointestinal hypermotility, nausea, vomiting

What is the most common underlying medical condition in which thyroid storm occurs?

Graves' disease most commonly, and less commonly multinodular goiter

What are the precipitants of thyroid storm?

Most often a thyroid event in a patient with preexisting thyroid disease:

Thyroid manipulation—surgery, radioiodine therapy, iodinated contrast or withdrawal of antithyroid medication

Systemic insult/stress:

Infection, MI, trauma, surgery, DKA, parturition

Do thyroid hormone levels correlate with illness severity?

No, and they are often not significantly greater than those in clinically milder forms of thyrotoxicosis.

In general terms, how is thyroid storm managed?

1. Supportive care usually in the ICU: oxygen, mechanical ventilation if needed, BP control, fluids, cooling blankets, antipyretics.
2. Treat thyrotoxicosis.
3. Search for and treat the underlying cause and precipitant if possible—e.g., infection, MI.

How is thyroid hormone synthesis blocked?

Propylthiouracil (PTU) is the preferred drug (600- to 1000-mg load, then 200 to 300 mg PO q6h). An alternative is methimazole (60- to 100-mg load, then 30 to 60 PO mg q8h).

How is the release of preformed thyroid hormone blocked?

Inorganic iodine 2 hours after giving PTU/methimzole (e.g., saturated solution of potassium iodide, 5 drops PO q6h)

What do steroids do in the treatment of thyrotoxicosis?

Steroids block the release of thyroid hormone, decrease conversion of T_4 to T_3, and cause immunomodulation in Graves' cases (dexamethsone 2 mg PO q6h or hydrocortisone 100 mg IV q6h to q8h).

How are beta blockers used?

Propranolol (40 to 80 mg PO q6h), labetalol, esmolol drip, oppose beta-adrenergic effects and reduce conversion of T_4 to T_3 (propranolol).

Why is PTU advantageous over methimazole in thyroid storm?

At high doses it inhibits conversion of T_4 to T_3.

Which drug is safer to use in pregnancy and lactation—PTU or methimazole?

PTU—it is less likely to cross the placenta and enter breast milk, but it should still be used with caution.

What is myxedema coma?

The term is used to describe progressive dysfunction of the cardiovascular, respiratory, and central nervous systems as a result of critical hypothyroidism; however, patients do not usually present in myxedema or coma.

What is myxedema?

Generalized skin and soft tissue swelling characterized as harder, generally nonpitting edema, sometimes associated with periorbital edema, macroglossia, and ptosis.

What causes myxedema?

Decreased clearance of glycosaminoglycans in interstitial fluid as a result of severe hypothyroidism.

What are the systemic manifestations of myxedema coma or severe hypothyroidism?

Hypothermia and altered mental status

Delayed relaxation phase of deep tendon reflexes

Bradycardia, hypotension, pericardial effusion

Hypoventilation

Constipation, ileus, megacolon

Decreased GFR and hyponatremia

Who is at greatest risk for myxedema coma?

The elderly with preexisting hypothyroidism during the winter months

What are some precipitants of myxedema coma?

Cold exposure

Trauma, burns, surgery

Infection, sepsis

Medications—CNS depressants, anesthetics, narcotics

What are the 5 H's of myxedema coma and their supportive treatments?

Hypothermia—passively rewarm (blanket, warm room)

Hypoventilation—oxygen, mechanical ventilation

Hypotension—Isotonic IVF, blood if anemia

Hyponatremia—free water restriction and saline infusion

Hypoglycemia—IV dextrose with isotonic fluid

Why is active rewarming contraindicated?

It can result in vascular collapse from vasodilatation.

What is the hormonal therapy for myxedema coma?

1. Thyroid replacement—T_4 500 μg IV loading dose, followed by 50 to 100 μg daily thereafter
2. Empiric steroids—hydrocortisone 100 mg IV q8h or dexamethasone (2 to 4 mg IV q8h) until adrenal insufficiency is ruled out

What initial hormone levels should be checked?

TSH, free T_4, and random cortisol (if <25, continue steroids; if >25, can discontinue steroid replacement)

Once therapy for myxedema coma is started, what is the time course for improvement?

Improvement is usually seen within hours.

ADRENAL EMERGENCIES

How does acute adrenal insufficiency or Addisonian crisis present?

Acute circulatory failure and hypotension

Fever, nausea, vomiting, and abdominal pain

Who is at greatest risk for adrenal crisis?

Patients with preexisting Addison's disease or adrenal insufficiency subjected to sudden stress or those who omit glucocorticoid therapy

What are some precipitants of adrenal crisis ...
    In patients with known adrenal insufficiency?

Omission of steroid therapy, failure to increase dose in stressful settings, or undiagnosed disease in the setting of an illness or systemic stressor

Infection, surgery, trauma, burns

    In patients without known adrenal insufficiency?

Bilateral adrenal hemorrhage or infarction

Pituitary apoplexy

What lab tests should be ordered if acute adrenal insufficiency is suspect?

Simultaneous ACTH and cortisol, plasma electrolytes, and blood glucose

What electrolyte abnormalities will be present in primary adrenal insufficiency?

In primary adrenal insufficiency aldosterone secretion is also deficient, so hyponatremia and hyperkalemia are usually both present.

What electrolyte abnormalities will be present in secondary (pituitary) adrenal insufficiency?

In secondary adrenal insufficiency, aldosterone is intact, so potassium and salt regulation will be relatively normal, although hyponatremia will still occur from glucocorticoid absence.

What "stress" cortisol level suggests an appropriate response?

A random cortisol of >25 μg/dL in the setting of significant stress is generally accepted as adequate, although there is some controversy about what constitutes a normal cortisol response to stress.

What doses of steroids are used to treat an adrenal crisis?

Hydrocortisone 100 mg IV or IM q6h (or dexamethasone 4 mg IV q12h if unable to draw blood samples for cortisol prior to treatment).

During an adrenal crisis, what other treatment is needed?

1 L of D5 0.9% saline immediately, then 3 to 4 L in the next several hours with continued fluids as per patient's condition and needs (electrolytes, volume status)

What is the next critical step in the treatment of an adrenal crisis?

Evaluate and treat the underlying illness (e.g., infection, adrenal hemorrhage).

What defines diabetic ketoacidosis (DKA)?

Blood glucose >250 mg/dL

Arterial pH <7.3

Serum bicarbonate <15 meq/L

Moderate ketonemia or ketonuria

What defines the hyperosmolar hyperglycemic state (HHS)?

Blood glucose >600 mg/dL

Serum total osmolality >330 mOsm/kg

Arterial pH $\geq$7.3

Serum bicarbonate >18 meq/L

Mild ketonemia or ketonuria

What types of diabetics present with DKA and HHS?

Type 1 and type 2 diabetics can present with either—depending on the relative degree of insulin deficiency and counterregulatory hormone excess.

Type 1 classically associated with DKA.

Type 2 classically associated with HHS.

What are the general features of a hyperglycemic crisis?

Altered mental status, variable degrees of lethargy, dehydration, polyuria and polydipsia

What features are more characteristic of DKA?	Abdominal pain, sweet "acetone breath," rapid and deep Kussmal respirations
What features are more characteristic of HHS?	More severe dehydration and hypovolemia; also electrolyte disturbances
	Focal neurologic deficits, movement disorders, and seizures
What are the three most common precipitants of hyperglycemic crises (DKA and HHS)?	Infections (30% to 50% of which are pneumonias or UTIs)
	Omission of, or inadequate, insulin therapy
	Myocardial ischemia or infarction
What are the typical total body water deficits in DKA and HHS?	~6 L in DKA
	~9 L in HHS
What are the five major components of management for DKA and HHS?	Volume replacement
	Insulin replacement
	Potassium and electrolyte management
	Acidosis/bicarbonate management
	Treatment of precipitating event or cause
How are the following managed in both DKA and HHS? **Volume replacement:**	
First hour	Give 1 L of NS within first hour of treatment prior to starting insulin.
Hours 2 to 4	Continue IVF at 500 to 1000 mL/hr of 0.45% or 0.9% saline depending on hydration and volume status—avoid exceeding 50 mL/kg in the first 4 hours.
Why should 50 mL/kg be the limit in the first 4 hours?	To reduce risk of cerebral edema

Insulin therapy:

IV bolus of regular insulin (0.15 U/kg), then

0.1 U/kg/hr IV infusion until resolution of DKA or HHS

What is the general goal of insulin therapy with regard to the fall in blood glucose?

Goal is a fall in blood glucose of 50 to 70 mg/dL/hr. If this does not occur, either fluid resuscitation or insulin dosing is inadequate. If fluids are adequate, double the amount of infused insulin.

When should dextrose be added to the fluid resuscitation?

Add dextrose to fluid when blood glucose is $\leq$250 mg/dL in DKA and $\leq$300 mg/dL in HHS.

What signs signal the resolution of DKA?

No gap, pH >7.3, HCO_3^- >18 meq/L

What signs indicate the resolution of HHS?

Total serum osmolality <315 mOsmol/kg and good mental status

Potassium:

What is the first step if the potassium is <3.3 meq/L?

Hold insulin therapy and replace K+ with 40 meq K+ (2/3 as KCL + 1/3 as Kphos or Kacetate)/L IVF until K+ >3.3 meq/L. Then initiate insulin.

What is the first step if the potassium is >5.5 meq/L?

Check q2h and replace when K+ <5.5 meq/L.

What is the first step if the potassium is 3.3 to 5.5 meq/L?

Replace with 20 to 30 meq K+/L IVF to maintain serum K+ at 4 to 5 meq/L.

Phosphate:

When does phosphate need to be replaced?

Phosphate usually does not need to be replaced unless it goes below 1 mg/dL.

How is phosphate replaced?

Can give 20 to 30 meq/L fluid over several hours and must monitor calcium levels

Sodium bicarbonate:

When is it reasonable to use sodium bicarbonate?

When arterial pH is <7.0

How should bicarbonate replacement be given?

If pH is 6.9 to 7.0, give 1 amp HCO_3^- in 250 mL sterile water + 15 meq KCl over ~1 hour

If pH is <6.9, give double the amount over 2 to 3 hours (with total 30 meq KCl).

How is the corrected sodium calculated?

Not all sodium levels need to be corrected; however, add 1.6 to 2.4 meq Na+ to measured sodium for every 100 mg/dL of glucose over 100 mg/dL (e.g., for blood glucose 300 mg/dL and Na+ 134, corrected Na+ is ~137.2 to 138.8).

How is the water deficit calculated?

$(0.6 \times \text{weight in kg}) \times [(Na^+/140) - 1] =$ water deficit (in L). This formula uses corrected sodium.

How is the water deficit repleted?

Restore volume status first with 0.9% saline during the first 6 to 8 hours, then 0.45% saline can be used over the next 24 hours to correct any remaining water deficit.

How is total plasma osmolality calculated?

$2 (Na^+) + (\text{glucose}/18) + (BUN/2.8)$, with the normal range being 285 to 295 mOsm/kg

How is effective osmolality calculated?

$2 (Na^+) + (\text{glucose}/18)$

Urea is an ineffective osmolar agent and passes in and out of cells; true tonicity is reflected by effective osmolality.

ANTERIOR PITUITARY

DISEASES OF THE ANTERIOR PITUITARY

What six hormones are produced in the anterior pituitary?

Prolactin, GH, TSH, ACTH, FSH, and LH. The secretion of those hormones is controlled by both releasing hormones from the hypothalamus and feedback from target-organ products.

Prolactinomas

How common are prolactinomas?

They account for ~40% of pituitary tumors.

What are the symptoms of prolactin excess?

Symptoms include amenorrhea (90%), galactorrhea (80% in women and rarely in men), infertility, and impotence in men (75%).

How do prolactinomas present in women?

Women tend to present with microadenomas (<1 cm) and signs of prolactin excess, most commonly amenorrhea, galactorrhea, and infertility, but rarely with neurologic signs.

How do prolactinomas present in men?

Men tend to present with macroadenomas (>1 cm) and signs of mass effect such as headache, visual loss, crainial nerve dysfunction, and hypopituitarism.

How is a prolactinoma diagnosed?

Elevated serum prolactin level and the absence of secondary causes, with confirmation by gadolinium-enhanced MRI of the pituitary. A serum prolactin >200 ng/dL is almost always indicative of a prolactinoma.

What are secondary causes of elevated prolactin levels?

Hypothyroidism, pregnancy, ovarian tumors, medications (including estrogens, phenothiazides, amitriptyline, metoclopramide, calcium channel blockers, histamine H2 blockers), renal failure, stress, cirrhosis, drugs (cocaine, opioids)

What is the medical treatment for a prolactinoma?

First-line therapy is medical with dopamine agonist bromocriptine or cabergoline. Medical therapy is successful in decreasing tumor size and prolactin levels in the majority of cases (>70%).

What is the surgical therapy for a prolactinoma?

TSS

What are the indications for surgery in patients with a prolactinoma?

If medical therapy fails, if the tumor is rapidly growing, if symptoms such as headache or vision changes persist or worsen despite medical therapy. Radiation therapy is rarely indicated.

What are the side effects of bromocriptine?

Nausea, fatigue, nasal stuffiness, postural hypotension

GH/ACTH-Secreting Tumors

What percent of pituitary tumors secrete GH and ACTH?

~15% each

What causes acromegaly?

GH excess after closure of the epiphyseal plates

What does GH stimulate?

Elevated GH stimulates secretion of IGF-1, which results in the insidious onset of symptoms (unfortunately, slow onset of symptoms often delays diagnosis for years).

What symptoms are associated with acromegaly?

Arthralgias, jaw enlargement and pain, macroglossia, sleep apnea, glucose intolerance, prominent forehead, increased hand and shoe sizes, carpal tunnel syndrome, cardiomegaly, increased sweating, hypogonadism and impotence, acanthosis/skin tags, and increased colon polyps

How are GH-secreting adenomas diagnosed?

Check IGF-1 levels. A level >3 U/mL suggests adenoma. Confirm with glucose suppression test.

How is a glucose suppression test performed?

Measure growth hormone levels during a 2-hour period after a standard 75-g oral glucose load. A positive test is failure to adequately suppress GH levels (GH nadir of >0.05 μg/L after glucose load is abnormal).

What are the first-line therapies for a GH adenoma?

Transsphenoidal surgery

Conventional pituitary radiation (4500 cGy), is also effective and has been shown to decrease GH levels to <5 ng/mL in 50% of cases after 5 years.

Gamma knife radiation focused to pituitary gland

What medical therapeutic options are available for GH adenomas?

Carbergoline, a dopamine agonist, may cause clinical improvement with a decline in IGF-1 levels in 50% of patients, but this is a temporary effect.

Octreotide, a synthetic somatostatin analog, reduces GH secretion in most patients but has variable effects on tumor size. Generally second line in patients who cannot undergo surgery or radiation and were unable to tolerate bromocriptine or cabergoline.

Pegvisomant, a GH receptor antagonist, has been approved for treatment of acromegaly that has not responded to other treatments. This medication is administered as a subcutaneous daily injection.

What is the cure rate for TSS of a GH adenoma?

The cure rate for TSS is 75% if the preoperative GH level is <40 ng/mL and 35% if the preoperative GH level is >40 ng/mL. These results vary with the experience of the neurosurgeon.

What is the difference between Cushing's syndrome and Cushing's disease?

Patient's with Cushing's syndrome manifest symptoms and signs attributable to excess glucocorticoid exposure regardless of origin—exogenous versus endogenous.

In Cushing's disease, the cause of Cushing's syndrome is pituitary-dependent (e.g., adenoma).

What are the three major steps in the diagnosis of Cushing's disease?

1. Establish the presence of Cushing's syndrome with the measurement of 24-hour urinary free cortisol (values >250 μg/24 hr are diagnostic) or a low-dose dexamethasone suppression test.
2. Determine the origin of hypercortisolism—either ACTH-dependent or independent—by measuring an ACTH level.
3. Differentiate between a pituitary and ectopic source of ACTH. An inappropriately elevated ACTH level should be followed up with a high-dose dexamethasone suppression test; serum cortisol will be suppressed by >50% in those with pituitary tumors but not in those with ectopic ACTH production.

What is the best time of day to measure an ACTH level in evaluating for causes of Cushing's syndrome?

Between 11 P.M. and 1 A.M. This is the time of day when ACTH secretion is at its lowest.

What ACTH values are significant?

Values above 5 pmol/L in the setting of hypercortisolism confirm an ACTH-dependent cause.

What test can be done if the high-dose dexamethasone test is inconclusive?

Inferior petrosal sinus sampling (IPSS)

How is IPSS done?

A catheter is placed in each inferior petrosal sinus, an IV bolus of CRH (100 μg) is given, and simultaneous samples of bilateral inferior petrosal sinus blood and one peripheral venous site are collected at regular intervals.

How is IPSS interpreted?

A petrosal sinus/peripheral ACTH ratio of >3.0 has a sensitivity of 97% and specificity of 100% in diagnosing Cushing's disease; a ratio of <1.4 is found in patients with ectopic ACTH syndromes.

What is the cure rate for TSS in Cushing's disease?

90% for patients with microadenomas, 50% for those with macroadenomas.

How is cure assessed after TSS?

With cortisol levels every 6 hours for 24 hours after surgery. If cure has been achieved, the patient's cortisol will be <5 μg/dL. "Normal" levels may indicate a surgical failure.

What are three options for treatment in patients who are not cured after TSS?

Repeat TSS, pituitary irradiation, and medical or surgical adrenalectomy

What is the treatment for ACTH LH, FSH, and TSH adenomas?

TSS, with a cure rate of 80% to 90%. If TSS is unsuccessful, treatment includes adjuvant conventional pituitary radiation or gamma knife radiation.

What is Nelson's syndrome?

Progressive enlargement of an ACTH-producing pituitary tumor after bilateral adrenalectomy due to lack of cortisol-mediated pituitary suppression

What is Sheehan's syndrome?

A postpartum infarct of the pituitary that results in a decrease in all anterior pituitary hormones and is often accompanied by the onset of DI

POSTERIOR PITUITARY GLAND

PHYSIOLOGY

What hormones are released by the posterior pituitary?

Vasopressin (or ADH) and oxytocin. Hormone release is controlled by direct nerve stimulation from the hypothalamus.

What are the physiologic stimuli for the release of ADH?

Osmolality (increases dramatically at plasma osmolality >285 to 290 mOsmol/kg)

Nonosmotic factors: BP and volume status, nausea, angiotensin II, acute hypoxia and/or hypercapnia, and hypoglycemia

What defines SIADH?

1. Decreased effective plasma osmolality (<275 mOsmol/kg)
2. Inappropriate urinary concentration at some level of hypoosmolality (urine osmolality >100 mOsmol/kg)
3. Clinical euvolemia with absence of signs of hypo- or hypervolemia
4. Elevated urinary sodium (usually >40 meq/L) with a normal salt and water intake
5. Absence of another cause like hypothyroidism, adrenal insufficiency, diuretics, or pituitary ACTH deficiency

What are the neoplastic causes of SIADH?

Bronchogenic carcinoma, lymphoma, sarcoma, and cancer of the duodenum, pancreas, brain, prostate, or thymus

What are the nonmalignant pulmonary causes of SIADH?

Pneumonia, TB, lung abscess, viral pneumonitis, empyema, chronic obstructive pulmonary disease, asthma, pneumothorax, and positive-pressure ventilation

What are the intracranial causes of SIADH?

Stroke, trauma, anterior pituitary diseases, hemorrhage, infections, brain tumors, and hydrocephalus or other pathology that increases intracranial pressure

What medications can cause SIADH?

Chlorpropamide, vincristine, vinblastine, cyclophosphamide, carbamazepine, oxytocin, narcotics, selective serotonin reuptake inhibitors, clofibrate, thiazides

What is the treatment for SIADH?

Correction of the underlying cause of SIADH.

Water restriction to 800 to 1000 mL/day.

Demeclocycline (interferes with renal action of ADH).

If severe symptomatic hyponatremia is present, 3% saline can be administered slowly over several hours and is generally given with a loop diuretic.

Conivaptan, an ADH inhibitor that works at both isotypes of the vasopressin receptor (V1a and V2).

At what rate should the sodium be corrected?

Rate of correction should not exceed 10 meq/L in the first 24 hours or 18 meq in the first 48 hours.

What is the indication to use conivaptan?

Treatment of hospitalized patients with euvolemic hyponatremia resulting from inappropriate or excessive secretion of ADH

What is cerebral salt wasting (CSW)?

A syndrome resulting from salt loss that is similar to SIADH based on laboratory measures and has most commonly been described after subarachnoid hemorrhage or other CNS insult

How can one differentiate SIADH from CSW?

1. Clinical history or status with evidence of hypovolemia
2. Trial of isotonic saline infusion

How can isotonic saline infusion help differentiate the cause of hyponatremia in CSW versus SIADH?

In CSW, isotonic saline will normalize the serum sodium because it will restore volume status, suppress physiologic ADH, and result in the excretion of excess water as dilute urine.

In SIADH, saline will not improve serum sodium and instead will likely make it worse.

What are the neurogenic (central) causes of DI?

Autosomal dominant familial inheritance, CNS injury, infection, cancer, and vascular (Sheehan's syndrome)

How is neurogenic DI treated?

DDAVP is the drug of choice in most cases (either SQ, intranasally, or orally). Worse cases are occasionally treated with chlorpropamide.

How is the release of oxytocin controlled?

Through neuroregulation by the hypothalamus, which is stimulated by estrogen or manipulation or distension of breasts or the female genital tract

What is the function of oxytocin?	It acts on membranes of myometrial cells to increase the force of contraction, exerts contractile effects on the myometrium postpartum, and contracts the myoepithelial cells of mammary alveoli to cause expulsion of milk.
What are the clinical uses of oxytocin?	For induction of labor and control of hemorrhage after delivery.

HYPOPITUITARISM

What are the symptoms and signs of the following: **GH deficiency?**	In children, decreased linear growth; in adults, fine wrinkling around eyes and mouth, decreased muscle mass, increased fat mass
Gonadotropin deficiency?	Amenorrhea, infertility, altered libido, decreased facial hair growth in men
TSH deficiency?	Hypothyroidism with fatigue, cold intolerance, and constipation in the absence of goiter
ACTH deficiency?	Cortisol deficiency manifest by fatigue, decreased appetite, weight loss; abnormal response to stress characterized by fever, hypotension, hyponatremia; and a high mortality rate
How is the diagnosis of GH deficiency made?	Insulin tolerance test (ITT). Insulin is injected and GH measured at specific time intervals thereafter.
What is a normal response of GH to insulin?	GH should normally rise to >9 ng/mL after insulin injection.
What other stimulation studies are available to detect GH deficiency?	Oral L-dopa and arginine infusion for adults and oral clonidine and intramuscular glucagon for children
How is the diagnosis of ACTH deficiency made?	ITT

What is the normal cortisol response to the ITT?	The cortisol level should be >20 μg/dL after adequate hypoglycemia.
What is empty sella syndrome?	The sella has little if any obvious normal pituitary tissue and is filled with cerebrospinal fluid.
What are the causes of the empty sella syndrome?	This is likely either the result of a prior pituitary tumor (that spontaneously regressed) or is congenital.
What is the pituitary function in empty sella syndrome?	In most cases, normal pituitary function is observed, but some patients do have pituitary hormone deficiencies.

ADRENAL GLAND

CUSHING'S SYNDROME

How is the dexamethasone suppression test performed?	Dexamethasone, 1 mg, is taken at 11 P.M., and a serum cortisol is measured at 8 A.M. the next morning. Normal response is suppression of cortisol to <5 μg/dL.
What are the causes of abnormal screening tests?	Pathologic hypercortisolism, noncompliance, stress, obesity, depression, alcoholism, increased metabolism of dexamethasone by anticonvulsants or rifampin
How is pathologic hypercortisolism confirmed?	Low-dose dexamethasone suppression test
How is a low-dose dexamethasone suppression test performed?	After measuring basal 24-hour urine free cortisol, 8 A.M. plasma cortisol, and ACTH, dexamethasone 0.5 mg is given PO every 6 hours for 48 hours. A 24-hour urine for free cortisol is collected during the second day, and serum cortisol is measured at 48 hours. In patients with pathologic hypercortisolism, urine free cortisol and cortisol levels are not suppressed.

A suppressed ACTH (<5 pg/mL) suggests what causes of endogenous Cushing's syndrome?

Primary adrenal tumor or nodular dysplasia

How is a high-dose dexamethasone suppression test performed?

Dexamethasone (2 mg) PO is taken every 6 hours for 48 hours. Urine is collected for free cortisol on the second day, and serum cortisol is drawn 6 hours after the final dose of dexamethasone is given.

Why is a chest CT obtained in some cases in which there is suppression of cortisol by high-dose dexamethasone?

Some ACTH-secreting bronchial carcinoid tumors can be suppressed with dexamethasone, thereby mimicking Cushing's disease.

Name four adrenal inhibitors and their site of inhibition.

1. Aminoglutethimide—blocks side-chain cleavage enzyme needed for conversion of cholesterol to pregnenolone
2. Metyrapone—inhibits 11β-hydroxylase, which catalyzes the final step in cortisol and aldosterone syntheses
3. Ketoconazole—blocks both side-chain cleavage enzyme and 11β-hydroxylase
4. Mitotane—a cytotoxic drug that preferentially destroys cells of the zona fasciculata and zona reticularis

ADRENAL INSUFFICIENCY

What are some differences in how patients with primary versus secondary adrenal insufficiency (AI) present?

For primary failure aldosterone is lost as well and ACTH levels are usually elevated, resulting in salt wasting, hyperkalemia, hypotension and hypovolemia, and hyperpigmentation.

For secondary failure or a pituitary lack of ACTH, aldosterone is intact and potassium and volume status is usually normal. There is also no associated hyperpigmentation.

How much adrenal function must be lost for primary AI to develop?

>90%

How much cortisol is normally produced at baseline?	~8 to 15 mg/day
How much cortisol is normally produced under stressful situations such as major surgery?	75 to 200 mg/day
When should plasma cortisol and ACTH be collected in evaluation of AI?	8 A.M.
What levels of cortisol suggest primary AI?	8 A.M. value of <3 μg/dL or <6 μg/dL under stress, with an elevated ACTH in this setting
What AM cortisol level virtually excludes AI?	$\geq$20 μg/dL
What diagnostic test is commonly used to diagnose or exclude primary AI?	The high-dose cosyntropin stimulation test
How is this test performed?	Injection of 250 μg of synthetic ACTH, IV or IM, measure cortisol at baseline, at 30 minutes, and at 60 minutes
What constitute normal and abnormal results?	A plasma cortisol at 30 or 60 minutes of $\geq$18 μg/dL excludes adrenal cortisol deficiency. An 8 A.M. ACTH should be collected to confirm the diagnosis (one would expect ACTH to be high).
How can a stimulated aldosterone measurement be helpful?	A postcosyntropin aldosterone level of <18 suggests deficiency.
What is the most common cause of ACTH deficiency?	Exogenous glucocorticoid use and abrupt withdrawal of chronic glucocorticoids can precipitate acute AI.
What happens to the adrenal gland when ACTH is chronically suppressed or absent?	It atrophies.

For patients who stop long-term (>1 year) glucocorticoids or those with a history of treated Cushing's disease, how long does it take for the function of the HPA axis to return to normal?

It can take up to a year or more. The individual response is variable, and the effect will depend on the total dose over time as well.

How is secondary AI evaluated?

A morning ACTH level, cosyntropin stimulation test, and then an insulin tolerance test if deficiency is still suspected despite a normal cosyntropin-stimulation test

How is an insulin tolerance test done?

0.1 to 0.15 U of insulin per kilogram of body weight is given as an IV bolus; baseline and serial cortisol levels are measured along with blood glucose.

A blood glucose of <40 mg/dL and signs of neuroglycopenia should be achieved.

What cortisol level excludes secondary AI?

A peak cortisol of ≥ 18 μg/dL excludes deficiency.

What test differentiates secondary from tertiary adrenal insufficiency?

The CRH stimulation test

What is the expected ACTH response to CRH in secondary AI?

Patients with secondary adrenal insufficiency have little or no ACTH response to CRH.

What is the expected ACTH response to CRH in tertiary AI?

Patients with tertiary adrenal insufficiency have an exaggerated ACTH response to CRH.

How should AI be treated?

Evaluate underlying cause and treat if possible.

Replacement cortisol doses range from ~10 to 20 mg in the A.M. and 5 to 10 mg in the P.M., to try to mimic physiologic secretion.

Fludricortisone at 0.05 to 0.2 mg/day, but this is not needed if ACTH deficiency is the cause.

DHEA 50 mg/day for women.

How should cortisol dosing be adjusted for mild stress?

Mild illness like a cold or a dental procedure—no adjustment.

How should cortisol dosing be adjusted for moderate stress?

Moderate illness such as fever, minor trauma, or minor surgery—double daily dose.

How should cortisol dosing be adjusted for severe stress?

Severe stress—hydrocortisone 150 to 200 mg divided in q6h to q8h dosing, then taper by 50% per day when stress is no longer present.

How is relative AI defined in septic shock?

By failure to increase cortisol by >9 μg/dL after a 250-μg cosyntropin stimulation test

What time of day should cortisol be measured in septic shock and other critical illness?

Any time; it loses diurnal variation in the setting of severe stress and should be elevated.

How should patients be selected for steroid treatment in septic shock?

Begin with baseline cortisol: If <15 μg/dL, initiate treatment; if 15 to 34 μg/dL, do cosyntropin stimulation test and treat if there is a failure to increase cortisol level by $\geq$9 μg/dL; if >34 μg/dL, it is reasonable not to treat as cortisol response is likely adequate.

How is relative AI treated in septic shock?

Hydrocortisone 50 mg IV q6h and fludrocortisones 0.5 mg once daily, both for 7 days

What are the clinical manifestations of polyglandular autoimmune syndrome type I?

Adrenal insufficiency, hypoparathyroidism, and mucocutaneous candidiasis

What is the inheritance pattern of polyglandular autoimmune syndrome type I?

Autosomal recessive

What are the clinical manifestations of polyglandular autoimmune syndrome type II?

Adrenal insufficiency, autoimmune thyroid disease (Hashimoto's or Graves' disease), autoimmune diabetes, gonadal failure, and alopecia

ALDOSTERONE

What aldosterone and renin levels are suggestive of an adrenal cause of hyperaldosteronism?

A ratio of plasma aldosterone to plasma renin activity >30 along with an aldosterone level >20 ng/dL is suggestive of either an aldosteronoma or bilateral adrenal hyperplasia and warrants further investigation. Also, secondary hyperaldosteronism is dependent on volume status. Renin secretion and levels of aldosterone should decline with saline infusion or blockade of converting enzyme (i.e., with captopril).

How do aldosterone-secreting adenomas and bilateral hyperplasia differ in their response to upright posture?

After 4 hours of upright posture, plasma aldosterone increases significantly in bilateral hyperplasia. Aldosterone does not rise in patients with adenomas and may even paradoxically decrease.

What diagnostic procedures can aid in localization of an aldosterone-secreting adenoma?

CT or MRI and adrenal venous sampling

What is the incidence of nonsecretory incidental adrenal masses detected on abdominal CT scan?

1%

How is adrenal venous sampling performed?

Both adrenal veins and a peripheral site are catheterized. A continuous infusion of ACTH is administered while samples for aldosterone and cortisol are obtained from all three sites.

What results would be expected with an adenoma?	The concentration of aldosterone from the adenoma-containing adrenal gland is typically 10 times greater than that of the opposite adrenal.
What medical therapies can be used in primary aldosteronism that has failed surgical management or in the nonsurgical candidate?	Spironolactone (200 to 400 mg/day), amiloride, and calcium channel blockers

PHEOCHROMOCYTOMA

What are the classic and most common presenting features of pheochromocytoma?	Paroxysmal episodes of severe headache, palpitations, and diaphoresis; >90% of cases present with at least two of these three features.
How common are pheochromocytomas in hypertensive patients?	0.1% to 0.6% in some studies
What is the "rule of 10s"?	10% of pheochromocytomas are extra-adrenal, 10% bilateral, 10% familial, 10% malignant, 10% recurrent, 10% incidental.
Which patients with hypertension should be screened for pheochromocytoma?	1. Patients with severe, sustained, or paroxysmal hypertension or grade 3 or 4 retinopathy 2. Patients with MEN 2 syndromes and their first-degree relatives 3. Patients with hypertension during labor, anesthesia, or receipt of radiographic contrast 4. Patients with worsening hypertension on beta-adrenergic blockers, guanethidine, or ganglionic blockers 5. Patients with unexplained pyrexia and hypotension 6. Patients with supra-adrenal masses

What special diet or medication adjustments are necessary before urinary catecholamines are measured?

Products containing vanilla and caffeine, acetaminophen (Tylenol) and beta-adrenergic blockers must be withheld for 72 hours.

How are plasma catecholamines measured?

The patient should be supine and resting in a comfortable setting. Plasma is best drawn from an indwelling catheter, as the stress of venipuncture may elevate catecholamines in some patients.

What factors affect plasma catecholamine levels?

Anxiety, pain, dehydration, congestive heart failure, smoking, and beta-adrenergic blockers

What is the clonidine suppression test?

Plasma catecholamine levels may be elevated in both essential hypertension and with pheochromocytomas. Clonidine (0.3 mg PO) suppresses the blood pressure in both groups and brings the plasma catecholamine levels back to the normal range in patients with essential hypertension but not in those with pheochromocytoma.

What is the treatment for pheochromocytomas?

Surgical removal of the tumors. All patients should be given alpha-adrenergic blocking agents. Calcium channel blockers may also be helpful, and beta-adrenergic blockers should be considered before surgery.

Why should alpha-adrenergic blockade be established before the use of beta-adrenergic blockers in patients with pheochromocytoma?

Administration of beta-adrenergic blockers before alpha-adrenergic blockade may precipitate a hypertensive crisis.

THYROID GLAND

What is the difference between thyrotoxicosis and hyperthyroidism?	Thyrotoxicosis encompasses all causes of thyroid hormone excess; hyperthyroidism is a form of thyrotoxicosis that occurs from increased thyroid hormone production.
How can one separate hyperthyroidism from other forms of thyrotoxicosis?	By doing a 24-hour radioiodine uptake scan
What conditions will result in increased uptake suggestive of hyperthyroidism?	Diffuse uptake: Graves' disease, TSH-producing pituitary adenomas, trophoblastic disease (from hCG-mediated thyroid stimulation)
	More focal uptake: Toxic adenoma, toxic multinodular goiter (usually mildly increased uptake)
What conditions result in low radioiodine uptake?	Subacute thyroiditis, radiation thyroiditis, amiodarone toxicity, exogenous thyroid intake, metastatic follicular thyroid cancer, and struma ovarii (thyroid tissue in an ovarian tumor, often teratoma)
What is the most common cause of hyperthyroidism?	Graves' disease
What forms of thyrotoxicosis are postpartum women at greatest risk for?	1. Postpartum thyroiditis—usually develops 3 to 6 months after delivery, then goes through a hypothyroid phase and finally returns to normal
	2. Graves' disease 3 to 9 months postpartum, in some cases transient, some recurrent, and some new
How is Graves' disease diagnosed?	Evidence of thyrotoxicosis, goiter, and infiltrative orbitopathy are enough to make the diagnosis.
	When the diagnosis is in question, an uptake scan should be performed, and one can test for TSH receptor antibodies.

What is the pathogenesis of Graves' orbitopathy?

There is buildup of glycosaminoglycans in the extraocular and adipose tissues as a result of cytokine-stimulated fibroblast activation. The immune system, via T cells and antibodies, appears to recognize a common antigen, most likely the TSH receptor, present in retro-orbital tissues.

What are the strategies for treatment of the following:
Graves' disease?

PTU or methimazole—it will take 2 to 6 weeks to see improvements, but larger doses may be needed for more severe disease. These drugs block the synthesis of new thyroid hormone but will not inhibit the release of hormone already present. Beta blockers can be used for symptoms, along with iodine for more severe cases.

Surgery.

Radioiodine ablation—most often recommended.

Subacute thyroiditis?

NSAIDs or corticosteroids for more severe disease

Postpartum thyroiditis?

Observation ± beta blockers for symptoms, and then many will need thyroid replacement during the hypothyroid phase

Toxic multinodular goiter?

Radioiodine therapy; surgery if mass effects from the goiter itself

Toxic adenoma?

Radioiodine versus surgery, depending on symptoms and nodule size

When should a low TSH be treated in the setting of mild thyrotoxicosis?

At <0.1 U/mL the risks of cardiac dysfunction, dementia, osteoporosis, and fractures is increased.

Why is radioiodine ablation preferred for Graves' disease?

PTU and methimazole therapy results in ~20% to 30% success in long-term treatment of Grave's disease; however, there are rare but serious side effects of agranulocytosis and hepatotoxicity.

What is the most common cause of hypothyroidism?

Hashimoto's thyroiditis

What are some other causes of hypothyroidism?

Iodine deficiency, drugs such as lithium, sulfonamides, and large doses of iodine in patients with preexisting thyroid disease and cystic fibrosis infiltrative disease (sarcoid, hemochromatosis, scleroderma, amyloid), postablation or surgery, central (hypothalamic or pituitary), and congenital causes

What is subclinical hypothyroidism?

It is seen in an asymptomatic patient with a slightly elevated TSH (5 to 15 mU/mL).

When is it reasonable to treat based on TSH alone?

Some suggest if TSH is >10 mU/mL; others recommend checking for TPO and antithyroglobulin antibodies first. If these are positive or the patient has goiter, the risk of developing overt hypothyroidism is great enough to treat empirically. If negative, it may be reasonable to follow TSH every 6 to 12 months.

How may lipid levels be helpful in evaluating the need to treat subclinical hypothyroidism?

For persistently elevated or increasing lipid levels, it would be reasonable to treat subclinical hypothyroidism.

What is the starting dose of levothyroxine?

In elderly patients or patients with cardiac disease, a low dose is given to start, then the dose is increased very gradually (e.g., a 25-μg dose is increased by 25 to 50 μg every 4 weeks until thyroid function tests normalize, which usually occurs at a dose of 125 μg/day).

In younger patients, a dose of 1.6 μg/kg/day is reasonable to start with.

What is the incidence of solitary thyroid nodules?

They occur in up to 5% of the population, with a female-to-male ratio of 4:1.

Incidence increases with age.

What percent of thyroid nodules are malignant?

2% to 5%

How are thyroid nodules evaluated?

1. Determine thyroid status by history, exam, and labs.
2. If normal or hypothyroid, a fine needle aspiration or biopsy should be done; most often an ultrasound is done for guidance as well as determination of size and consistency.
3. If hyperthyroid, an iodine uptake scan is done to evaluate for hyperfunction.

What are the two most common thyroid cancers?

Papillary—most common

Follicular—second most common

What three cancers of the thyroid present as solitary, cold nodules?

Papillary, follicular, and medullary carcinoma

What cancers of the thyroid present as rapidly enlarging masses or goiter?

Anaplastic—rapidly enlarging mass, 90% present with metastases

Thyroid lymphoma—rapidly enlarging goiter

What are the risk factors for the following cancers:
    Papillary

Radiation exposure of the head and neck, especially as a child.

    Follicular

Iodine deficiency

    Medullary carcinoma

80% sporadic, other associated with MEN2 A and B.

    Anaplastic

Previous (20%) or coexisting (20% to 30%) differentiated thyroid cancer (often papillary)

    Thyroid lymphoma

Chronic Hashimoto's thyroiditis (~50%) and history of hypothyroidism with goiter (~10% to 20%)

What are the approximate 10-year survivals for the following cancers:

Papillary	98%
Follicular	92%
Medullary	80%
Anaplastic	13%

What are therapies for thyroid cancer?

For follicular and papillary cancers, debate continues as to the most effective therapies. Patients with small lesions usually undergo partial or near-total thyroidectomies, depending on the preference of the surgeon. The larger malignant lesions, follicular cancers and medullary carcinoma, likely need near-total thyroidectomies, as they are more likely advanced or multifocal. For metastatic disease, radioactive iodine can be used.

What is the nonthyroidal illness (NTI) syndrome?

A range of thyroid hormone abnormalities encountered in critical illness or starvation

What are the typical thyroid function tests in the NTI syndrome?

Abnormalities progress with more severe illness through several stages:
1. With mild illness, there is a decrease in T_3 and no change in other parameters.
2. With progressive illness, T_3 is further reduced, T_4 is increased from reduced clearance, and TSH is normal.
3. With more severe illness, normal TSH secretion is lost and all parameters decrease.

What lab test may be useful in diagnosing this syndrome?

rT_3. Reverse T_3 will be elevated in the first two stages but may begin to decrease in the most severe stage.

What two drugs commonly used in ICUs directly suppress TSH release?	Dopamine and high-dose corticosteroids
What are the physical and chemical features of amiodarone that result in its ability to alter thyroid function and action?	It provides a high iodine load—it is 37% iodine by weight.
	It resembles T_4 structurally and inhibits T_4 deiodination to T_3; this results in higher T_4 levels, lower T_3, and a rise in TSH. These effects usually resolve in a few weeks.
	It may compete for the T_3 receptor in tissues.
	It has direct toxic effects on the thyroid gland.
Who is likely to become hypothyroid versus thyrotoxic on amiodarone?	In areas of iodine sufficiency, it most often causes hypothyroidism; in areas of iodine deficiency, it most often causes thyrotoxicosis.

MULTIPLE ENDOCRINE NEOPLASIA SYNDROMES

What gene is mutated in MEN1?	The *MEN1* gene is believed to be responsible—with a loss-of-function mutation.
What are the most common endocrine tumors in MEN1?	Parathyroid, pancreatic, pituitary
What gene is mutated in MEN2?	The *RET* oncogene—with a gain-of-function mutation
What are the most common endocrine tumors in MEN2 A?	Medullary thyroid carcinoma, pheochromocytoma, and parathyroid
What distinguishes MEN2 B?	Medullary thyroid carcinoma, pheochromocytoma, and multiple mucosal neuromas

BONE AND MINERAL DISORDERS

HYPOCALCEMIA

What are the clinical manifestations of acute hypocalcemia?	Predominantly neuromuscular irritability, which is manifest as tetany, perioral paresthesias, tingling in the hands and feet, and muscle cramps. If severe it can cause seizures, generalized tonic muscle spasm, laryngospasm, papilledema, emotional instability, and psychosis.
What are Chvostek's and Trousseau's signs?	Chvostek's sign: tetany of the ipsilateral facial muscles elicited by tapping on the facial nerve anterior to the ear. Contraction is seen in the corner of the mouth, the nose, and the eye.
	Trousseau's sign: carpal spasm after 3 minutes of occluding arm blood flow with a blood pressure cuff. Often the spasm is painful.
What is the classic ECG finding in hypocalcemia?	Prolonged QT interval
What is the differential diagnosis for hypocalcemia if ...	
It is PTH-related?	Postparathyroid, thyroid, or radical neck surgeries
	Congenital absence of PTH glands, DiGeorge's syndrome, autoimmune polyglandular syndrome I
	Hypomagnesemia, respiratory alkalosis
	Hemochromatosis, Wilson's disease, metastatic disease
	Pseudohypoparathyroidism types I and II
Vitamin D–related?	Deficiency, fat malabsorption syndromes
	Liver disease/failure (impaired 25-hydroxylation)
	Renal failure (hyperphosphatemia and impaired 1 alpha-hydroxylation)
	Vitamin D–dependent rickets types I and II

Other causes?	Critical illness (sepsis, pancreatitis, toxic shock)
	Chelation (phosphate infusion, citrated blood products)
	HIV infection (drug therapy and vitamin D deficiency)
How does serum albumin relate to total calcium measurement?	There is a decrease in total serum calcium of ~0.8 mg/dL for every 1 g/dL decrease in albumin.
What is the best test for calcium in acute or critical illness?	Ionized calcium
What is hungry bone syndrome?	Severe and prolonged hypocalcemia after parathyroid removal in a patient with preexisting hyperparathyroidism and bone disease. Thought to result from sudden increase in bone calcium uptake upon withdrawal of excessive PTH.
What is the treatment for acute symptomatic hypocalcemia?	Calcium gluconate 100 mg IV (~10 mL of 10% solution) over 15 to 20 minutes, then 100 mg over 24 hours if symptoms persist. Once symptoms resolve, replacement is with oral calcium carbonate (1.5 to 3.0 g of elemental calcium) in three to four divided doses daily, usually along with vitamin D (400 to 800 IU/day).

HYPERCALCEMIA

What are the clinical manifestations of hypercalcemia?	Nausea, vomiting, abdominal pain, and constipation
	Fatigue, weakness, altered mental status.
	Polyuria and polydipsia.
	In severe or acute cases it can lead to lethargy and coma.
What is the classic ECG finding in hypercalcemia?	Shortened QT interval

What are the most common causes of hypercalcemia?

1. Hyperparathyroidism (mainly outpatients).
2. Malignancy (most common in inpatient setting). Can be related to osteolytic disease from metastases, PTHrP, or excess 1, 25(OH)$_2$-vitamin D (B-cell lymphoma).

What are some other causes of hypercalcemia?

Vitamin D–mediated:

Sarcoid and granulomatous disease (excess 1α-hydroxylation of vitamin D by macrophages)

Vitamin D intoxication

Other:

Hyperthyroidism, adrenal insufficiency

Rhabdomyolysis, immobilization (e.g., after spinal cord injury, calcium peaks at ~4 months)

Drugs—thiazides in the setting of hyperparathyroidism, chronic lithium, milk-alkali syndrome, excess vitamin A

Paget's disease

What are some important lab tests in hypercalcemia of malignancy?

PTHrP, PTH, and 1, 25(OH)$_2$-vitamin D levels.

What is milk-alkali syndrome?

Hypercalcemia, metabolic alkalosis, and renal failure after ingestion of large amounts of calcium and alkali

What is a common cause of this syndrome?

Ingestion of excessive calcium carbonate (up to several grams a day)

What are the treatments for acute symptomatic hypercalcemia?

1. Normal saline (0.9%) at 2 to 4 L/day initially.
2. IV Pamidronate 60 to 90 mg once a day over 4 to 24 hours (restores calcium to normal in 2 to 3 days)
3. Calcitonin (human) 0.5 mg SQ every 12 hours (reduces calcium in hours but the effect lasts for only a few days)

4. Lasix—if vigorous hydration fails to improve hypercalcemia or volume overload occurs. Otherwise it risks volume contraction and aggravation of renal failure.

OSTEOPOROSIS

How does osteoporosis differ pathologically from osteomalacia?	Osteoporosis is characterized by the disruption of normal bone architecture; there are fewer, thinner, and less connected trebeculae as well as thinned and more porous cortices. There is no gross defect in collagen structure or mineralization.
	Osteomalacia is characterized by a lack of mineral in newly formed bone matrix as well as a reduced rate of bone growth. There are obvious defects of increased osteoid and decreased mineralization.
What is a T score?	The standard deviation (SD) from the bone mineral density (BMD) of a young normal population.
What is a Z score?	The SD away from an age- and gender-matched group.
How is osteoporosis defined?	T score <-2.5
What defines normal and low bone mass?	Normal is T score >-1 Low is T score -1 to -2.5
When is treatment for osteoporosis generally indicated?	T score <-2.0 T score <-1.5 and risk factors Women over age 70 with multiple risk factors
What is the most common cause of secondary osteoporosis?	Corticosteroid use—bone loss after 1 year approaches 20%.

What is the incidence of fractures in patients on corticosteroids for greater than 6 months?	30% to 50%
How can steroid-induced osteoporosis be prevented or treated?	Calcium (1500 mg/day elemental), vitamin D (800 IU/day), bisphosphonates, teriparatide, calcitonin
What is the lifetime risk of osteoporosis in a man over age 50?	13%
How is the action of selective estrogen receptor modulators (SERMs) different from that of hormone replacement therapy?	Estrogen-like drugs, such as SERMs, have estrogen-agonist activities at bone but antagonist actions at breast and uterus. The single agent in this class is raloxifene (Evista).
How do bisphosphonates work and how are they dosed?	Bisphosphonates inhibit bone resorption; they include etidronate (cyclic therapy), alendronate (continuous or weekly therapy), risedronate (continuous or weekly therapy) and ibandronate (monthly or given IV every 3 months).
What is an added benefit of calcitonin?	Calcitonin can stabilize bone mass and may have additional beneficial actions on reducing bone pain from fractures.
How is human PTH administered?	Daily SQ injections of recombinant human PTH can increase BMD and reduce spine fractures; it is approved for the treatment of postmenopausal osteoporosis.
What are some causes of osteomalacia?	Vitamin D deficiency with resulting calcium and phosphate deficiency caused by malabsorption syndromes, hepatic disease with fat malabsorption, pancreatic disease with exocrine insufficiency, and renal disease

PAGET'S DISEASE

What is the epidemiology of Paget's disease?

Paget's disease is most common in persons above 50 years of age, with a slight male predominance. There may be a genetic component in that 15% to 30% of patients have a family history of Paget's disease.

How is the diagnosis of Paget's disease made?

Biochemically, Paget's disease is characterized by an increase in markers of bone turnover, including increased urinary excretion of hydroxyproline, an elevated serum alkaline phosphatase, and osteocalcin.

What are the radiographic findings in Paget's disease?

Affected bones show cortical thickening, expansion, and areas of mixed lucency and sclerosis. The skull of affected patients is often described as having a cotton-wool appearance.

What is the therapy for Paget's disease?

Therapy is directed at suppressing the activity of the osteoclasts. These medications include calcitonin, etidronate, alendronate, risedronate, and plicamycin. Calcitonin is given as a subcutaneous injection. Unfortunately tachyphylaxis has been reported. Etidronate is very effective but may alter normal mineralization and must be given on an intermittent regimen. Plicamycin is a very potent inhibitor of resorption but has a number of toxicities and should be reserved for refractory cases.

REPRODUCTIVE ENDOCRINOLOGY

FEMALE

What disorders cause or present as primary amenorrhea?

Genotype disorder (e.g., testicular feminization and 5-α reductase deficiency)

Anatomic defect [e.g., Müllerian agenesis, Asherman's syndrome (intrauterine adhesions), and imperforate hymen]

Ovarian failure (e.g., gonadal dysgenesis and autoimmune disease)

Metabolic (e.g., weight loss and chronic illness)

Hormonal (e.g., polycystic ovary disease, congenital adrenal hyperplasia, hyperprolactinemia, and hypopituitarism)

What is the first test that should be done in evaluating secondary amenorrhea?

A pregnancy test

What are some causes of secondary amenorrhea?

Pregnancy, Asherman's syndrome (outflow obstruction as a result of uterine instrumentation), premature ovarian failure, hyperprolactinemia, hypothalamic causes

What other diseases are associated with premature ovarian failure?

Autoimmune diseases such as Hashimoto's thyroiditis, type 1 diabetes, and Addison's disease

Why does hypothyroidism cause elevated prolactin?

Because of increased levels of TRH, which directly stimulate prolactin production

What is hypothalamic amenorrhea?

It results from impaired GnRH release, which occurs in the setting of stress, severe weight loss, fat loss, and excessive exercise.

Women with amenorrhea are often at risk for osteoporosis; is this true for women with PCOS?

Generally, no. Women with PCOS are generally overweight and have high androgen levels, both of which appear to protect bone mass.

What are some of the adverse effects that have been associated with postmenopausal hormone replacement therapy?

26% higher rate of cardiac events during the first 5 years (Women's Health Initiative), increased breast cancer risk (RR 1.2 to 1.3), increased risk of dementia in women over age 65 (hazard ratio of 2.0)

What hormones have these adverse effects been associated with?

Estrogen-progesterone combination therapy

What are the recommendations for treating osteoporosis, vasomotor symptoms, and vaginal dryness?	Nonestrogen therapy for osteoporosis and the shortest duration and lowest doses of estrogen for menopausal symptoms

MALE

What are the features of childhood hypogonadism?	Puberty is delayed or does not occur.
What are some symptoms and signs of adult male hypogonadism?	Decreased libido, energy, and infertility
What are some physical features of adult male hypogonadism?	Soft, smooth skin, loss of body hair, gynecomastia, and a decrease in size of prostate and testes—these signs are usually detectable if androgen deficiency has been present for years.
How should the cause of hypogonadism be evaluated?	Measure a morning serum testosterone; if low, then check LH and FSH to separate central versus primary gonadal disease.
What are the feedback signals for LH and FSH?	Testosterone, estradiol, and inhibin-B
What hormone will be elevated in milder forms of gonadal failure?	FSH—regulated by inhibin-B from the Sertoli cells; they are more sensitive to damage than the Leydig cells, which secrete testosterone and estradiol.
What is the most common congenital cause of primary testicular failure?	Klinefelter's syndrome: 47 XXY
How frequently does it occur?	1 in 500 to 1000 men
How is it diagnosed?	Usually in teenagers with incomplete pubertal development, gynecomastia, or small testes

What malignancies afflict men with Klinefelter's syndrome?

Testicular or extragonadal germ cell tumors—particularly in the mediastinim

What immune diseases afflict men with Klinefelter's syndrome?

Lupus, systemic sclerosis, thyroiditis

What psychiatric disorders afflict men with Klinefelter's syndrome?

Depression, anxiety, poor verbal skills

What vascular disorders afflict men with Klinefelter's syndrome?

Varicose veins and leg ulcers

What are some other causes of primary testicular failure?

Cryptorchidism, orchitis, chemotherapy

What is hypogonadotropic hypogonadism?

Hypothalamic or pituitary dysfunction resulting in abnormal LH secretion and hypogonadism

What is the key laboratory test in hypogonadal men?

Testosterone, because LH is secreted in pulses

What lab abnormalities would be expected in hypogonadotropic hypogonadism?

Low serum testosterone and low to low-normal LH

What are some causes of hypogonadotropic hypogonadism?

Congenital—sporadic (75%) and familial. Mutations in LH and FSH beta subunits, GnRH receptor gene, and mutations of transcription factors PROP-1 or HESX1

Acquired—pituitary or suprasellar tumor (craniopharyngioma), illnesses such as cancer and AIDS as a result of low GnRH

What lab test(s) should be ordered if hypogonadotropic hypogonadism is found?

Prolactin—because prolactinomas are the most common functional pituitary tumors. Other pituitary hormones should be checked as well.

What disorder is associated with anosmia or other midline defects and hypogonadotropic hypogonadism?	Kallmann's syndrome
When should free testosterone be measured?	In obesity and hyperinsulinemic states
Why are those two conditions associated with low testosterone?	Because these states are associated with low sex hormone–binding globulin levels, which will result in low total testosterone and mimic hypogonadotropic hypogonadism.

ENDOCRINE TUMORS OF THE PANCREAS AND GUT

What are the various pancreatic and gut endocrine tumors?	1. Insulinoma 2. Glucagonoma 3. Gastrinoma 4. Somatostatinoma 5. VIPoma 6. Carcinoid
What are the symptoms of an insulinoma?	Most often postexercise hypoglycemia and sometimes hypoglycemia after overnight fasting
Besides imaging, how is an insulinoma diagnosed?	Inappropriately high insulin and C-peptide in the setting of spontaneous or induced (72-hour fast) hypoglycemia (blood glucose <50 mg/dL) and the absence of other precipitants, such as sulfonylurea therapy or insulin antibodies
What are the symptoms of a glucagonoma?	Necrolytic migratory erythema—a raised erythematous rash beginning at the groin and perineum with occasional bullae
Besides imaging, how is a glucagonoma diagnosed?	Pancreatic mass and a glucagon level >1000 pg/mL are virtually diagnostic; most have >500 pg/mL. However, the classic syndrome can rarely manifest with high-normal glucagon levels.

What are the symptoms of a gastrinoma?

Abdominal pain, diarrhea, and heartburn; refractory peptic ulcers leading to perforation and hemorrhage.

Besides imaging, how is a gastrinoma diagnosed?

Fasting gastrin >200 pg/mL and gastric acid secretion of >15 meq/h in the absence of antisecretory therapy (ppi/H2 blockers). Most have gastrin >500 pg/mL. Diagnosis can be confirmed with a secretin stimulation test for levels 200 to 500 pg/mL. A rise in serum gastrin >200 pg/mL from baseline or doubling in 15 minutes after a bolus of IV secretin.

What are the symptoms of a somatostatinoma?

Mild diabetes, steatorrhea, and cholelithiasis. Arises in pancreas and duodenum.

In addition to imaging, how is a somatostatinoma diagnosed?

Found as either a pancreatic or duodenal mass or, if suspected based on symptoms, a somatostatin level >160 pg/mL is suggestive.

What are the symptoms of a VIPoma?

Intermittent watery diarrhea, hypokalemia, and achlorhydria

Besides imaging, how is a VIPoma diagnosed?

History of severe, recurrent, diarrhea and fasting plasma VIP >200 pg/mL

What are the symptoms of a carcinoid?

Flushing, diarrhea, right heart fibrosis and failure, and—less commonly—bronchial constriction

Besides imaging, how is a carcinoid diagnosed?

Clinical features and urinary 5-HIAA >100 μmol in 24 hours. Not elevated in hindgut carcinoid, and a number of foods/substances may result in false positives. Avoiding certain foods prior to testing and using multiple less specific markers may be needed (chromogranin A, fasting blood serotonin, plasma substance P, hCG-α).

DIABETES MELLITUS

How is diabetes diagnosed?	Any of the following: 1. Symptoms of polyuria, polydipsia, and unexplained weight loss, plus a random plasma glucose of ≥ 200 mg/dL 2. Fasting plasma glucose of ≥ 126 mg/dL (no food intake of ≥ 8 hours) 3. A 2-hour plasma glucose concentration ≥ 200 mg/dL after a 75-g oral glucose tolerance test
What ethnic groups have a high risk of developing diabetes?	Hispanic Americans, African Americans, Asians, Pacific Islanders, and Native Americans
What defines the metabolic syndrome?	Abdominal obesity (waist circumference > 102 cm in men and > 88 cm in women) Triglycerides ≥ 150 mg/dL HDL < 40 mg/dL in men and < 50 mg/dL women Blood pressure $\geq 130/85$ Fasting blood glucose ≥ 110 mg/dL
What are five general forms of diabetes mellitus?	1. Type 1 diabetes—split into types 1A and 1B—both characterized by severe insulin deficiency. −1A refers to autoimmune-mediated diabetes and is the most common of this type. −1B refers to other forms of severe insulin deficiency (e.g., pancreatitis associated insulin deficiency). 2. Type 2 diabetes accounts for ~90% of cases globally and is characterized by insulin resistance, obesity, and impaired pancreatic insulin secretion. 3. Latent autoimmune diabetes of adulthood—patients can be thin or phenotypically appear like type 2 diabetics but have autoimmune beta-cell destruction and diabetes diagnosed as adults.

4. MODY (maturity-onset diabetes of youth) five forms due to impaired β-cell function resulting from genetic defects.

5. Gestational diabetes—glucose intolerance with onset at or first recognized during pregnancy.

What are the major autoantibodies in autoimmune (Type 1A or LADA) diabetes?

1. Anti-GAD65 (The 65-kDa form of glutamic acid decarboxylase)
2. Islet-cell autoantibodies (ICA512)
3. Insulin autoantibodies (less common in adults)
4. Autoantibodies to tyrosine phosphatases IA-2, IA-2B (less common in adults)

What is the 10-year risk of diabetes among first-degree relatives of type 1 diabetics based on number of antibodies present?

For ≥ 2 antibodies, 90%

For 1, only ~20%

What is the function of GAD65?

It is the enzyme involved in the synthesis of GABA from glutamic acid. Beta-cell GABA may play a role in the regulation of insulin and/or glucagon secretion.

What rare neurologic syndrome is associated with anti-GAD65 antibodies?

Stiff-man syndrome—as a result of GAD autoantibodies to neuronal epitopes, these patients also have a higher incidence of type 1A diabetes.

Are there genetic linkages in type 1A diabetes mellitus?

HLA haplotypes (e.g., DR3 and DR4) are associated with a higher incidence of type 1 diabetes mellitus. There is a 50% concordance in identical twins.

Are there genetic linkages in type 2 diabetes mellitus?

There is nearly a 100% concordance in identical twins. There are no HLA markers.

What are the two most common forms of MODY and their causes?

MODY 3 is the most common (25% to 50%). The defect is in hepatic nuclear factor 1α, resulting in defective insulin synthesis and beta-cell function.

MODY 2 is the second most common (10% to 40%) and is due to defects in glucokinase, a rate-limiting step in beta-cell glucose sensing.

How common is gestational diabetes?

5% to 10% of pregnancies

How is gestational diabetes diagnosed?

Oral glucose tolerance test, random blood glucose ≥200 mg/dL, or fasting glucose ≥126 mg/dL. The latter two should be confirmed on a subsequent day.

What is the risk of developing diabetes in patients with a history of gestational diabetes?

~50% at 10 years after delivery

HYPERGLYCEMIA IN THE HOSPITAL

What is stress hyperglycemia?

Hyperglycemia that may occur in both nondiabetics and diabetics as a result of the stress hormone response (catecholamines, cortisol, etc.) to a severe systemic stressor.

What is the physiologic role of increased glucose production and insulin resistance in acute stress?

To maintain a constant supply of glucose to the CNS under conditions where nutrient intake and tissue delivery may be impaired

What are some conditions that cause stress hyperglycemia?

Hypoxia (PaO_2 <30 to 40 mm Hg), hypotension/shock, recovery from hypoglycemia, hypothermia, surgery, trauma, burns, sepsis, myocardial infarction

How should stress hyperglycemia be managed when CNS perfusion is in question?

When CNS perfusion is in question (hypotension, hypoxia, cerebrovascular occlusive disease), one should be careful to avoid hypoglycemia and correct the underlying pathology before measures for tight glycemic control are initiated.

How should stress hyperglycemia be managed when CNS perfusion is not in question?

When CNS glucose delivery is not in question or in cases of surgery, burns, cold stress—when nutrient requirements are increased—the use of insulin to control glucose should be initiated as needed.

What levels of hyperglycemia are associated with adverse effects on wound healing and the vascular, hemodynamic, and immune systems?

Blood glucose levels >200 to 250 mg/dL. These require prompt treatment and control.

When should a hemoglobin A_1C be measured in hospitalized patients?

For known diabetics, on admission to assess recent control and intervention needs

For hyperglycemic patients without a previous diagnosis of diabetes, to assess for the presence of undiagnosed diabetes

What level of hemoglobin A_1C suggests previously undiagnosed diabetes?

>7%

What are the blood glucose goals for patients in the ICU?

As close to 110 mg/dL as possible and <180 mg/dL overall

What are the blood glucose goals for patients on a general medical ward?

As close to 90 to 130 mg/dL as possible and <180 mg/dL after meals

What are some benefits of tight glucose control in the ICU?

Fewer bloodstream infections, shorter duration of mechanical ventilation and ICU stay, less antibiotic use, and less critical-illness polyneuropathy, renal failure, and need for hemodialysis (This is from surgical ICU data.)

What mortality benefit has been shown with tight glucose control in the ICU?	10% absolute risk reduction in mortality for those treated in the ICU >5 days (This is from surgical ICU data.)

HYPOGLYCEMIA

How is hypoglycemia most reliably diagnosed?	The most reliable method is Whipple's triad: Low plasma glucose concentration, symptoms of hypoglycemia, and relief of symptoms with restoration of normal glucose concentration.
What blood glucose level defines hypoglycemia?	<50 mg/dL after an overnight fast indicates postabsorptive hypoglycemia. However, it is not possible to define an exact number below which symptoms occur, as patients with chronically elevated blood glucose may experience symptoms at levels that would be considered normal for others.
What are the two major groups of hypoglycemic symptoms?	Autonomic/neurogenic, which can be divided further into adrenergic symptoms and paresthesias Neuroglycopenic
What are the adrenergic symptoms?	Palpitations, tremor, and anxiety, and cholinergic symptoms of sweating, and hunger
What are the neuroglycopenic symptoms?	A direct result of glucose deprivation resulting in altered mental status, dizziness, confusion, visual changes, fatigue, headache, weakness, and seizures
What diabetics are at greatest risk of hypoglycemia?	Type 1 diabetics, the elderly, and those with acute renal failure or on hemodialysis
What are some causes of hypoglycemia?	Drugs: Insulin, sulfonylurea, alcohol, sulfonamides Critical illness: Sepsis, renal failure, liver failure

Hormonal deficiency: Adrenal, growth hormone, glucagon, epinephrine

Tumor: Insulinoma, large non-insulin-secreting tumor burden

Autoimmune: Insulin antibodies, insulin receptor antibodies

What is the classic diagnostic test for hypoglycemia?

A supervised 72-hour fast: Fast until blood glucose <45 mg/dL with symptoms or signs of hypoglycemia. Measure baseline and hypoglycemic parameters.

What are the three standard tests to order in the setting of acute hypoglycemia or after a 72-hour fast?

1. Insulin level (may be falsely elevated if insulin antibodies are present)
2. C peptide
3. Sulfonylurea level

What results would one expect from exogenous insulin administration?

Elevated insulin, low C peptide, and negative sulfonylurea level

What results would one expect from an insulinoma?

Elevated insulin and C peptide but negative sulfonylurea level

What results would one expect from sulfonylurea ingestion?

All three elevated—insulin, C peptide, and sulfonylurea

What are the treatments for acute hypoglycemia?

1. Oral glucose if able to eat (4 to 8 oz fruit juice or 2 to 3 glucose tablets)
2. IV glucose D5% infusion or 50 mL of D50% IV push
3. IM glucagon (0.5 to 1 mg for one dose, can repeat in 25 minutes)

TREATMENT OF DIABETES

What are the daily glycemic goals in type 1 diabetes?

Premeal glucose, 80 to 120 mg/dL

2-hour postmeal glucose, <160 mg/dL

Bedtime glucose, 100 to 140 mg/dL

What does intensive insulin therapy include?

A long-acting insulin such as glargine to mimic basal pancreatic insulin secretion, and then rapid-acting insulin to mimic prandial insulin secretion with or without a correction dose for premeal hyperglycemia. This type of regimen requires more frequent monitoring and injections but allows for greater flexibility in dietary intake and glucose correction.

What are the three components of intensive insulin therapy?

1. Basal insulin such as glargine
2. Meal-based insulin depending on body weight or carbohydrate counting
3. Correction doses or sliding scale that can be given along with meal based doses to adjust for premeal hyperglycemia

How are the morning and evening doses calculated in a split-mixed regimen?

The total amount of insulin required for most patients with type 1 diabetes mellitus is 0.5 to 1.0 U/kg/day and, for patients with type 2, 1 to 2 U/kg/day (or more). Two thirds of the total is given in the morning and one third in the evening. Of the morning dose, two thirds is given as NPH (or Lente) and one third as regular insulin. In the evening, the amounts of regular and NPH are usually even. If using a glargine-based regimen in type I DM, approximately 40% to 50% of the total daily dose is given as glargine and the remainder as rapid-acting insulin.

When should type 2 diabetics begin pharmacotherapy?

When lifestyle modification fails to maintain a hemoglobin A_1C of <7%

What drug is the only agent shown to reduce both microvascular (e.g., retinopathy) and macrovascular (e.g., MI and death) diabetic complications?

Metformin—the major action of which is to reduce hepatic glucose output/hepatic insulin resistance

When should metformin not be used?

For creatinine ≥ 1.5 mg/dL in men and ≥ 1.4 mg/dL in women; a better estimate would be a calculated creatinine clearance of <50 mL/min (by Cockroft-Gault equation).

Alcoholics

Patients with symptomatic heart failure

24 to 48 hours prior to IV contrast (it can be resumed 48 hours or later after contrast)

What drugs act predominantly as peripheral insulin sensitizers?

The thiazolidinediones—pioglitazone and rosiglitazone

What are some potential side effects of these drugs?

Edema and weight gain; there is some suggestion they may increase cardiac events and mortality.

What drugs stimulate insulin secretion (secretagogues)?

The sulfonylureas (glyburide, glipizide, glimepiride), meglitinides (repaglinide), and nateglinide, a derivative of phenylalanine

How are the different secretagogues used?

Glipizide and glimepiride are long-acting and can be taken once daily.

Repaglinide and nateglinide are rapid-acting and are taken with meals.

What are the new incretin mimetics and enhancers?

Mimetics: Exenatide (Exendin-4), a GLP-1 receptor agonist

Enhancers: DPP-IV (dipeptidyl peptidase) inhibitors, which block the breakdown of GLP-1. These include sitagliptin and vildagliptin.

What are the effects of GLP-1?

GLP-1 is a gut-derived hormone that enhances glucose-induced insulin secretion, reduces glucagon secretion, slows gastric emptying, and may preserve and promote beta-cell life and growth.

How is exenantide used?

Subcutaneously twice per day; it is approved for the treatment of type II DM in conjunction with sulfonylurea and or metformin therapy.

When should type 2 diabetics initiate insulin therapy?

Upon failure to maintain a hemoglobin A_1C of <7% on two oral agents and lifestyle modifications. Addition of a third agent may reduce A_1C by 0.9% to 1.3%; therefore an A_1C of >8.3% on two agents will require insulin.

How should insulin therapy for type 2 diabetics be initiated?

Starting with a single daily dose (most often bedtime) of long-acting insulin may reduce hemoglobin A_1C to <7%; however, as beta-cell failure progresses, the insulin regimen may progress toward that of a typical regimen in type 1 diabetes.

DIABETIC NEPHROPATHY

How many stages are there in the progression of diabetic nephropathy?

Five

What happens in the kidney at each stage of diabetic nephropathy and what is the timing of the occurrence?

    Stage 1

Glomerular hyperfiltration, increased GFR (up to 140% normal), and renal enlargement

    Stage 2

Early glomerular lesions. Expansion of the glomerular mesangium and thickening of the glomerular basement membrane occurs from 4 or 5 years to 15 years after onset of diabetes mellitus.

    Stage 3

Incipient diabetic nephropathy. Microalbuminuria (defined as urinary protein excretion between 30 and 200 mg/day) develops and precedes later nephropathy and the development of

| **Stage 4** | Clinical nephropathy with proteinuria and declining GFR. GFR declines below normal, and proteinuria >300 mg/day develops. Signs of reduced oncotic pressure (e.g., anasarca) become evident. Hypertension is universal. Overt nephrotic syndrome with proteinuria, hypoproteinemia, and hyperlipidemia can develop. Nearly all patients with azotemia from diabetic nephropathy have coincident retinopathy. End-stage renal disease usually develops within 5 years of clinical proteinuria. |
| **Stage 5** | End-stage renal disease. Uremic signs and symptoms are apparent and "renal replacement therapy" is necessary. |

end-stage renal disease. GFR begins to decline once the microalbuminuria exceeds 70 μg/min. Hypertension often is noted.

MAJOR TRIALS IN ENDOCRINOLOGY

The following is a list of the pivotal trials in endocrinology with references.

DIABETES

DCCT: The Diabetes Control and Complications Trial evaluated the importance of strict glycemic control. Groups were divided into intensive therapy (average blood glucose of 155 mg/dL) versus conventional therapy on long-term microvascular complications in type 1 diabetes mellitus. Compared with conventional therapy: the risk of development of retinopathy declined by 76%; the risk of progression of retinopathy declined by 54%; the occurrence of microalbuminuria declined by 39%; the occurrence of overt proteinuria declined by 54%; and the risk of development of neuropathy declined by 60% in the intensive therapy group. The major adverse event was a twofold to threefold increase in severe hypoglycemia. *N Engl J Med* 1993;329:977–986.

UKPDS: Like the DCCT, the United Kingdom Prospective Diabetes Study investigated the incidence of complications in patients with type 2 diabetes receiving intensive therapy versus conventional therapy. The intensive therapy group had a significant 25% decrease in incidence of microvascular complications. *Lancet* 1998;352:837–852.

ABBREVIATIONS

ALF	Acute liver failure
AFP	Alpha-fetoprotein
AIDS	Acquired immunodeficiency syndrome
AMA	Antimitochondrial antibody
ANA	Antineutrophil antibodies
ANCA	Antineutrophil cytoplasmic antibody
Anti-HCV	Antibodies to hepatitis C
APACHE II	Acute Physiology and Chronic Health Evaluation II test
ARDS	Adult respiratory distress syndrome
ATP	Adenosine triphosphate
Anti-HBc	Antibodies to hepatitis B core antigen
Anti-HBe	Antibodies to hepatitis B e antigen
ASMA	Antismooth muscle antibody
AVM	Arteriovenous malformation
BMI	Body mass index
BRBPR	Bright red blood per rectum
BUN	Blood urea nitrogen
CBC	Complete blood count
CBD	Common bile duct
CD	Crohn's disease
CEA	Carcinoembryonic antigen
CLO	*Campylobacter*-like organism
CMV	Cytomegalovirus
CRC	Colorectal cancer
CREST	Calcinosis, Raynaud's, esophageal dismobility, sclerodactyly, and telangectasia
CT	Computed tomography
DES	Diffuse esophageal spasm
DIC	Disseminated intravascular coagulopathy
DILI	Drug-induced liver injury
EGD	Esophagogastroduodenoscopy
ELISA	Enzyme-linked immunosorbent assay
ERCP	Endoscopic retrograde cholangiopancreatography
EUS	Endoscopic ultrasound
FAP	Familial adenomatous polyposis
GB	Gallbladder
GERD	Gastroesophageal reflux disease
GI	Gastrointestinal
HAV	Hepatitis A virus
HBV	Hepatitis B virus
HBcAg	Hepatitis B core antigen
HBeAg	Hepatitis B e antigen
Anti-HBs	Antibodies to hepatitis B surface antigen
HBsAg	Hepatitis B surface antigen

HCC	Hepatocellular carcinoma
HCV	Hepatitis C
HDV	Hepatitis delta virus
HIDA	Hepatobiliary iminodiacetic acid
HIV	Human immunodeficiency virus
HLA	Human leukocyte antibody
HNPCC	Hereditary nonpolyposis colon cancer
HPS	Hepatopulmonary syndrome
HRS	Hepatorenal syndrome
H2RA	H2-receptor antagonist
IBD	Inflammatory bowel disease
IBS	Irritable bowel syndrome
INR	International normalized ratio
LES	Lower esophageal sphincter
LGI	Lower gastrointestinal (distal to ligament of Treitz)
MALT	Mucosal-associated lymphoid tissue
MEN	Multiple endocrine neoplasia
MRCP	Magnetic resonance cholangiopancreatography
MRI	Magnetic resonance imaging
NAC	N-acetyl cysteine
NAFLD	Nonalcoholic fatty liver disease
NAPQI	N-acetyl-p-benzoquinoneimine
NSAID	Nonsteroidal anti-inflammatory drug
OCP	Oral contraceptive pills
PBC	Primary biliary cirrhosis
PCR	Polymerase chain reaction
PPHTN	Portopulmonary hypertension
PPI	Proton pump inhibitor
PSC	Primary sclerosing cholangitis
PSE	Portosystemic encephalopathy
PT	Prothrombin time
PTT	Partial thromboplastin time
PUD	Peptic ulcer disease
PVT	Portal vein thrombosis
RBC	Red blood cell
RDA	Recommended daily allowance
SBP	Spontaneous bacterial peritonitis
SLE	Systemic lupus erythematosus
SRMD	Stress-related mucosal disease
TIPS	Transjugular intrahepatic portosystemic shunt
UC	Ulcerative colitis
UGI	Upper gastrointestinal (proximal to ligament of Treitz)
VIP	Vasoactive intestinal peptide
VOD	Veno-occlusive disease
WBC	White blood cell
ZES	Zollinger-Ellison syndrome

NUTRITION

What is normal energy metabolism?

Adults require 25 to 30 kcal/kg body weight per day (i.e., 2100 kcal/day in a 70-kg person). A typical American derives 40% to 45% of calories from carbohydrates, 40% to 45% from lipids, and 10% to 15% from protein.

What nutrients do humans require?

Macronutrients, the major part of the diet, include proteins, carbohydrates, lipids, water, and electrolytes.

Micronutrients, which are often used in minute amounts, include trace elements and vitamins.

What are the clinical consequences of marasmus?

Emaciation, growth retardation, wasting of subcutaneous fat, severe constipation, dry skin, and thin, sparse hair

What are the clinical consequences of kwashiorkor?

Decreased protein synthesis with muscle atrophy and normal or increased body fat. Accompanying are anorexia, anasarca, edema, "moon face," distended abdomen as a result of dilated bowel loops and hepatomegaly, dry skin, and hypopigmented, dry hair. Edema may mask true malnutrition.

What is the RDA and how has it changed?

The recommended daily allowances are different for men and women and vary with age. In addition, although the RDA nomenclature has been used for several decades to define a set of standards for nutrient and energy intake, a major revision occurred in 1997 to create a broader set of dietary guidelines than the RDA. The revised nomenclature is known as the dietary reference intakes (DRI).

What are the most common deficiencies associated with intestinal disease?

Folate, calcium (duodenum and jejunum), magnesium (ileum and jejunum), vitamin B12 (terminal ileum), zinc

What laboratory tests suggest malnutrition?

Low serum albumin, prealbumin, carotene, transferrin, total lymphocyte count, negative nitrogen balance, and delayed hypersensitivity skin response to common antigens are useful indices for visceral protein status.

How much should healthy adults be fed?

20 to 25 kcal/kg, 0.8 to 1.0 g protein/kg

How much should obese adult patients or patients adapted to "starvation" be fed?

20 to 25 kcal/kg, 1.0 to 1.5 g protein/kg

How much should adult patients experiencing mild to moderate stress be fed?

25 to 30 kcal/kg, 1.3 to 1.5 g protein/kg

How much should adult patients experiencing moderate to severe stress be fed?

30 to 35 kcal/kg, 1.6 to 2.5 g protein/kg

What is the general rule of thumb for nutrition?

If the gut works, use it.

Clinical pearl

Recovery is slow. It is much easier to prevent malnutrition than to treat it.

How are potassium, magnesium, and phosphorus levels maintained during starvation?

By depleting the intracellular stores of these minerals. Phosphorus levels are maintained by mobilization of bone stores and enhanced renal resorption.

What causes the mineral depletion seen in refeeding syndrome?

On refeeding, metabolism increases as the body attempts to replenish its stores of ATP and increase protein synthesis, body cell mass, and glycogen synthesis. Phosphate, magnesium, and potassium are retained by cells during these processes; thus the corresponding serum level may fall. Also, after carbohydrate ingestion, the resulting increase in serum insulin can cause intracellular shifts of potassium and phosphate, contributing to the low serum levels.

What factors contribute to the fluid overload and cardiac insufficiency in some patients with refeeding syndrome?

With chronic starvation, cardiac mass, end-diastolic volume, and stroke volume all decrease. Bradycardia and fragmentation of cardiac myofibrils may occur. In addition, increased insulin levels (resulting from carbohydrate ingestion) lead to sodium and water retention. Ventricular arrhythmias, often preceded by a prolonged QT interval, may result from hypokalemia and hypomagnesemia.

What GI changes occur with chronic starvation and subsequent refeeding syndrome?

Decreased mucosal epithelial cell mass and regeneration, decreased digestive pancreatic enzymes, and impaired absorption of amino acids. Diarrhea is not uncommon.

How long does it take for the changes to reverse?

They usually reverse within 1 to 2 weeks on refeeding.

What BMI is considered normal?

Between 18.5 and 24.9 kg/m^2

What BMI defines a person as being obese?

30 kg/m^2

How many calories should overweight and obese people exclude from their diet to lose weight?

Dietary changes must be individualized, ideally with the guidance of a nutritionist or other trained professional. A low-calorie diet (1000 to 1500 kcal/day) can produce an 8% weight loss over 4 to 6 months. Very low calorie diets have greater initial yield but are associated with more complications (e.g., electrolyte abnormalities, gallstones, and arrhythmias) and greater rates of weight regain.

How much of an energy deficit is needed to lose weight?

On average, a 7500-kcal deficit is needed to lose 1 kg of adipose tissue (the average adult expends approximately 3500 kcal after walking 35 miles).

What are some examples of medications that have been used to treat obesity?

Appetite suppressants (e.g., amphetamines, fenfluramine, phentermine, sibutramine, selective serotonin reuptake inhibitors), phenylpropanolamine, opioid antagonists, dietary fat substitutes (e.g., Olestra, Simplesse), carbohydrase inhibitors (e.g., Acarbose), lipase inhibitors (e.g., orlistat), thermogenic agents (e.g., thyroid hormone, ephedrine), and other hormones (e.g., human chorionic gonadotropin, cholecystokinin-octapeptide). Currently, only sibutramine and orlistat are approved for long-term use.

For which patients is surgical treatment of obesity considered?

Patients with a BMI >40 kg/m^2 or a BMI >35 kg/m^2 with medical comorbidities. Patients should have failed nonsurgical weight-loss strategies.

GASTROINTESTINAL BLEEDING

What are symptoms and signs of acute, severe GI bleeding?

Hemodynamic instability (i.e., tachycardia, tachypnea, orthostatic hypotension, angina, mental status change or coma, and cold extremities)

What additional signs may be present in a cirrhotic patient with GI bleeding?

Hepatic encephalopathy or HRS

What are the more common causes of UGI bleeding?

Peptic ulcer (related to *Helicobacter pylori* or NSAID use), hemorrhagic gastritis, Mallory-Weiss tear, erosive esophagitis, and varices. Also consider neoplasm, angiectasia (formerly known as angiodysplasia), Dieulafoy's lesion, gastric vascular ectasia, aortoenteric fistula, and hemobilia.

What are the more common causes of LGI bleeding?

Hemorrhoids and fissures (rarely require hospitalization), AVMs, diverticulosis, ischemia, neoplasms, IBD, infectious colitis, radiation colitis, and Meckel's diverticulum

How much blood must be present to produce melena?

At least 100 mL of blood must be present in the GI tract for melena to occur. Note: Iron, bismuth, and some foods can cause black stools.

Does bright red blood per rectum always indicate a LGI bleed?

Bright red blood per rectum usually indicates a LGI source, but 10% to 15% of cases result from vigorous UGI bleeding.

How much bleeding from the UGI is necessary to cause BRBPR?

Need 1000 mL blood for hematochezia

Is NG aspiration necessary in LGI bleeding?

In all patients with GI bleeding, NG aspiration and lavage should be considered. Some 10% to 15% of patients presenting with hematochezia will have UGI sources.

How is NG aspiration helpful?

Continuous bright red blood demonstrates active, vigorous bleeding, whereas "coffee grounds" are more consistent with bleeding that is slower or has stopped.

Is there a false-negative rate with NG aspiration?

There is a 16% false-negative rate for NG lavage (even if bile is visualized) in patients with endoscopically active UGI bleeding.

Is a rectal examination needed for UGI bleeding?

Yes; character and color of stool can help determine the severity and source of bleeding.

Why might the BUN be elevated in the setting of an UGI bleed?

The BUN becomes elevated due to the digestion of blood proteins and absorption of nitrogenous compounds in the small intestine.

What additional testing should be considered in patients with a UGI source of bleeding?

For UGI sources, consider urgent endoscopy.

What is the treatment for bleeding associated with PUD?

Medical therapy includes supportive care, transfusions when needed, correction of any coagulopathy, and acid suppression (with PPIs or H_2RAs). An intravenous PPI should be initiated in the acute setting; it acts to minimize further PUD progression and promote more effective coagulation.

What is the medical treatment for acute esophageal varices that are causing GI bleeding?

For intermediate- and high-risk lesions, endoscopic thermal coagulation, with or without preceding epinephrine injections, is frequently performed.

Intravenous octreotide is used to "decompress" the portal venous system without the significant cardiovascular side effects of vasopressin and nitroglycerin.

Broad-spectrum antibiotics are indicated (generally ciprofloxacin is used), as there is increased morbidity and mortality directly attributable to infectious complications of variceal bleeding in a cirrhotic patient.

What percent of patients with compensated cirrhosis develop esophageal varices?

Approximately 40%

What percent of patients with decompensated cirrhosis develop esophageal varices?

Approximately 85%

What is the mortality associated with an esophageal variceal bleed?

Approximately 30%

What is a TIPS procedure?

Transjugular intrahepatic portosystemic shunt

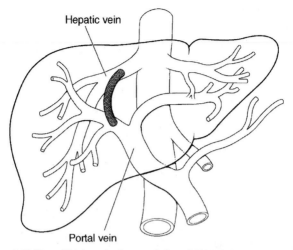

Hepatic vein

Portal vein

(From Yamada T, Alpers DH, Laine L, Owyang C, Powell DW: *Textbook of Gastroenterology,* 3rd ed. Philadelphia: Lippincott Williams & Wilkins, 1999:723.)

What oral medications may decrease the risk of variceal bleeding?

Beta-adrenergic blockers. Nitrates are sometimes used.

How are beta blockers titrated?

Propranolol or nadolol is started at a relatively low dose and then titrated to achieve a 25% reduction in resting heart rate or a resting heart rate of 50 to 60 bpm.

Do beta blockers decrease the incidence of the development of esophageal varices in patients with portal hypertension?

No, they only decrease the incidence of bleeding from existing esophageal varices by reducing the hepatic venous pressure gradient.

Which factors predict the progression of esophageal varices?

A higher Child-Pugh score, alcohol as an etiology of the varices, and the presence of red wale marks

Are gastric varices treated the same as esophageal varices?

Unlike esophageal varices, gastric varices do not respond optimally to band ligation; novel therapies for gastric varices, such as the injection of various glue-like materials into the varices, are being investigated.

How are antisecretory agents—H$_2$ antagonists, PPIs, and antacids—useful in GI bleeding?

They neutralize pathogenic gastric acid after UGI bleeding. Maintaining intragastric pH >4.0 reduces the direct harmful effects of acid and pepsin on the bleeding lesion and allows platelets to aggregate.

What is a simple rule for quantifying the amount of blood loss a patient has experienced?

Tachycardia = 10%

Orthostatic hypotension = 20%

Hypotension = 30%

What are the adverse prognostic factors for GI bleeding?

Severe persistent bleeding.

Onset of bleeding after admission or rebleeding in the hospital (>30% mortality in some series).

Mortality doubles in patients >60 years of age and in those with concomitant central nervous system, hepatic, pulmonary, or neoplastic disease. It triples in patients with renal disease, and it increases several-fold in patients with cardiac or pulmonary disease.

Urgent surgery for UGI bleeding carries a 25% mortality compared to 2% for elective surgery.

Should an adherent clot be removed or left alone?

Recent studies demonstrate decreased recurrences of bleeding and better outcomes with removal of adherent clots and subsequent thermal coagulation or epinephrine injection.

Name a medication that could be of benefit in stabilizing a bleeding ulcer prior to definitive therapy.

Octreotide, which decreases splanchnic blood flow and decreases acid secretion.

ESOPHAGUS

DYSPHAGIA, REFLUX, AND MOTILITY

What does dysphagia with solid foods suggest?

Solid food > liquid suggests structural abnormality.

What does dysphagia with either suggest?

Solids = liquids suggests neuromuscular (motility) origin.

Does the location of the patient's symptoms accurately predict the location where the food or liquid is getting "stuck"?

No, particularly for distal esophageal lesions

Name the disorder from these defining characteristics:

    Intermittent dysphagia

Schatzki's ring

    Progressive dysphagia for solids and liquids

Scleroderma or achalasia

    Regurgitation of undigested food

Achalasia or Zenker's diverticulum

    Patients often have undergone workup for angina

Nutcracker esophagus or diffuse esophageal spasm

What is the characteristic appearance of achalasia on barium swallow?

Bird's beak appearance

What is the treatment for achalasia?

Achalasia can be treated with pneumatic balloon dilation of the LES or surgical myotomy. Injection of botulinum toxin into the LES can be utilized for patients who are not good surgical candidates, but repeat injections are generally required every 6 months.

What is pseudoachalasia?

A tumor in the distal esophagus producing findings similar to those of achalasia on imaging and manometry

How are DES and nutcracker esophagus diagnosed?

Manometry demonstrates >20% simultaneous contractions in DES and high-amplitude contractions in nutcracker esophagus. Barium swallow may demonstrate a "corkscrew" esophagus in DES (although this is not diagnostic).

What is the treatment for DES and nutcracker esophagus?

These motility disorders can be difficult to treat, and antidepressants (including tricyclic antidepressants), calcium channel blockers, nitrates, and antispasmodics are often used to attempt to alleviate symptoms.

GASTROESOPHAGEAL REFLUX

How common is esophageal reflux?

Common. More than 33% of Americans have intermittent symptoms; 10% have daily heartburn.

What is the nonpharmacologic treatment of GERD?

Lifestyle changes—elevation of the head of the bed (6 to 8 inches), weight loss, avoidance of tight-fitting clothes, smoking cessation, decreased caffeine consumption, avoidance of foods and medications that decrease LES pressure, minimizing oral intake for a few hours before lying supine, and consumption of frequent small, high-protein meals

What is the pharmacologic treatment of GERD?

PPIs, H_2 receptor antagonists, and prokinetics. Metoclopramide increases LES pressure and improves esophageal and gastric emptying.

What are the interventional treatments for GERD?

Open or laparoscopic Nissen fundoplication, which is usually reserved for patients who have failed medical therapy. Endoscopic suturing and radiofrequency treatment are newer, less invasive techniques.

Clinical pearl

The character of the pain does not help to differentiate cardiac from noncardiac sources. Pain of esophageal origin may radiate to the neck, arm, or jaw and can be aggravated by stress and exercise. Therefore an adequate cardiac evaluation is often first required to exclude potentially life-threatening processes.

What type of cancer may arise in Barrett's esophagus?

Adenocarcinoma

How frequent is dysplasia and adenocarcinoma in the setting of Barrett's esophagus?

Dysplasia and adenocarcinoma have a prevalence of 3% to 9%. The risk of developing adenocarcinoma is about 0.5% to 0.8% per year in patients with Barrett's esophagus.

How should Barrett's esophagus be followed up?

Patients without evidence of dysplasia should undergo endoscopy with multiple biopsies every 2 to 3 years. Patients with evidence of low-grade dysplasia should have more frequent surveillance.

What is the treatment for Barrett's esophagus with severe or high-grade dysplasia?

Surgical esophagectomy is often recommended. If a patient is not a surgical candidate, endoscopic ablation with photodynamic therapy can be considered.

What additional risk factors exist for development of adenocarcinoma of the esophagus?

Male gender, Caucasian race, obesity, chronic GERD, and smoking (possibly)

What is tylosis?

A rare autosomal dominant disease associated with hyperkeratosis of the palms and soles of the feet

How is the staging of esophageal carcinoma performed?

CT and endoscopic ultrasound (EUS) with fine needle aspiration. EUS is particularly good at determining depth of invasion and local lymph node metastases.

What is the typical EGD appearance of esophageal infection with each of the following?
    Candida

Confluent or nodular white-yellow plaques

    Herpes

Vesicles and ulcers

    CMV

Diffuse ulceration or a giant esophageal ulcer

What is the treatment of esophageal infection with each of the following?

    Candida?

Fluconazole, ketoconazole, nystatin, or amphotericin B

    Herpesvirus?

Acyclovir. Foscarnet can be used for resistant herpes infections.

    CMV?

Ganciclovir or foscarnet

What are the risk factors for developing pill esophagitis?

Poor esophageal motility, large pills, gelatin capsules, and advanced patient age.

Which class of medications is associated with high-risk pill esophagitis?

Bisphosphonates, because of their potential to produce severe esophageal erosion.

What is the treatment for pill esophagitis?

Patients should be in an upright position to take the pills, and a full glass of liquid should be taken with them. Viscous lidocaine or sucralfate may be tried for symptomatic relief.

STOMACH

GASTRITIS, GASTROPARESIS, AND DUMPING SYNDROME

What percentage of gastric ulcers are related to *H. pylori?*

50% to 70%

What are infectious causes of gastritis?

Bacterial infections (e.g., tuberculosis, syphilis, phlegmonous or emphysematous gastritis caused by systemic bacterial infections), viral infections (e.g., CMV, herpesviruses), fungal infections (e.g., *Candida*, histoplasmosis, mucormycosis), and parasitic infections (e.g., anisakiasis, *Cryptosporidium*)

What are noninfectious causes of gastritis?

CD, eosinophilic gastritis, graft-versus-host disease, sarcoidosis, pernicious anemia, and Ménétrier's disease

How is the diagnosis of gastroparesis made?

The diagnosis is largely clinical, but clinicians generally utilize the confirmation of a gastric emptying study. This study can define the degree of delayed emptying; however, it is difficult to standardize. A half-life >90 minutes suggests delayed gastric emptying.

Clinical pearl

An exacerbation of gastroparesis may be caused by severe hyperglycemia that then resolves when the blood sugar is adequately controlled.

Can erythromycin be used for long-term treatment of gastroparesis?

No, patients develop tachyphylaxis within weeks.

Does gastric pacing normalize gastric motility?

No, it is thought to reduce symptoms by feedback to the central nervous system, reducing symptoms of fullness and nausea.

What occurs during the early (hyperosmolar) phase of dumping syndrome?

Approximately 1 hour after eating, dumping of hyperosmolar food draws water into the small bowel lumen, stimulating intestinal motility and release of vasoactive peptides. Hypotension, dizziness, and tachycardia result.

What occurs in the late (hypoglycemic) phase of dumping syndrome?

Approximately 1 to 3 hours after eating, rapid absorption of large amounts of glucose stimulates excessive insulin release. This causes hypoglycemia, which results in tachycardia, light-headedness, and diaphoresis.

PEPTIC ULCER DISEASE

What are symptoms of PUD?

Dyspepsia, nausea, bloating, and belching

What causes PUD?

The vast majority of PUD is related to *H. pylori* (70% to 90%) or NSAID use (15% to 30% of gastric ulcers). Zollinger-Ellison syndrome, malignancy, CD, radiation, and infectious etiologies (e.g., CMV and TB) account for <10% of cases.

What if a gastric ulcer is found by EGD?

Gastric ulcers (but not duodenal ulcers) should be reassessed with a repeat EGD after 8 weeks of therapy because of the potential for an underlying gastric malignancy. If *H. pylori* is present, the treatment of PUD should include *H. pylori* eradication.

What medical conditions have been associated with *H. pylori*, other than PUD?

Gastritis (both acute and chronic forms), intestinal metaplasia of the gastric mucosa, gastric adenocarcinoma, and MALT lymphoma (thus *H. pylori* is classified as a class I definite gastric carcinogen in humans). The contribution of *H. pylori* to dyspepsia in the absence of PUD remains controversial. It may be a cause of unexplained iron-deficiency anemia.

What is the epidemiology of *H. pylori*?

It is the most common chronic bacterial infection throughout the world, with at least 50% of the world's population affected. Prevalence increases with age, and *H. pylori* is more common in blacks and Hispanics, owing to socioeconomic and possibly genetic factors. In the United States, about 50% of people >60 years of age have serologic evidence of infection. In developing nations, >80% of those >50 years of age test seropositive. Most infections are acquired during childhood. Incidence is 0.1% to 1% per year for adults in developed countries.

What is the natural history of *H. pylori* infection?

Typically, it is a chronic lifelong infection unless medically eradicated. The majority of people with *H. pylori* remain asymptomatic and never develop PUD or cancer.

Are all *H. pylori* infections the same?

Probably not. Some *H. pylori* organisms have a cytotoxin-associated gene A (CagA strains). Compared with CagA(–) strains, CagA(+) strains appear to result in more severe inflammation and epithelial injury, are more likely to be associated with gastric or duodenal ulcers, and may impart a greater risk of gastric adenocarcinoma.

Which patients should undergo testing for *H. pylori?*

Patients with active PUD, a documented history of PUD, or gastric MALT lymphoma

Should asymptomatic patients undergo *H. pylori* testing?

In general, asymptomatic patients should not undergo testing. Consider it for patients with a family history, particularly descendants of high-risk populations, such as Japanese, Korean, or Chinese patients or those with a personal fear of gastric carcinoma.

Should patients with "functional dyspepsia" undergo *H. pylori* testing?

Although many physicians are testing the utility of this approach, it is controversial.

What are the diagnostic tests for *H. pylori*?

H. pylori serology (ELISA), ^{13}C bicarbonate assay, CLO test (rapid urease test), histology, breath tests (^{13}C, ^{14}C), *H. pylori* culture, and stool assays. Note: PPI therapy may affect the results of the noninvasive tests.

What are the uses and advantages of the most common tests?

    H. pylori serology (ELISA)

IgG antibody against *H. pylori* is detected. The test is noninvasive and inexpensive.

    Stool antigen assays

ELISA assay—useful for initial diagnosis of *H. pylori* and documentation of eradication after treatment

    Breath tests (^{13}C, ^{14}C)

It is safe, noninvasive, and involves very low radiation exposure. It is the test of choice to document successful eradication of *H. pylori* but should be performed at least 4 weeks after completion of the eradication regimen and after PPI discontinuation.

CLO test (rapid urease test)	Results are available within hours.
Histologic study	
***H. pylori* culture**	Useful when antimicrobial resistance is suspected to allow sensitivities to be determined
PCR of mucosal biopsies	Excellent sensitivity and specificity; can be performed even if biopsy specimen is not fresh

What are the disadvantages of each?

***H. pylori* serology (ELISA)**	Titers remain high for a year or more, so it cannot accurately confirm recent *H. pylori* eradication. May be less accurate in patients >50 years of age and in those with cirrhosis.
Stool antigen assays	Limited availability. Sensitivity may be reduced in patients taking PPIs or bismuth-containing products. May not be accurate in evaluating for successful *H. pylori* eradication, particularly if performed 1 month after treatment.
Breath tests (^{13}C, ^{14}C)	Require minimal amounts of radiation exposure if ^{14}C (but not ^{13}C) is used. Sensitivity is reduced in patients taking PPIs or H_2RAs.
CLO test	Requires EGD. Sensitivity is reduced in patients with recent GI bleeding and in patients taking PPIs, H_2RAs, antibiotics, or bismuth-containing products.
Histologic study	Requires EGD. Sensitivity is reduced in patients taking PPIs or H_2RAs.
***H. pylori* culture**	Technically complex and requires strict transport conditions because of *H. pylori*'s fastidious nature. An academic tool—not widely available.

PCR of mucosal biopsies	Limited availability, and not practical for routine use. False positives may occur from contamination of specimen at the laboratory (given the high sensitivity of PCR).
What is the current standard therapy for *H. pylori*?	Bismuth, metronidazole, and tetracycline. Noncompliance with this regimen is common (owing to side effects and the number of pills). One common easier regimen involves a 2-week course of twice-daily amoxicillin, clarithromycin, and a PPI. Antimicrobial resistance is an emerging problem.
What is the current resistance pattern of *H. pylori* in the United States?	35% to 40% resistance to metronidazole and 10% to 12% resistance to clarithromycin
What percentage of patients who are treated with triple therapy have eradication of their *H. pylori*?	About 75%
What should be done if *H. pylori* is detected in the setting of PUD?	Eradication (cure) of *H. pylori* should be attempted, as 1-year ulcer recurrence rates are 6% to 80% without and <10% with eradication of *H. pylori*. Eradication should be confirmed in patients with a history of bleeding ulcers because 30% may develop recurrent bleeding ulcers.
Should eradication of *H. pylori* always be confirmed?	Confirmation of *H. pylori* cure is not mandatory in uncomplicated PUD.
Does *H. pylori* offer any protective effects?	*H. pylori* in the stomach can inhibit acid secretion and may offer some protection against esophagitis.
What are the causes of elevated gastrin?	Hypochlorhydric and achlorhydric conditions (e.g., pernicious anemia, *H. pylori* infection, gastric atrophy, and medications such as PPIs)
	Hypersecretory conditions (e.g., ZES, retained antrum syndrome, antral G-cell

hyperplasia, gastric outlet obstruction, short bowel syndrome, systemic mastocytosis, basophilic granulocytic leukemia)

Decreased clearance (e.g., renal failure)

List some distinguishing features of ZES.

Multiple ulcers, ulcers in unusual locations, recurrence after treatment, or MEN 1 features. Close to 40% of patients will have accompanying diarrhea.

What is the epidemiology of ZES?

Majority of patients between 30 to 50 years old. Occurs in men more frequently than women. May be sporadic or associated with MEN I (genetic defect in chromosome 11).

What is the "gastrinoma triangle"?

Defined by the junctions of the CBD and cystic duct, the second and third portion of the duodenum, and the neck and body of the pancreas

Are gastrinomas in ZES considered malignant?

60% to 90% are malignant, typically determined by the tumor's behavior (e.g., metastases) rather than histology. Approximately 30% will have metastases (generally to liver or bone). Sporadic gastrinomas tend to be malignant more often than those associated with MEN I.

How is the diagnosis of ZES made?

Elevated fasting gastrin (most patients have levels >150 pg/mL; some have levels >1000 pg/mL, which is virtually diagnostic in the correct clinical setting).

Elevated basal acid output (98% of cases).

If the gastrin level is equivocal, a secretin stimulation test can confirm the diagnosis.

After intravenous administration of 2 U/kg of secretin, there is an increase in serum gastrin of >200 pg/mL above the basal gastrin level.

Calcium stimulation test may also be useful (as intravenous calcium stimulates gastrin secretion).

| What are common metastatic sites for gastrinomas? | Bone, liver, and lung |

| What is the treatment of ZES? | High-dose PPIs should be used to decrease gastric acid hypersecretion. When feasible, surgical excision of the primary gastrinoma should be attempted, as this is the only curative option. Rarely, more radical surgeries, such as antrectomy with vagotomy or total gastrectomy, are required. Surgery for ZES in the setting of MEN 1 is controversial. Other interventions—including octreotide, chemotherapy, and embolization of tumors—have not yet been shown to have consistent benefit. |

| What is the prognosis for ZES after surgical excision? | Up to a 30% surgical cure rate may be achieved with an aggressive approach to tumor localization. ZES tends to be indolent and survival can be quite long. Octreotide or hepatic artery embolization can be utilized for metastases. |

SMALL AND LARGE INTESTINE

DIARRHEA

| List the most common etiologies of inflammatory diarrhea. | Infectious, IBD, ischemic, and radiation |

| What are common causes of traveler's diarrhea? | *Escherichia coli, Salmonella, Giardia lamblia,* and *Entamoeba histolytica* |

| What are the infectious causes of chronic diarrhea? | *Giardia, E. histolytica* (people in institutions), *Mycobacterium tuberculosis, Clostridium. difficile* (pseudomembranous colitis), and *Cryptosporidium, Microsporidium,* or *Isospora* (most common in people with AIDS) |

| What are the inflammatory causes of chronic diarrhea? | UC, CD, microscopic colitis, and ischemia |

Which infectious agents are a common cause of bloody stool?	Think **CHESS:** *Campylobacter* **H**emorrhagic *E. coli* (serotype 0157:H7) **E.** *histolytica* **S**almonella **S**higella
Clinical pearls	Avoid antibiotic therapy in enteric *Salmonella* infection because a prolonged carrier state may be induced. Antimotility agents must be used with caution in patients with inflammatory diarrhea (e.g., IBD, pseudomembranous colitis, *Shigella, Salmonella*).
What chronic diarrheal state may be missed on colonoscopy?	Microscopic colitis is not usually apparent on gross examination of colonic mucosa and requires random biopsies.

MALABSORPTION

What is celiac sprue?	T cell–mediated inflammatory reaction to dietary gluten (wheat, barley, rye, oats) that causes injury to the small bowel—genetic predisposition. Also known as gluten-sensitive enteropathy.
Who is affected by celiac sprue?	Can occur at any age. Serologic testing of blood donors suggests a prevalence of 1:250 in the United States. HLA DQ II is found in 95%.
What dermatologic manifestation is associated with celiac sprue?	Dermatitis herpetiformis
What diseases are associated with celiac sprue?	Type 1 diabetes, autoimmune thyroiditis, PBC, sclerosing cholangitis, and IgA nephropathy

What serologic markers should be checked for?

IgA antiendomysial antibodies (sensitivity >90%, specificity >95%) or ELISA for tissue transglutaminase (sensitivity >90%, specificity >95%), which is the antigen for the antiendomysial antibody. Antigliadin antibodies can also be measured.

Are these markers helpful during treatment?

These markers are not sensitive for diagnosis if the patient has already initiated a gluten-free diet; they can be used to assess response to or compliance with a gluten-free diet.

Clinical pearl

2% to 3% of patients with celiac sprue have IgA deficiency. Thus, IgA levels should be obtained to minimize false-negative serologies.

What does a small bowel biopsy show in celiac sprue?

Biopsy is the "gold standard" for diagnosis, showing blunt, flattened villi and an inflammatory infiltrate in the lamina propria, with intraepithelial lymphocytes.

What else confirms the diagnosis of celiac sprue?

Response to gluten-free diet. Small bowel biopsies should be repeated after 4 to 6 months of a gluten-free diet. If no histologic improvement is seen, the diagnosis should be questioned.

What vitamin deficiencies are most commonly seen?

Folic acid, iron, calcium, and vitamin D

What other risks are associated with celiac sprue?

Lymphoma, esophageal cancer, melanoma, splenic atrophy, liver function test abnormalities, and sequelae of vitamin deficiencies (e.g., anemia, coagulopathy, osteomalacia, or osteoporosis)

What is the treatment of celiac sprue?

Lifelong gluten-free diet and nutritional supplementation as needed (calcium/vitamin D, iron, and folate). These interventions can decrease the risk of cancer, infertility, and osteoporosis associated with celiac sprue.

What is the treatment of dermatitis herpetiformis?

Dapsone, in addition to a gluten-free diet

On treatment, how long should it take for dermatitis herpetiformis to resolve?

Can take up to a year for improvement in symptoms

What is tropical sprue?

An acquired form of sprue of unclear etiology but thought to be bacterial in nature, infrequently encountered in the continental United States. It often improves with antibiotic therapy.

What vitamin deficiency is often seen in tropical sprue?

Folic acid

What is Whipple's disease?

Systemic disorder typically affecting middle-aged men. Protean manifestations include diarrhea, weight loss, abdominal pain, and arthralgias. There may also be anemia, fevers, myalgias, intra-abdominal lymphadenopathy, serositis, and central nervous system involvement.

What are other causes of intrinsic small bowel disease that result in malabsorption?

CD, lymphoma, parasitic infection, radiation enteritis, abetalipoproteinemia, and ischemia

What are the causes of pancreatic exocrine insufficiency?

Chronic pancreatitis, pancreatic resection, pancreatic cancer, and cystic fibrosis

What nutrients are not absorbed properly with exocrine insufficiency?

Fat, protein, and carbohydrates

What are the causes of bile acid insufficiency?

Any disorder of bile acid enterohepatic circulation (e.g., severe intrinsic liver disease, biliary obstruction, and disorders of the terminal ileum)

How does malabsorption occur in bile acid insufficiency?

Insufficient bile acids impair the formation of intraluminal micelles.

What nutrients are not absorbed properly in bile acid insufficiency?

Fat and fat-soluble vitamins (A, D, E, K).

Why does malabsorption of fat and fat-soluble vitamins occur with small bowel bacterial overgrowth?

Bile salt deconjugation occurs, resulting in impaired micelle formation.

What vitamin B12/folate levels are characteristic of bacterial overgrowth?

Low vitamin B12, elevated folic acid (due to bacterial production)

What are the symptoms and signs of malabsorption?

Steatorrhea

Weight loss

Bone pain or tetany (calcium deficiency)

Glossitis or stomatitis (iron and riboflavin deficiency)

Edema (hypoalbuminemia)

Bleeding and easy bruisability (vitamin K deficiency)

Night blindness (vitamin A deficiency)

What is the bile acid breath test used for?

To establish the presence of small bowel bacterial overgrowth

How is the test performed?

^{14}C-glycocholate is ingested. Normally, 95% is absorbed in the terminal ileum and 5% enters the colon and is deconjugated by bacteria to $^{14}CO_2$, which is absorbed and exhaled in expired air.

How is a positive test determined?

With bacterial overgrowth, earlier bacterial deconjugation occurs and a larger amount of $^{14}CO_2$ is measured.

What is the treatment for malabsorption?

Therapy is directed at the specific cause of malabsorption.

Dietary modification is frequently necessary—low-fat diets (restriction of long-chain fatty acids) or ingestion of medium-chain triglycerides (which do not require bile acids for absorption) may be used.

Bile acid binders (cholestyramine) may improve bile salt–induced diarrhea but can significantly worsen steatorrhea.

IRRITABLE BOWEL SYNDROME

What key symptoms are virtually diagnostic for IBS?

Diarrhea does not awaken the patient from sleep, the patient denies weight loss, and symptoms related to stress.

What are the subgroups of IBS?

Constipation-predominant, diarrhea-predominant, and alternating diarrhea/constipation.

What organic conditions can cause symptoms similar to IBS?

Lactase deficiency, IBD, colon cancer, microscopic colitis, enteric infections, and endometriosis. In a recent study of 300 patients with newly diagnosed IBS, 5% were found to have celiac sprue.

In addition to emotional and dietary therapy, what medications can be used to treat IBS?

1. Medications—tegaserod (constipation and bloat predominant) and alosetron (diarrhea-predominant) are the only two specific therapies for IBS. Other therapies aimed at controlling symptoms include antispasmodics when abdominal pain and constipation predominate, antidiarrheals (loperamide) when diarrhea predominates, laxatives when constipation predominates, and antidepressants (e.g., tricyclics).
2. Antibiotics—Recent studies show that a 10-day course of rifaximin produces a significant improvement in symptoms for at least 6 months.

Clinical pearl

Some patients with IBS report a past history of physical or sexual abuse in childhood. In some cases this can be correlated with the severity of symptoms.

ISCHEMIC BOWEL

What is the most common region affected in ischemic bowel?	Ischemic colitis (i.e., colonic ischemia)
What age group is typically affected with ischemic colitis?	Most cases (>90%) of noniatrogenic ischemic colitis occur in patients >60 years of age.
What are the causes of ischemic colitis?	In the majority of cases, no specific cause or trigger is identified. Potential causes include mesenteric artery or vein occlusion, vasospasm, vasculitis, systemic circulatory insufficiency, trauma, medication-induced (e.g., digoxin may cause mesenteric vasospasm; also vasopressors, psychotropic drugs, danazol, gold, estrogens), hematologic disorder, volvulus, and strangled intestinal hernias.
What is the treatment for acute ischemic colitis?	In the absence of gangrene or evidence of perforation, management is conservative. This usually includes intravenous fluid, bowel rest, and broad-spectrum antibiotics.
What is the usual prognosis for patients with ischemic colitis?	In uncomplicated cases, symptoms resolve in 24 to 48 hours and the colon heals itself in 1 to 2 weeks; however, it can progress to chronic colitis and stricture formation.
What is acute mesenteric ischemia?	Acute ischemia of the mesentery and small bowel. It may lead to intestinal perforation if not diagnosed and treated early.
What are some nonocclusive conditions that can result in acute mesenteric ischemia?	Hypovolemia, sepsis, congestive heart failure, recent myocardial infarction, arrhythmias; mesenteric ischemia has also been seen after cardiac surgery or dialysis.

What conditions may cause occlusive vascular disease and subsequent acute mesenteric ischemia?

Factors that predispose to thrombotic (e.g., polycythemia or hypercoagulable states) or embolic disease (e.g., atrial fibrillation or endocarditis)

What are symptoms and signs of acute vascular occlusion?

Pain out of proportion to exam (20% to 30% are painless).

Decreased or absent bowel sounds.

Occult blood that rapidly progresses to frankly bloody stool.

Hypotension, tachycardia, fever, elevated WBC count, and acidosis may occur if transmural infarction occurs and peritonitis develops.

What serum markers are available?

Lactic acid (causing an anion gap acidosis) can point to the diagnosis. However, an elevated lactic acid indicates that infarction is already occurring.

What are the CT findings?

Portal venous gas or pneumatosis intestinalis may occur late. CT angiography or magnetic resonance angiography may be helpful.

What is the treatment for acute mesenteric ischemia?

Potential options include surgical revascularization, percutaneous angiography–guided revascularization, intra-arterial infusion of thrombolytic or vasodilator agents, or systemic anticoagulation. In patients with nonocclusive disease, attempts to optimize blood flow are important.

What venous disorder can cause intestinal ischemia?

Mesenteric venous thrombosis causes approximately 10% of cases of intestinal ischemia. Predisposing factors include hypercoagulable states and cirrhosis. It may present as acute or chronic disease.

What is the treatment for mesenteric venous thrombosis?

If there is no evidence of complication, anticoagulation is preferred.

What causes chronic mesenteric ischemia?	Atherosclerosis is the most common cause. The pain is usually postprandial because of the increased blood flow required for digestion.
How is the diagnosis of chronic mesenteric ischemia made?	Doppler ultrasounds, magnetic resonance angiography, or spiral CT may be helpful. If these are abnormal or if clinical suspicion is very high, angiography should be performed.
What does abdominal angiography show in patients with chronic mesenteric ischemia?	Complete or near-complete occlusion of at least two of the three major splanchnic arteries
What are treatment options for chronic mesenteric ischemia?	Percutaneous transluminal angioplasty or arterial bypass or endarterectomy

DIVERTICULAR DISEASE

What is the incidence of diverticular disease?	Colonic diverticula are common, occurring in approximately 50% of patients >60 years of age.
Where do small bowel diverticula most commonly arise?	In the proximal duodenum, near the ampulla of Vater
How common are small bowel diverticula?	Common, occurring in approximately 20% of the population
What is Meckel's diverticulum?	A persistent omphalomesenteric duct—the most common congenital abnormality of the GI tract
What is the rule of 2s?	Meckel's diverticulum occurs in 2% of the population, it is found approximately 2 feet from the ileocecal valve, and it is approximately 2 cm long.
What is unusual about the composition of the Meckel's diverticulum?	Approximately 50% of all Meckel's diverticula contain heterotopic tissue (e.g., functional gastric mucosa, pancreatic tissue, colonic epithelium, and even biliary epithelium).

What are the most common complications of a Meckel's diverticulum?

Those containing gastric mucosa can cause ileal ulceration with bleeding. Other complications include diverticular inflammation, perforation, or obstruction.

How is the diagnosis of a Meckel's diverticulum made?

A Meckel's scan (with technetium-99m) may help if gastric mucosa is present, particularly in children with bleeding. However, this test is less helpful in adults, even if they present with bleeding. Small bowel follow-through is rarely diagnostic. Angiography may be helpful.

Clinical pearl

90% of patients with colonic diverticula are asymptomatic.

DIVERTICULITIS[1]

What is the most common location for diverticulitis to occur?

Sigmoid colon, secondary to increased intraluminal pressures

How is the diagnosis of diverticulitis made?

Often based on symptoms and physical examination alone. Abdominal CT scan may be useful. Colonoscopy should be avoided because of the risk for perforation.

What CT findings are characteristic of diverticulitis?

Characteristic findings include fat stranding, bowel wall thickening, and air seen in the diverticula.

What is the treatment for diverticulitis?

Patients with mild disease may be managed with a liquid diet and broad-spectrum antibiotics with anaerobic coverage (generally ciprofloxacin and metronidazole), whereas patients with more severe disease will require bowel rest and intravenous fluids in addition to broad-spectrum antibiotics.

---

[1] In collaboration with V. Shami, N. Thielman, and C. Sable.

| **What if a patient doesn't respond to adequate therapy?** | Patients generally begin to improve within 48 hours. If no improvement is noted, complicated diverticulitis (e.g., abscess, perforation, or fistula) should be suspected. |

DIVERTICULAR BLEEDING

| **How does diverticular bleeding usually present?** | Bleeding is usually painless. Some 70% of diverticular bleeds are localized in the right colon. Bleeding stops spontaneously in 80% of cases. |

| **How are bleeding diverticula localized and treated?** | A tagged red blood cell scan helps localize the site, angiography allows for the option of embolization if a bleeding source is found. Colonoscopy allows for localization and therapy with epinephrine injection if the bleeding does not obscure visualization of the colon. Surgical resection of involved areas may be required. Long-term therapy involves prevention of progression of disease with a stool-softening regimen. |

| **What are some other complications of colonic diverticular disease?** | Spastic diverticular disease—episodic or constant constipation, crampy lower quadrant abdominal pain, and postprandial abdominal distension

Strictures—secondary to chronic inflammation |

INFLAMMATORY BOWEL DISEASE

| **What is the geographic distribution of IBD?** | Incidence rates for IBD show geographic variation, with higher rates in northern countries (e.g., United States, United Kingdom, Norway, and Sweden) than in southern countries. Within the United States, rates are greater in northern states. |

| **What socioeconomic classes and ethnicities are commonly affected?** | The highest incidence is in developed countries. Greater incidence in higher socioeconomic groups.

Whites are affected more than nonwhites.

More frequent in Jewish populations. |

Which genders are more frequently affected?

Overall, men and women are affected equally. However, CD itself (excluding UC) is slightly more common in women.

What is the age distribution for IBD?

Peak incidence is between ages 15 and 30 years, with a second smaller peak between ages 60 and 80 years (particularly CD).

What are some risk factors for IBD?

Genetic susceptibility: with CD, the risk of IBD for first-degree relatives is about 4%, which is 13-fold higher than in control populations. Children of a person with CD have a 10% risk of developing CD.

Smoking appears to increase the risk of CD but may actually decrease the risk of UC.

Oral contraceptives may increase risk of IBD, particularly CD.

Dietary and infectious factors may also contribute.

What are the bowel differences between CD and UC?

UC: typically involves the rectum, continuous inflammation of the mucosal layer

CD: affects any segment of the GI tract, often discontinuous and transmural inflammation

What are the extraintestinal manifestations of IBD (see Table 5-1)?

    What manifestations occur _concurrently_ with intestinal disease activity?

Uveitis

Episcleritis

Erythema nodosum

Arthritis/arthropathies (peripheral)

    What manifestations occur _independently_ of intestinal disease activity?

Ankylosing spondylitis

Pyoderma gangrenosum

PSC

Other extraintestinal manifestations include gallstones, kidney stones, and demineralizing bone diseases.

Table 5–1. **Differences between CD and UC**

	Crohn's Disease	**Ulcerative Colitis**
GI tract involvement	Mouth to anus	Colon
Gross inflammation	Skip lesions	Continuous from rectum
Rectal involvement	Rectal sparing	99%
Histologic inflammation	Transmural	Mucosal or submucosal
Histology	Focal inflammation and granulomas	Diffuse inflammation
Fistulae	Common	Rare
Ulcers	Linear or transverse	Diffuse or superficial
Bleeding	20%	98%
Abdominal pain	Common	Uncommon
Perianal disease	80%	25%
Abdominal mass	Common	Uncommon
Carcinoma	Uncommon	Common
Toxic megacolon	Rare	More likely
Postsurgical recurrence	Frequent (70%)	Rare
Smoking	Exacerbates CD	May be protective

What is the medical treatment for IBD?	Therapy of IBD depends on the severity of inflammation and the site of involved bowel. Mild disease may be treated with the 5-acetylsalicylic acid derivatives. Immunosuppressive therapy (e.g., azathioprine, 6-mercaptopurine, cyclosporine, and methotrexate) and biologic therapies (e.g., infliximab) are utilized as chronic therapy for moderate to severe disease. Corticosteroids are generally used for acute flares but may be required as chronic therapy in more refractory cases.
What supplement should be given in prescribing 5-acetylsalicylic acid derivatives?	Folic acid, because the 5-acetylsalicylic acid derivatives inhibit folic acid absorption
How can the side effects of the 5-acetylsalicylic acid derivatives be minimized?	Many of the side effects of the 5-acetylsalicylic acid derivatives arise from the sulfa group, so newer

formulations that lack the sulfa group may be tolerated better.

What is budesonide?

A corticosteroid that undergoes extensive first-pass hepatic metabolism after it is absorbed in the gut and thus has a lower incidence of systemic manifestations than conventional steroids.

How should antibiotics be used in treatment of IBD?

They are useful for fistulas or perianal disease as well as colitis. Antibiotics used include ciprofloxacin and metronidazole.

How should immunosuppressive therapies be used in treatment of IBD?

They may be used for treating patients with active disease who have not responded to corticosteroids, for maintenance of remission, and as steroid-sparing agents. However, because of their delayed onset of action, they have limited usefulness in treating severe acute disease.

How is infliximab used in treatment of CD?

May be useful as a steroid-sparing agent or as a "bridge" to other immunosuppressive medications because it can result in rapid improvement. It is also useful for fistulizing CD and in some cases for maintenance of disease remission. Overall, approximately two thirds of patients respond to therapy.

What are contraindications to using infliximab?

Infliximab should not be used in stricturing CD. Also, it may result in disseminated tuberculosis; thus all patients should be screened prior to initiation.

Does diet affect disease activity in patients with CD?

No specific diet has been consistently shown to change outcomes in CD. However, initiation of total parenteral nutrition or elemental tube feeds may actually induce remission in some patients. Unfortunately, relapse is the rule on resuming a normal diet.

Crohn's Disease

What are the causes in CD of:

    Diarrhea?

Fat malabsorption, bile salt malabsorption, decreased absorptive surface area, bacterial overgrowth, and decreased fluid and electrolyte absorption.

    Gallstones?

Impaired ileal resorption of bile salts (gallstones occur in 15% to 30% of patients)

    Kidney stones (oxalate)

These occur due to reduced intraluminal concentrations of free calcium (because the calcium is bound by free fatty acids, which are poorly absorbed in patients with small bowel CD), allowing more unbound oxalate to be absorbed by the colon into the systemic circulation.

How is the diagnosis of CD made?

The clinical symptoms and signs—combined with endoscopic or radiographic evidence of ulcerations, strictures, and skip areas—suggest CD. A biopsy demonstrating noncaseating granulomas and chronic inflammation also supports the diagnosis. Anti-*Saccharomyces cerevisiae* antibodies, or ASCA, may help make the diagnosis in patients with unclear histology; they are found in >60% of patients with CD.

When is surgical treatment used for CD?

Surgery may be required in symptomatic obstruction, fistulous disease, abscess, toxic megacolon, and for patients who experience intolerable drug toxicity. The goal is to preserve as much bowel as possible. Postoperative recurrence in CD is high (approximately 70%).

ULCERATIVE COLITIS

What are the clinical features of proctitis or left-sided colitis?	Rectal bleeding and tenesmus. Systemic symptoms are usually absent, and diarrhea is variably present. Extension of disease can occur but is uncommon. There is little or no malignant potential.
What are the clinical features of mild UC?	Fewer than four bowel movements per day with minimal blood; mild anemia but no fever or tachycardia
What are the clinical features of severe UC?	Six or more bloody stools per day, with fever, tachycardia, and significant anemia
What are the clinical features of fulminant colitis?	Severe bloody diarrhea (at least 10 episodes per day). Fever, hypovolemia, and anemia are common, and occur in 5% to 15% of UC patients.
What are possible precipitating factors for toxic megacolon?	Barium enemas, colonoscopy, medications (e.g., antidiarrheals, anticholinergics, and opiates), and rapid tapering of corticosteroids in patients with colitis
What is the medical treatment of toxic megacolon?	Complete bowel rest, NG tube suction, stress ulcer prophylaxis, electrolyte replacement, and corticosteroids (if active, noninfectious colitis is present)
When is surgery considered?	If resolution does not occur within 24 to 72 hours
How should colon cancer screening be done in patients with UC?	Annual colonoscopy with random mucosal biopsies to look for dysplasia is recommended after 8 to 10 years of UC.
When is colectomy recommended?	If significant dysplasia or carcinoma is found
What is the surgical treatment for UC?	The goal of surgery in UC is cure; it is indicated for medical failure and complications such as perforation or toxic megacolon.

MICROSCOPIC COLITIS

What is microscopic colitis?	Includes collagenous colitis and lymphocytic colitis, considered variants of IBD. Findings include either a thickened collagen basement membrane in the colonic epithelium or a lymphocytic infiltrate in the mucosa. Often the gross appearance on endoscopy is normal.
Who is affected by microscopic colitis?	It predominately affects middle-aged women.
What is the treatment for microscopic colitis?	There is no curative therapy. Medications, to varying degrees, include 5-ASA products, steroids, antidiarrheal agents, antibiotics, fiber, or cholestyramine. Minimizing caffeine, NSAIDs, dietary fats, and lactose may help some patients.

APPENDICITIS

What are symptoms and signs of appendicitis?	Poorly localized periumbilical pain (secondary to visceral irritation) is followed within several hours by a more steady, localized right-lower-quadrant pain (secondary to parietal peritoneal irritation). Anorexia, nausea, and vomiting usually ensue.
What indicators suggest appendiceal perforation?	Perforation is suggested by fever $>38°C$ and leukocyte count $>15,000/mL$.
What is the treatment of acute appendicitis?	Generally, emergent appendectomy is desirable.
What is the risk of perforation in acute appendicitis?	25% by 24 hours after the onset of symptoms 50% by 36 hours 75% by 72 hours

COLORECTAL POLYPS, CRC, AND COLONIC POLYPOSIS SYNDROMES

Describe the "adenoma-carcinoma" model.	In most cases of CRC, an area of normal mucosa first undergoes a genetic mutation

(mutations in the *APC* gene, which is a tumor suppressor gene, account for approximately 80% of first hits). When this occurs, the previously normal mucosa may, as aberrant clones accumulate, develop into an early adenomatous polyp. The adenomatous cells then experience additional mutations, leading to various molecular abnormalities, such as loss of heterozygosity, deletions/mutations of other tumor suppressor genes (such as *K-ras*, *p53*, or the "deleted in colon cancer" gene, or DCC), methylation abnormalities, and/or mismatch repair genes abnormalities. Over time, these changes may cause progression from benign adenomas to frank CRC.

Clinical pearl

If a polyp is found at flexible sigmoidoscopy, there is a 10% to 15% chance of finding a more proximal synchronous polyp; therefore colonoscopy is recommended.

What is the treatment if a resected polyp is benign?

Endoscopic surveillance should be performed regularly. Hyperplastic polyps do not progress to CRC and should not affect screening parameters.

What are the screening recommendations for the following patients?

An average-risk patient with no family history of CRC?

Begin screening at age 50 with colonoscopy every 10 years or fecal occult blood testing annually with sigmoidoscopy every 5 years.

An average-risk patient found to have a few benign adenomatous polyps that were successfully removed?

A 3- to 5-year interval between colonoscopies is commonly recommended. This may change as we learn more about the natural history of adenomatous polyps and their progression into CRC.

A patient with a first-degree relative with CRC?

Begin screening at age 40 or 10 years before the age of onset of the involved relative (normal intervals between colonoscopy for one involved relative, 5-year intervals if two first-degree relatives are affected).

A patient with IBD?

Initiate annual colonoscopy 8 years after onset of pancolitis or 15 years after left-sided colitis. Random biopsies must be performed.

A patient at risk for familial adenomatous polyposis?

Annual sigmoidoscopy starting at 10 years of age.

When can screening colonoscopy be discontinued?

When a patient has a life expectancy of <10 years.

After a person has adenomatous polyps removed, what are some factors that influence the frequency with which surveillance colonoscopies should be performed?

Presence of preexisting high-risk factors (e.g., personal or family history of CRC or hereditary CRC syndromes), number of polyps identified on previous endoscopic studies, and adequacy of previous attempts at removing polyps

How common is colon cancer?

It is the second most common cancer overall in the United States, with a 6% lifetime risk in the general population.

How does age affect the risk of colon cancer?

The incidence doubles every decade from 40 years of age to 80 years of age.

What other factors may be associated with an increased risk of CRC?

Personal history of colorectal adenomas or colon cancer (relative risk = 2 to 4)

Personal or family history of polyposis syndrome

Familial cancer syndromes (see below)

First-degree relatives with colon cancer

Personal history of IBD (particularly UC)

Personal history of gynecologic cancers

If a person has family members with a history of adenomatous polyps or CRC, how much greater is his or her personal risk of adenomatous polyps or CRC?	One first-degree relative with CRC: two- to threefold increased risk Two first-degree relatives with CRC: three- to six fold increased risk One first-degree relative with CRC at an early age (<50 years): three- to sixfold increased risk One first-degree relative with adenomatous polyp: about twofold increased risk
What other factors might increase the risk for CRC?	High-red-meat diet, high-fat diet, pelvic irradiation, alcohol, cigarette smoking, and obesity
What are factors that might protect against CRC?	High-fiber diet with fruits and vegetables, exercise, NSAIDs, high calcium and folate intake, and postmenopausal hormone replacement therapy
Are any serum tumor markers useful in CRC?	CEA is a nonspecific tumor antigen associated with colon cancer. It is not diagnostic and is used only to monitor for recurrence after treatment or metastatic spread.
What is the disadvantage to barium enema?	About one third of tumors and polyps are missed, particularly if smaller than 1 cm in size.
What are the 5-year survival rates of colon cancer by Dukes' staging?	
Dukes' A	95% to 100%
Dukes' B1	67%
Dukes' B2	50%
Dukes' C1	40%
Dukes' C2	20%
Dukes' D	0%

How much has survival changed over the last 20 years?	Survival rates have changed little in the last 20 years.
What is the presurgical evaluation of CRC patients with potentially resectable disease?	Radiographs, including a chest radiograph, and liver CT scan (particularly with an abnormal hepatic panel)

HEREDITARY CRC SYNDROMES

What is the genetic basis for HNPCC?	HNPCC is an autosomal dominant condition with incomplete penetrance. It is caused by inherited or germ-line mutations in various DNA mismatch-repair genes.
What is the lifetime risk of colon cancer in HNPCC patients?	>80%. As with most colon cancers, HNPCC tumors arise from adenomatous precursors (see adenoma-carcinoma model).
Is HNPCC a polyposis syndrome?	No. Although HNPCC predisposes people to CRC, they typically have relatively few adenomatous polyps.
Where are the CRCs located in patients with HNPCC?	About 60% to 70% are proximal to the splenic flexure.
What extracolonic cancers are associated with HNPCC?	There is a 40% to 60% lifetime risk of developing an extracolonic malignancy. Common sites include the small intestine, stomach, ovaries, genitourinary tract, and pancreas.
What are the clinical features required for the diagnosis of HNPCC?	The criteria, referred to as the Amsterdam criteria, are as follows: 1. At least three first-degree relatives with cancer of the colorectum, endometrium, small bowel, ureter, or renal pelvis 2. At least two successive generations affected

3. At least one case diagnosed before 50 years of age

When these criteria are met, 50% of families are found to have a disease-causing mutation.

How often should screening colonoscopies be performed in patients with an HNPCC mutation?

At least every 2 years starting at age 25 years (or 10 years earlier than the youngest family member found to have a CRC)

What is the treatment for patients with HNPCC found to have adenomatous polyps or CRC?

Colectomy is recommended when cancer or an adenomatous polyp with advanced histologic features is found. Prophylactic colectomy for carriers of HNPCC-associated mutations remains controversial.

What are the major hereditary polyposis syndromes?

FAP, Gardner's syndrome, Turcot's syndrome, Peutz-Jeghers syndrome, juvenile polyposis, neurofibromatosis, Cowden's syndrome, and Cronkhite-Canada syndrome

What are the modes of inheritance and the genes involved in these polyposis syndromes?

FAP and Gardner's syndrome?

Autosomal dominant; disorders result from mutations in the *APC* gene on the long arm of chromosome 5. However, both *APC* alleles must be mutated to result in expression of the syndrome (i.e., "two-hit" hypothesis).

Turcot's syndrome?

Usually results from *APC* mutations (autosomal dominant), but some cases result from mutations in mismatch-repair genes (autosomal recessive).

Peutz-Jeghers syndrome?

Autosomal dominant with incomplete penetrance; involves mutations in the *STK* gene on chromosome 19.

Cowden's syndrome?

Autosomal dominant; juvenile polyposis syndrome involves mutations in the *PTEN* gene on chromosome 10.

Cronkhite-Canada syndrome?

A noninherited syndrome (it is acquired)

What is FAP and Gardner's syndrome?

Hereditary polyposis syndromes in which numerous adenomatous polyps develop and there is a very high risk of cancer

What is the difference between FAP and Gardner's syndrome?

Once believed to be separate diseases, FAP and Gardner's syndrome are caused by mutations in the same gene (the *APC* gene) and have similar GI manifestations. Patients with Gardner's syndrome tend to have more prevalent extraintestinal manifestations (dental abnormalities, osteomas, thyroid cancer, and desmoid tumors) than do patients with classic FAP.

What types of polyps are found in FAP and Gardner's syndrome?

Adenomas of the colon, stomach, and small bowel. Benign fundic gland polyps may also be seen in the stomachs of these patients.

How is the diagnosis of FAP and Gardner's syndrome made?

There are specific tests to evaluate for the presence of the abnormal mutated APC protein (i.e., protein truncation testing) or the mutated gene itself.

What is the risk of colon cancer in FAP and Gardner's syndrome?

100% (adenocarcinoma)

Are there any medical therapies that are effective in treating the colonic polyps in FAP and Gardner's syndrome?

NSAIDs (e.g., sulindac, celecoxib) have been shown to decrease the size and number of polyps in FAP patients. However, polyps and cancer still develop; thus surgery remains the only definitive treatment.

What is Turcot's syndrome?

A syndrome of familial polyposis associated with primary central nervous system tumors (e.g., brain tumors)

What types of polyps are seen in Turcot's syndrome?

Adenomas, similar to those seen in FAP and Gardner's syndrome

What is the risk of CRC for patients with Gardner's and Turcot's syndrome?

100% (adenocarcinoma), as in FAP. Proctocolectomy is recommended for patients who have developed multiple colonic polyps or for people who are found to have the genetic defect.

What is Peutz-Jeghers syndrome?

A syndrome involving mucocutaneous pigmentation (buccal mucosa, hands, feet, and perianal skin) with bladder, nasal and GI polyposis

What types of polyps are seen in Peutz-Jeghers syndrome?

Hamartomatous polyps (mostly small bowel, but also colon and stomach)

What complications are associated with Peutz-Jeghers syndrome?

Polyps can cause intussusception or obstruction. They can also infarct, causing bleeding and abdominal pain.

What is the risk of CRC in patients with Peutz-Jeghers syndrome?

<3% risk of cancer

What is juvenile polyposis syndrome?

A rare syndrome resulting in nonneoplastic, hamartomatous GI tract polyps (mostly colonic, some gastric and small bowel) usually occurring in children between 4 and 14 years of age

What is the risk of colon cancer with juvenile polyposis syndrome?

At least 10%, possibly higher. They arise from adenomatous changes within the hamartomatous polyps. Other cancers—such as gastric, duodenal, and pancreatic—can also occur.

What is Cronkhite-Canada syndrome?

An acquired, nonfamilial syndrome, involving GI polyposis and cutaneous hyperpigmentation, hair loss, nail atrophy, diarrhea, weight loss, abdominal pain, and malnutrition in middle-aged patients

What is the cancer risk in Cronkhite-Canada syndrome?	It develops in 15% as a result of adenomatous changes within hamartomatous polyps.

PANCREAS

DISEASES OF THE PANCREAS

Acute Pancreatitis

How frequently is an elevated serum amylase seen in patients with acute pancreatitis?	The most sensitive indicator of pancreatitis, it is present in 75% of patients with acute pancreatitis.
How quickly does the amylase elevate?	Within 24 hours; it resolves in 3 to 5 days in the absence of ongoing pancreatic injury.
What are other causes of hyperamylasemia?	Renal insufficiency, salivary gland disorders, acidemia, and macroamylasemia (amylase binds to proteins and cannot be filtered), as well as other pancreatic, biliary, or intestinal processes (pseudocyst, trauma, obstruction or ischemia)
When are falsely low amylase levels seen?	With hypertriglyceridemia or a history of chronic pancreatitis
How specific is an elevation of serum lipase?	The most specific indicator of pancreatitis, it is elevated in 70% of patients with acute pancreatitis. It remains elevated longer than amylase.
What complications are seen with acute pancreatitis?	Shock, ARDS, acute renal failure, hypocalcemia, and GI hemorrhage can all be seen in severe pancreatitis.
How is abdominal CT helpful in acute pancreatitis?	It can be used to determine the size and appearance of the pancreas (i.e., diffuse inflammation, necrosis, fluid collections), spread of inflammation, and presence of biliary abnormalities. CT is far superior to transabdominal ultrasound in visualizing the pancreas.

How is the severity of pancreatitis graded on CT?

The Balthazar score:

Grade A: Normal appearance

Grade B: Focal or diffuse enlargement of the pancreas

Grade C: Grade B plus peripancreatic inflammation

Grade D: Single peripancreatic fluid collection

Grade E: Two or more collections of fluid or gas in the pancreas or retroperitoneum

What is the treatment for acute pancreatitis?

NPO, fluid resuscitation (often requiring large volumes secondary to third spacing), and provision of analgesia while determining the cause

What are the Ranson criteria?

Prognostic indicators determined at presentation and within 48 hours of admission (see Table 5–2).

What is the predicted mortality rate based on the Ranson criteria?

1 to 2 risk factors, <1%

3 to 5 risk factors, 10% to 20%

6 to 7 risk factors, nearly 100%

What is another model for calculating severity of pancreatitis?

APACHE II is a scoring system that ranks various clinical parameters and may be more accurate than the Ranson criteria, but it is more complex and requires computer calculation.

Table 5–2. Ranson Criteria for Severity of Acute Pancreatitis

At Presentation	Within 48 Hours
Age >55 years	Base deficit >4 meq/L
WBC >16,000/:L	BUN increase >5 mg/dL
Glucose >200 mg/dL	Fluid sequestration >6 L
AST >250 IU/L	Serum calcium <8 mg/dL
LDH >350 IU/L	Hct decrease >10%
	Po_2 <60 mm Hg

Note: Amylase level is not one of the Ranson criteria!
AST, aspartate transaminase; LDH, lactate dehydrogenase; Hct, hematocrit.

What structures are potentially affected in the inflammatory process?

Bile duct, duodenum, mesenteric vessels, spleen, posterior mediastinum, and diaphragm

What is the most frequent complication of pancreatitis?

Fluid collections occur in approximately 30% of cases; however, 50% of these respond without intervention.

What are pseudocysts?

Accumulations of necrotic tissue, pancreatic juice, blood, and fat within or near the pancreas, which occur several weeks after the onset of acute pancreatitis. They have an organized wall of fibrinous material without an epithelial lining.

When are empiric broad-spectrum antibiotics used in acute pancreatitis and what antibiotic is preferred?

The carbapenems have been shown to decrease the incidence of infection when pancreatic necrosis is identified.

What sites are involved when polyserositis develops in the setting of pancreatitis?

Pericardium, pleura, and synovial surfaces. Alveolar capillary membranes may also be disrupted, leading to noncardiogenic pulmonary edema or ARDS.

What is the cause of pancreatitis-induced DIC?

Circulating pancreatic enzymes

What causes cardiovascular shock in pancreatitis?

It is usually caused by hypovolemia or circulating vasodilators.

What is the etiology of gastric varices in acute pancreatitis?

Splenic vein thrombosis may result from the surrounding inflammation.

Chronic Pancreatitis

Describe autoimmune pancreatitis.

An autoimmune process, most common in Asian populations, that causes pancreatic ductal irregularities and pancreatic enlargement. Laboratory testing reveals hypergammaglobulinemia with elevated

IgG4 levels, with the frequent finding of other autoimmune markers (ANA). Can be associated with other autoimmune diseases such as Sjögren's or SLE.

What is the classic triad of chronic pancreatitis?

Steatorrhea, calcification of pancreas on radiographs or CT, and diabetes (<25% of cases)

What are symptoms and signs of chronic pancreatitis?

Abdominal pain, malabsorption, diabetes, and jaundice

The abdominal pain is typically steady, boring, achy, in the midepigastrium, upper quadrants, or periumbilical area, radiating to the back; worse when supine, better when sitting up and leaning forward. The pain is worst in the first 5 years after diagnosis, then may diminish or resolve in two thirds of patients.

What are possible laboratory findings in chronic pancreatitis?

Normal or slightly elevated amylase and lipase; elevated liver function tests (suggests concomitant liver disease, and biliary obstruction), elevated glucose (diabetes mellitus), elevated alkaline phosphatase (osteomalacia), and elevated PT (vitamin K malabsorption)

What radiographic finding may be seen on plain films in chronic pancreatitis?

One-third show diffuse pancreatic calcifications. CT scans can identify calcifications in three quarters of patients.

What does ERCP demonstrate in chronic pancreatitis?

ERCP is the gold standard to demonstrate pancreatic ductal anatomy. Ductal dilatation, cystic changes, strictures, and calculi may be visualized and potentially treated. Brushings to rule out pancreatic carcinoma can also be done.

What other modality is useful in identifying changes consistent with chronic pancreatitis?

EUS is the most sensitive modality for diagnosing chronic pancreatitis.

What measures are taken to manage pain in chronic pancreatitis?

Abstinence from alcohol, use of narcotics (addiction is common), celiac ganglion blockade with EUS or fluoroscopic guidance, use of ERCP for removal of ductal stones, dilatation and stenting of strictures, and providing duct drainage. Surgical resection or drainage procedures (e.g., pancreaticojejunostomy, or Puestow procedure) may be needed. Pancreatic enzyme replacement is useful in some but not all patients.

Pancreatic Neoplasia

What are the risk factors for pancreatic adenocarcinoma?

Smoking, African heritage, family history, chronic pancreatitis, exposure to carcinogens, increased age, and a history of diabetes

What genetic mutations are associated with pancreatic adenocarcinoma?

Mutations in the *K-ras* oncogene occur in 90% and mutations in the tumor suppressor genes *p16* and *p53* occur in 95% and 50% to 75% respectively.

What are the clinical manifestations of pancreatic adenocarcinoma?

Painless jaundice is classically associated with a pancreatic mass, but symptoms such as abdominal discomfort, anorexia, nausea, and weight loss occur more commonly. Symptoms usually are nonspecific or present late, such that the diagnosis is generally delayed until late in the disease process.

What imaging modalities are useful in the diagnosis of pancreatic adenocarcinoma?

Helical CT scan of the abdomen is the preferred modality for diagnosis and to evaluate for metastases. EUS is more accurate than CT for evaluating tumor size and nodal involvement. EUS also allows for biopsy if the diagnosis remains in question.

What tumor marker can be used for following the status of pancreatic adenocarcinoma?

CA-19-9 levels can be useful in monitoring status during treatment. CA-19-9 should not be used for diagnostic purposes as its specificity is too low.

What is the current optimal therapy for pancreatic adenocarcinoma?

Whipple procedure (resection of the pancreatic head, duodenum, first portion of jejunum, and gallbladder with CBD) followed by chemotherapy with 5-fluorouracil

What parameters delineate a resectable pancreatic adenocarcinoma?

No evidence of metastases, no involvement of the celiac or superior mesenteric arteries, and patent superior mesenteric and portal veins.

What is the treatment of choice for unresectable pancreatic adenocarcinoma?

Chemotherapy with 5-fluorouracil in combination with x-ray therapy is the preferred treatment for locally advanced disease. Gemcitabine is the preferred chemotherapeutic agent for metastatic disease.

What is the prognosis of pancreatic adenocarcinoma?

The prognosis is dismal, as even resectable cancer has a 2-year survival rate of only 20%.

What are the three main types of pancreatic cystic neoplasms?

Mucinous cystadenoma, serous cystadenoma, and intraductal papillary mucinous tumor

Describe characteristics of the intraductal papillary mucinous tumor.

A mucin-producing neoplasm that occurs most commonly in the main pancreatic duct in older men. Mucin production may cause obstruction leading to pancreatitis. The risk of invasive cancer is high and surgical resection should be performed.

Describe characteristics of the mucinous cystadenoma.

Mucinous cystadenomas usually occur as large macrocystic cysts that do not communicate with the pancreatic duct. Aspirates generally demonstrate elevated CEA levels with low amylase/lipase levels. Their malignant potential is high and surgical resection should be performed.

Describe characteristics of the serous cystadenoma.

Serous cystadenomas usually occur as a collection of multiple microcystic cysts that do not communicate with the pancreatic duct. Their malignant potential is low, and small, asymptomatic cystadenomas can be observed.

LIVER AND BILIARY TRACT

What happens to the amount of urobilinogen in the setting of CBD obstruction?

It decreases because bilirubin cannot get into the bowel to be metabolized into urobilinogen by the gut bacteria. Thus, in a patient with cholestatic liver enzymes and a large amount of urinary urobilinogen, it is less likely that CBD obstruction will be the cause of the cholestasis.

What are the causes of unconjugated hyperbilirubinemia?

Increased bilirubin production—hemolytic anemia, ineffective erythropoiesis, blood transfusions, resolving hematomas, defective conjugation (Gilbert's disease, Crigler-Najjar types I and II), and drugs

What is Gilbert's disease?

A benign, common cause of mild unconjugated hyperbilirubinemia, resulting from an autosomal dominant inherited partial deficiency in bilirubin glucuronyl transferase activity. Serum bilirubin is usually 1.3 to 3.0 mg/dL (rarely >5 mg/dL).

What are specific causes of conjugated hyperbilirubinemia?

Hereditary disorders (e.g., Dubin-Johnson syndrome, Rotor's syndrome)

Hepatocellular diseases

Infiltrative diseases (e.g., sarcoidosis, Hodgkin's lymphoma, tumor, infection, tuberculosis, and abscess)

Extrahepatic cholestasis (e.g., choledocholithiasis, PSC, biliary stricture or tumor, and obstructive pancreatic processes)

Intrahepatic cholestasis (e.g., pregnancy, sepsis, postoperative jaundice, PBC, and medications—thiazides, OCPs, NSAIDs)

CHOLELITHIASIS

What is the pathogenesis of cholesterol gallstones?	They are formed when the GB becomes supersaturated with cholesterol, leading to nucleation and stone formation.
What is the correlation between serum cholesterol levels and gallstones?	There is no straightforward correlation.
What are the characteristics of cholesterol gallstones?	The majority occur as multiple, mixed (>70% cholesterol) stones, whereas <10% occur as pure cholesterol (generally single stones).
What are risk factors for cholesterol gallstones?	Think **four Fs:** **F**emale **F**at **F**ertile **F**orty
What are some of the other risk factors for cholesterol gallstones?	Diabetes Diet—rapid weight loss or fasting, cholesterol-lowering diets Drugs—estrogen, clofibrate, octreotide, ceftriaxone Hyperlipidemia Heredity—especially Pima Indian women Bile salt malabsorption—pancreatic insufficiency, cystic fibrosis, ileal disease, ileal bypass or resection
What are the two types of pigmented gallstones?	Black and brown
What are the risk factors for black pigmented gallstones?	Chronic hemolysis, advancing age, long-term total parenteral nutrition, and cirrhosis
What are the risk factors for brown pigmented gallstones?	Seen mostly in biliary stasis associated with bacterial infection in bile ducts (e.g., *E. coli*)

What is biliary colic?

Relatively, rapid onset of steady epigastric or right-upper-quadrant pain, which may radiate to the interscapular area or the right shoulder and may be associated with nausea and vomiting. Episodes usually last 1 to 6 hours and may follow ingestion of a heavy meal or occur at night.

How is the diagnosis of cholelithiasis made?

Most commonly by ultrasound, which has a sensitivity and specificity of >90%. CT scan is less reliable.

How is the diagnosis of choledocholithiasis made?

Ultrasound has a sensitivity of only 50%. Elevations in AST, alkaline phosphatase, and bilirubin to greater than twofold normal values has a greater sensitivity but lower specificity than ultrasound. EUS and MRCP can be useful diagnostic tools if the clinical picture is unclear. ERCP should be utilized as both a diagnostic and therapeutic intervention in those patients with complications such as cholangitis or pancreatitis.

What are other complications of cholelithiasis?

Biliary stricture formation, gallstone ileus, fistulization, sepsis, perforation, and peritonitis

ACUTE AND CHRONIC CHOLECYSTITIS

What are causes of acute cholecystitis?

Approximately 90% of cases are associated with cholelithiasis.

How is the diagnosis of acute cholecystitis made?

The triad of sudden onset of right-upper-quadrant tenderness, fever, and leukocytosis is highly suggestive. Ultrasound reveals a stone in >90% of cases. Cholescintigraphy or HIDA scan is the most sensitive imaging modality.

What ultrasound findings are suggestive of acute cholecystitis?

Thickened GB wall, pericholecystic fluid, and elicitation of Murphy's sign with the ultrasound probe applying direct pressure over the GB. "Sonographic Murphy's" sign has a positive predictive value >90%.

What is the treatment of acute cholecystitis?

Conservative therapy includes nothing by mouth, NG tube placement if the patient has been vomiting, IV fluids, parenteral analgesics, and IV antimicrobial agents.

Cholecystectomy—open or laparoscopic—is the only definitive therapy.

Cholecystotomy—may be required in severe cases in which surgery is contraindicated.

What is the mortality rate of acute cholecystitis?

1%

What is acalculous cholecystitis?

Inflammation of the GB in the absence of gallstones. It is associated with a high incidence of complications (e.g., necrosis, gangrene, and GB perforation).

How common is acalculous cholecystitis?

It represents 5% to 10% of all cases of acute cholecystitis.

What is the mortality rate of acalculous cholecystitis?

50%; most affected patients are elderly or debilitated with coexisting disease or trauma.

How is the diagnosis of acalculous cholecystitis made?

Requires a high index of suspicion because symptoms (e.g., abdominal pain, nausea, and fever) and laboratory results (e.g., leukocytosis and elevated liver enzymes) are not always present and the disorder may present as an isolated fever in a ventilated patient.

Ultrasound or CT findings of a thickened GB wall, pericholecystic fluid, intramural gas, sloughed mucosal membranes, and sonographic Murphy's sign are supportive of the diagnosis.

Hepatobiliary scintigraphy (e.g., HIDA scan) has sensitivities ranging from 70% to 90%; false-positive results are frequent.

What is the treatment for acalculous cholecystitis?

Urgent cholecystectomy is required in those patients who are surgical candidates. Cholecystostomy may be utilized for high-risk surgical candidates.

What is emphysematous cholecystitis?	Infection of the GB by gas-producing organisms including anaerobes such as *Clostridium welchii* or *C. perfringens*.
What is a predisposing factor for emphysematous cholecystitis?	Diabetes
What is the evaluation and treatment of chronic cholecystitis?	Imaging via ultrasound or CT can demonstrate characteristic changes. Patients generally derive symptom relief with cholecystectomy. If chronic acalculous cholecystitis is suspected, evaluation with cholescystokinin (CCK) scintigraphy to determine GB ejection fraction can be helpful. Manometry via ERCP can confirm biliary dyskinesia and allows for stent placement.

CHOLANGITIS

What are complications of cholangitis?	Sepsis, hepatic abscess, biliary strictures
What is the treatment for cholangitis?	Relief of obstruction is essential (via ERCP, percutaneous transhepatic cholangiography, or surgery) and intravenous antibiotics with coverage for enteric organisms

ACUTE HEPATITIS

What are the causes of acute hepatitis that generate transaminases >1000?	The differential can generally be limited to viral, toxic ingestion, or ischemic causes. More rarely, autoimmune hepatitis can present in this manner.

VIRAL HEPATITIS

What viruses—other than HAV, HBV, and HCV—can cause acute hepatitis?	Several, including herpes simplex viruses, Epstein-Barr virus, and CMV

Hepatitis A

What is the mode of transmission for HAV?	Fecal–oral

Why is parenteral transmission of HAV rare?

Because the viremic phase is short

In the illustration below, the curves mark the appearance of the HAV, symptoms and signs, various antibodies, and laboratory tests. What antibody time course is illustrated by:

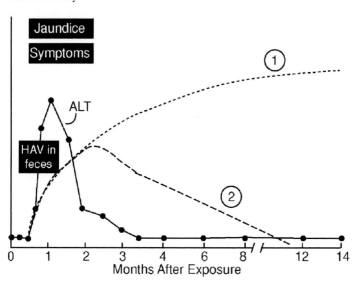

(From Hoofnagle JH, DiBisceglie AM. Serologic diagnosis of acute and chronic viral hepatitis. *Semin Liver Dis.* 1991;11:73.)

Curve 1?

Anti-HAV IgG

Curve 2?

Anti-HAV IgM

How is the diagnosis of acute HAV infection made?

Transaminitis (or cholestatic hepatitis) and the presence of anti-HAV IgM in the serum during acute illness. HAV IgG denotes previous infection and recovery or vaccination. It is present after 3 weeks of disease and persists indefinitely.

What complication other than fulminant hepatic failure can rarely be seen in acute HAV infection?

Aplastic anemia

Who should receive the HAV vaccine?

Travelers to endemic areas, patients with chronic liver disease and persons at high risk, such as day-care and health-care workers

Hepatitis B

What happens to hepatocytes after infection with HBV?

The virus is not cytopathic, but it generates a host immune response, resulting in lysis of infected hepatocytes.

What is the epidemiology of HBV infection?

In low-prevalence areas—such as the United States, western Europe, Australia, and New Zealand—the HbsAg carrier rates are 0.1% to 2%. In high-prevalence areas, including Southeast Asia and sub-Saharan Africa, HbsAg carrier rates are 10% to 20%. HBV accounts for 35% to 70% of all cases of viral hepatitis worldwide and nearly all cases of virus-induced fulminant hepatic failure.

What is the risk associated with blood transfusion?

Approximately 1 in 63,000, mostly because of the window period.

What is the rate of perinatal transmission?

Approximately 90% in HbeAg-positive mothers, while only 30% in HbeAg-negative mothers. Breast-feeding does not appear to be a risk factor and cesarean section is not protective.

What is the rate of HBV transmission after an occupationally related needle-stick injury?

Approximately 30% (in an unvaccinated health-care worker)

What is the incubation period for acute HBV (time from exposure to jaundice)?

1 to 6 months

In the illustration on the following page, the curves mark the appearance of the HBV symptoms and signs, various antibodies, and laboratory tests. What antibody time course is illustrated by:

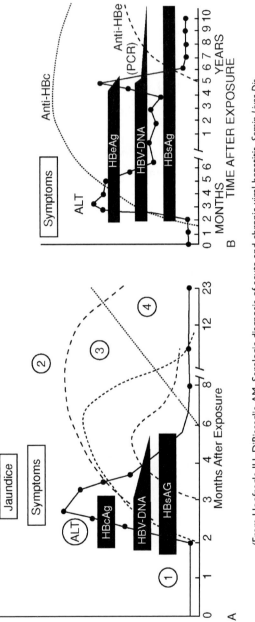

(From Hoofnagle JH, DiBisceglie AM. Serologic diagnosis of acute and chronic viral hepatitis. *Semin Liver Dis.* 1991;11:73.)

Curve 1?	HbsAg
Curve 2?	Anti-HBc IgG
Curve 3?	Anti-HBc IgM
Curve 4?	Anti-HBs IgG

What happens to markers of HBV during acute HBV infection?	Serum becomes positive for HbsAg and HBV DNA. HbeAg is detected in patients with high circulating levels of HBV; it signals active viral replication and infectivity.
What happens to the serologic markers in chronic HBV infection?	HbsAg persists for >6 months. Over time, anti-HBc IgM wanes and anti-HBc IgG develops.
What are the two main phases of chronic HBV infection?	Replicative and nonreplicative phases
Describe the replicative phase of chronic HBV infection acquired in adults.	There is usually HbeAg and HBV DNA in serum, active liver disease (elevated transaminases), and features of both active and chronic hepatitis on liver biopsy. Spontaneous seroconversion to a nonreplicative phase occurs at a rate of 10% to 20% per year. This is manifest by clearance of HbeAg and the development of anti-Hbe.
Describe the replicative phase of chronic HBV infection acquired in infancy or childhood.	These patients are more likely to have chronic HBV, but they often develop immune tolerance to the virus. When this happens, ongoing viral replication may occur with minimal hepatitis. A similar rate of seroconversion to a nonreplicative phase is seen (10% to 20% per year); but when it occurs, it is often heralded by a flare of hepatitis.
Describe the nonreplicative phase of chronic HBV infection.	During this phase, patients are HbeAg-negative and anti-Hbe–positive. Many of these patients have undetectable HBV DNA by PCR testing, and no

evidence of active liver disease, and they may remain in remission for years.

What happens to HbsAg after converting from a replicative to a nonreplicative phase?

In a minority of patients, the HbsAg titer may become undetectable over time.

What are extrahepatic manifestations of chronic HBV infection?

Circulating antigen–antibody complexes can result in various conditions, including serum sickness (fever, rash, arthralgia, and arthritis), glomerulonephritis, essential mixed cryoglobulinemia, papular acrodermatitis (Gianotti-Crosti syndrome), aplastic anemia, and polyarteritis nodosa (systemic vasculitis).

What percentage of all patients with polyarteritis nodosa are HbsAg-positive?

10% to 50%

What can cause a flare of hepatitis in chronic HBV-infected patients whose liver disease has been quiescent?

Reactivation of active liver disease can occur spontaneously. Also, cessation of immunosuppressive medications (e.g., chemotherapeutics or corticosteroids) can lead to reactivation of hepatitis (due to reconstitution of the immune system).

How common is cirrhosis in chronic HBV infection?

Develops in 10% to 30% without treatment

What factors are associated with increased risk of HCC in chronic HBV?

The risk increases with long-standing viral replication. Unlike many other causes of cirrhosis, HBV can lead to HCC even without the development of cirrhosis because of the integration of HBV DNA into host DNA.

What is lamivudine and how is it used in patients with chronic HBV?

A nucleoside analog, reverse transcriptase inhibitor, which has suppressive activity against HBV replication. Initially, HBV replication is suppressed in >90% of patients. However, loss of HbsAg is rare, and viral replication often resumes once therapy is discontinued. This may be associated with a flare of hepatitis.

What happens with continued treatment with lamivudine?

Over time, some patients convert back to the replicative phase even while continuing lamivudine. HBV mutants, such as the YMDD mutant, appear to develop more commonly with lamivudine therapy.

What is the YMDD mutant of HBV?

A genetic variant of HBV that develops in approximately 30% of patients receiving lamivudine. These mutants continue to replicate. Fortunately, they seem to be less virulent than the wild-type HBV.

What treatment options are available for lamivudine-resistant HBV?

Adefovir and entecavir, both nucleoside reverse transcriptase inhibitors, can be used in resistant cases but are more expensive than lamivudine and have a slower onset of action. Entecavir may also be used as an initial therapy.

What could explain a negative HbeAg but a PCR test that reveals moderate levels of viremia?

This suggests the presence of a mutant strain of the HBV virus, known as a "precore" mutant. This strain of HBV has a genetic mutation that makes the virus incapable of producing HbeAg even though the virus is still actively replicating.

What does superinfection in an HBV patient mean?

Infection with other hepatotropic viruses (e.g., HAV, HCV, HDV, and CMV) after acquiring HBV, which may lead to worsening hepatitis or decompensated liver disease

Who should receive the hepatitis B vaccine?

Members of high-risk groups, all infants, travelers at risk, and people with cirrhosis or chronic liver disease that is not caused by HBV

After sexual exposure to HBV, both hepatitis B immune globulin and the first of three hepatitis vaccines should be administered within 14 days of exposure. Follow-up doses are given at 1 and 6 months.

Hepatitis C

Are there different subtypes of HCV?

Six distinct genotypes with multiple subtypes have been identified worldwide. Subtypes 1a and 1b are most common in the United States and western Europe (and are the most difficult to eradicate), followed by genotypes 2 and 3. Genotypes 4, 5, and 6 are rarely seen in the United States.

What is the current risk of HCV infection from an HCV antibody-negative blood donation?

<1 in 1 million

What is the risk of HCV infection for a health-care worker after a needle-stick injury?

Approximately 3% (as high as 10%). The risk associated with a stick from a hollow needle is much higher than that with a solid needle.

What is the rate of sexual transmission of HCV?

Sexual transmission of HCV is much less efficient than that of HBV or HIV. Although the risk is increased in persons with high-risk sexual practices, persons in monogamous relationships with HCV-infected partners appear to have 0.1% annual risk of infection.

How often does chronic HCV develop?

Approximately 80% will progress to chronic infection. Once this occurs, spontaneous clearance is uncommon.

What is the rate of progression to cirrhosis in chronic HCV?

Approximately 25% of patients progress to cirrhosis, generally after at least 20 years of chronic HCV.

What is the incidence of HCC in HCV?

In patients with cirrhosis, the incidence is approximately 1% to 4% per year. HCC only rarely develops in cases of HCV without cirrhosis; thus routine screening is not warranted unless cirrhosis or fibrosis is present on biopsy.

What is essential mixed cryoglobulinemia?

Although most HCV patients with measurable cryoglobulins are asymptomatic, some develop a systemic disorder that can manifest with signs and symptoms of a vasculitis, such as arthralgias, weakness, purpura, petechiae, peripheral neuropathy, and Raynaud's phenomenon. In severe cases, glomerulonephritis may occur.

In the illustration below, the curves mark the appearance of the symptoms and signs, various antibodies, and laboratory tests of a patient with chronic active HCV.

What antibody time course is illustrated by curve 1?

Anti-HCV IgG

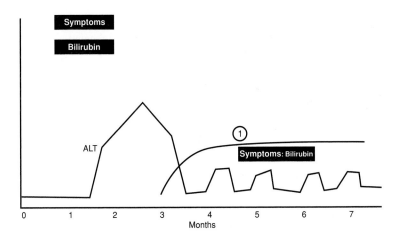

What conditions can cause a false-negative HCV antibody test?

Immunocompromised conditions, renal failure, and cases associated with essential mixed cryoglobulinemia

What is the treatment for acute HCV infection?

Supportive care

Which patients should be considered candidates for treatment of chronic HCV?

Patients with significant extrahepatic manifestations (e.g., glomerulonephritis) and those with persistent viremia, transaminitis, and significant necrosis, inflammation, or fibrosis on liver biopsy (because these patients are at high risk of disease progression). Patients with normal transaminases and no significant histologic evidence of disease are at less risk of disease progression. In such cases, the decision to treat must be tailored to the individual.

When should treatment be initiated after a patient contracts acute HCV?

Treatment should be initiated at 8 to 12 weeks following infection. Patients initiated on therapy at 8 weeks have a higher rate of sustained response, but early treatment leads to treatment of more patients who would have spontaneously cleared the infection.

How is response to treatment of HCV assessed?

HCV viral load is evaluated at week 12 of treatment for genotype 1 and week 4 of treatment for genotypes 2 and 3. One should expect at least a 1-log decrease in viral load at this time if there is to be an eventual meaningful response. If a 1-log decrease in viral load is not met, it is reasonable to discontinue therapy to avoid unnecessary side effects.

In attempting to eradicate the HCV virus, what are the usual durations of treatment?

Approximately 24 weeks for genotypes 2 and 3

Approximately 48 weeks for other genotypes

Of patients who attain a sustained virologic response, how many will remain PCR-negative?

Approximately 95% for at least 5 years. Many of these patients will also have improvement in their health-related quality-of-life scores and normal or improved histology on subsequent liver biopsies.

Hepatitis D

What is the epidemiology of HDV?

Its prevalence in an area correlates with that of HBV. Approximately 5% of HBV carriers have concomitant HDV infection. It is rare in Western countries, where most cases involve high-risk groups (e.g., intravenous drug users and those who have had multiple previous transfusions).

What is the mode of transmission of HDV?

Like that of HBV. Perinatal transmission is rare. The most important factor influencing transmission of HDV is the presence of an already established HBV infection.

What are clinical manifestations of acute HDV superinfection in patients with chronic HBV?

Superinfection often results in a flareup of hepatitis, often severe. Of the survivors, >90% will progress to chronic HDV with HBV. Less commonly, the HDV infection may resolve (while the HBV persists), or the HDV superinfection may result in clearance of HbsAg. Fulminant hepatitis is not uncommon.

What is the course of chronic HDV infection?

Variable. In most cases, the disease causes more rapid histologic progression to cirrhosis. Approximately 80% will progress to cirrhosis in 5 to 10 years. However, many of these patients remain clinically stable for many years before decompensated liver disease occurs. In a minority of patients, a rapidly progressive course to liver failure over months to years can occur; in another subset of patients, a benign, nonprogressive course may ensue.

During the early time period of chronic HDV, what may happen to the HBV?

During the early period of chronic HDV, the HDV may inhibit HBV replication, making HBV DNA undetectable.

How is the diagnosis of HDV made?

Detection of HDV RNA or HDV antigen in the serum or liver is the most accurate. Serologic tests to detect antibodies to

HDV are commonly used. In the acute phase of coinfection, antibodies to HDV might not be detectable; repeat serology in several weeks may be needed to confirm the diagnosis.

What is the prognosis of HDV?

Overall, cirrhosis develops in approximately 80% of cases during a 5- to 10-year period. In a minority of patients, the flareup of hepatitis caused by HDV superinfection can result in clearance of the HBV.

What is the outcome of HDV and HBV after liver transplantation?

Reinfection of the graft liver with HBV, and the severity of such recurrences, may actually be decreased by the presence of HDV. In some cases, a third form of HDV can occur—HDV can infect the transplanted hepatocytes but HBV reinfection is initially prevented by posttransplant use of HBV intravenous immune globulin; thus the HDV remains latent. However, over time, the HBV evades neutralization and reinfects the hepatocytes, allowing HDV to replicate. Clinical hepatitis can then occur.

What is the mortality associated with HDV?

15% mortality over 3 years

Hepatitis E

What serologic markers suggest infection with HEV?

HEV IgM is diagnostic of acute infection, whereas HEV IgG occurs months to years after infection.

How long does it take to recover from HEV infection?

Biochemical markers usually normalize over 1 to 6 weeks after symptoms manifest.

How is HEV prevented?

No vaccine is clinically available at this time. HEV intravenous immune globulin, for postexposure prophylaxis, has not shown consistent clinical benefit.

Hepatitis G

What is HGV?	An RNA virus currently being studied
How is it transmitted?	By blood transfusions. Approximately 2% of eligible donor samples contain HGV RNA.
How is HGV infection detected?	By detection of HGV RNA by PCR, or detection of antibodies by enzyme immunoassays. Presence of antibodies suggests clearance of infection and also immunity.
What is the clinical significance of HGV?	The significance of HGV infection is uncertain. There is conflicting literature regarding the pathogenicity of HGV infection. In cases of chronic liver disease in which HGV RNA is present, it is unclear whether the HGV is causative or not.

DRUG-INDUCED LIVER INJURY

What is the epidemiology of DILI?	It accounts for 10% of cases of adult hepatitis (40% of cases in patients >50 years of age) and 25% of all cases of fulminant hepatic failure.
What is the pathophysiology of DILI?	In most cases, the drug or drug metabolites cause direct hepatocellular injury and necrosis. In other cases, DILI arises from injury to the biliary epithelium, vascular endothelium, and autoimmune damage via hapten production on the surface of hepatocytes. Often the reactions are idiosyncratic (i.e., not dose dependent, and may occur long after the drug was started).
What are some drugs that cause liver injury via direct toxicity?	Ethanol, acetaminophen, certain NSAIDs, methotrexate, azathioprine, 6-mercaptopurine, intravenous tetracycline, and L-asparaginase
What are some drugs that cause liver injury via idiosyncratic reactions?	Phenytoin, sulfonamides, amoxicillin-clavulanate, halothane, dapsone, isoniazid, ketoconazole, amiodarone, and propylthiouracil

What are some common herbal remedies that may cause liver injury?	Jin bu huan, ma huang, valerian, germander, skullcap, chaparral leaf, comfrey, mistletoe, and herbal teas containing toxic alkaloids
Is liver biopsy helpful in the diagnosis of DILI?	Liver biopsy obtained early may be helpful in identifying the type and extent of injury. However, histologic findings are often not specific to DILI and may be seen in hepatitis from other causes.
What is the treatment of DILI?	Supportive care and avoidance or discontinuation of suspected agents. Most cases resolve.

ACETAMINOPHEN HEPATOTOXICITY

What happens to acetaminophen when ingested, and what causes the hepatic injury?	After ingestions of therapeutic doses, most ($>90\%$) is conjugated to glucuronide or sulfates into nontoxic metabolites. Approximately 4% is metabolized by the cytochrome P-450 system, resulting in N-acetyl-p-benzoquinoneimine (NAPQI), a toxic intermediate that normally is rapidly inactivated by conjugation to glutathione and then renally excreted. However, after large ingestions of acetaminophen, more NAPQI is produced and the stores of glutathione are overwhelmed, resulting in decreased clearance of the NAPQI, which causes hepatocyte injury.
What is the effect of malnutrition on the effect of acetaminophen hepatotoxicity?	Increases the risk of toxicity by the same mechanisms
How is the diagnosis of acetaminophen hepatotoxicity made?	Clinical suspicion and history, verified by laboratory testing
What are the initial symptoms of acetaminophen toxicity?	Manifestations in the first 24 hours include nausea, vomiting, malaise, and diaphoresis.

What are the lab findings of acetaminophen toxicity and when are they seen?

Liver enzyme abnormalities begin to appear at 24 hours and usually peak at 72 hours (transaminitis may be severe and evidence of hepatic synthetic dysfunction may develop).

Evidence of renal failure, hypoglycemia, and encephalopathy develops maximally at this stage.

How is the potential risk of hepatotoxicity after acetaminophen ingestion determined?

Serum acetaminophen levels should be drawn 4 hours and 24 hours after ingestion. These values should be evaluated using the Rumack-Matthews nomogram. This nomogram applies only to acute ingestions with an accurate, established time of ingestion.

What is considered to be a toxic acetaminophen dose?

Ingestion of >7.5 to 10 g (250 mg/kg) of acetaminophen over a 24-hour period

Ingestion of >4 g over a 24-hour period in a person with increased susceptibility to acetaminophen

What prognostic indicators are available for acetaminophen overdose?

The King's College Criteria and the APACHE II score (see discussion of acute liver failure, below)

What is the significance of hyperphosphatemia in acetaminophen overdose?

In one study, hyperphosphatemia was seen exclusively in nonsurvivors; signifying lack of hepatocyte regeneration (hepatocyte regeneration requires phosphate, generally leading to hypophosphatemia) and renal failure.

What is the mechanism of action for *N*-acetyl-cysteine?

Early on, it decreases the risk of severe hepatotoxicity by limiting the formation of NAPQI, increasing glutathione stores (which facilitate detoxification of NAPQI), and enhancing sulfation of acetaminophen to nontoxic metabolites. Once hepatotoxicity develops, *N*-acetyl-cysteine may be beneficial because it has antioxidant and anti-inflammatory activities. It may also improve blood and oxygen delivery to the liver.

ACUTE LIVER FAILURE

What are the main causes of ALF?	Acetaminophen is the leading cause (40%). Many other drugs (as outlined in the discussion of DILI) as well as toxins (*Amanita*) may cause ALF. Viral causes include HAV, HBV, HCV, HEV in pregnancy, HSV, EBV, adenovirus, and CMV. Autoimmune hepatitis, acute fatty liver of pregnancy and inherited disorders (Wilson's) along with vascular disease (VOD and Budd-Chiari) can also cause ALF.
What are the King's College Criteria?	The King's College Criteria are indicators of poor prognosis without liver transplantation. They have good specificity but relatively poor sensitivity.
What are the poor prognostic indicators of the King's College Criteria (immunosuppression)?	Arterial pH <7.3 following volume resuscitation or the combination of PTT >100 with creatinine >3.4 with at least grade III encephalopathy
What are the poor prognostic indicators of the King's College Criteria (nonacetaminophen)?	PTT >100 or any three of the following: drug toxicity, age <10 or >40, jaundice preceding coma by >7 days, PT >50, total bilirubin >17.5
What other prognostic indicators are available for evaluating ALF and the need for transplantation?	The APACHE II score has similar specificity to the King's College Criteria but better sensitivity. Unfortunately the APACHE score requires larger amounts of data, requires the use of a computer program, and thus is not as easily accessible.
What is the main cause of death in ALF?	Early mortality is most often related to cerebral edema. Once patients have survived the early stages of ALF, infection becomes the leading cause of death.
What lab markers signify recovery and hepatocyte regeneration?	Correction of transaminases does not necessarily imply recovery; it may only indicate a "burned-out" liver. Recovery of

synthetic function is essential to determine improving liver status. Hypophosphatemia is a marker of hepatocyte regeneration, as phosphate is required for cellular activity. Elevated AFP levels are also markers of hepatocyte regeneration.

OTHER HEPATOBILIARY DISORDERS

Primary Sclerosing Cholangitis

What are usual laboratory findings at the time of diagnosis?

Elevated alkaline phosphatase (>2 times normal), elevated serum transaminases (<5 times normal), and fluctuating bilirubin levels

Elevated serum IgM in 40% to 50% of cases

Positive p-ANCA in 65% of cases

What diseases have been seen in association with PSC?

70% have UC, but CD, autoimmune diseases, and infiltrating disorders can also be risk factors.

What is the medical therapy for PSC?

No medical therapy has yet consistently improved outcomes in PSC patients, including immunosuppressive medications, colchicine, and ursodeoxycholic acid.

Medical therapies directed at the manifestations of the disease include:

Antibiotics for ascending cholangitis

Cholestyramine, antihistamines, and ursodeoxycholic acid, which may improve pruritus

Replacement of fat-soluble vitamins

What is the surgical therapy for PSC?

Liver transplantation is the only lifesaving treatment for end-stage PSC. The 5-year survival is 85% to 90%.

What is the recurrence rate of PSC following liver transplantation?

Up to 20% of transplanted patients experience recurrence.

Clinical pearls

PSC can precede UC symptoms by several years, so colonoscopy should be performed despite the absence of bowel symptoms. In patients with known UC, do not be fooled by quiescent bowel symptoms, because PSC is not related to IBD disease activity.

Primary Biliary Cirrhosis

What is PBC?

An autoimmune destruction of intrahepatic bile ducts, leading to chronic cholestasis and cirrhosis. It may be in the spectrum of autoimmune liver disease.

What other conditions are associated with PBC?

Sjögren's syndrome and keratoconjunctivitis sicca are each found in up to 75% of patients. Scleroderma, CREST syndrome, and Hashimoto's thyroiditis are also seen.

What symptoms and signs may be seen on presentation of PBC?

Insidious fatigue and pruritus, with jaundice developing months or years later, occurs in 50% to 65% of cases.

Hyperpigmentation, hepatosplenomegaly, hirsutism, and xanthomata may be present.

25% of patients are diagnosed owing to asymptomatic elevations in alkaline phosphatase and other liver enzymes.

What are laboratory findings in PBC?

Elevation of alkaline phosphatase is the most characteristic abnormality (usually 2 to 20 times normal).

Transaminases are mildly elevated (1 to 5 times).

Hyperbilirubinemia is not common at diagnosis (only 10%), but significant rises may occur with progression of disease (and serve as a prognostic indicator).

Cholesterol and triglycerides are often elevated.

What are other laboratory findings in PBC?

Antimitochondrial antibody in 90% to 95% of cases (the subtype M2 is most specific for PBC).

Elevated serum IgM (4 to 5 times normal). These patients often fail to convert IgM to IgG following immunizations. Other autoantibodies (ANA, antihistone, antithyroid) may also be present.

What is seen on liver biopsy in PBC?

Granulomas are classic, but, more commonly there is inflammatory destruction of bile ducts, a paucity of bile ducts, and portal fibrosis.

What is the medical therapy specifically for PBC?

Ursodeoxycholic acid may delay progression of disease or the need for transplantation and may improve survival free of transplant. Colchicine or methotrexate have also been shown to improve survival.

How is hyperlipidemia in PBC treated?

Ursodeoxycholic acid and other cholesterol-lowering medications may help. However, there does not appear to be an increased risk of atherosclerosis in PBC patients.

How are fat malabsorption and steatorrhea in PBC treated?

With replacement of fat-soluble vitamins and medium-chain triglycerides as well as a low-fat diet

How is pruritus in PBC treated?

It may respond to ursodeoxycholic acid, antihistamines, cholestyramine, or naloxone.

What is the recurrence rate of PBC following liver transplantation?

With proper immunosuppression, there is no recurrence of disease following transplant.

What is the prognosis for PBC patients without transplantation?

Survival is 10 to 15 years in asymptomatic patients but only 7 years in symptomatic patients.

What are the poor prognostic indicators for PBC?

They include patient age, level of hepatic function (bilirubin, PT, albumin), and histologic scores. AMA levels do not affect prognosis.

Autoimmune Hepatitis

What are the main forms of autoimmune hepatitis and what groups do they affect?

Type I—classic autoimmune hepatitis, typically characterized by positive ANA (80%) or ASMA (70%). The majority have elevated levels of IgG.

Type II—defined by the presence of antibodies to liver and kidney microsomes, which typically develops in girls or young women.

Overlap syndromes—conditions in which the histologic features and serologic markers of both autoimmune hepatitis and PBC (or, less commonly, PSC) coexist.

What are the typical liver enzyme abnormalities seen in cases of autoimmune hepatitis?

Transaminitis is usually greater than alkaline phosphatase or bilirubin.

What is seen on liver biopsy in autoimmune hepatitis?

Portal inflammation with lymphocytes and plasma cells, erosion of the limiting plate, piecemeal necrosis, and rosette formation

What are treatment options for autoimmune hepatitis?

Corticosteroids are the mainstay of treatment and are generally given with a very gradual taper over a 2-year period. Other immunosuppressive medications, such as azathioprine, are sometimes used in addition to a steroid agent. Note: Decompensated liver disease is not an absolute contraindication to therapy; many of these patients will respond with significant clinical improvement.

What is the response rate to treatment of autoimmune hepatitis?

Remission is achieved in approximately 80% of cases, usually within several months. Up to 50% of cases remain in remission or have only mild inflammation for several months to years after discontinuation of therapy. However, over time, most patients will require repeat therapy as well as chronic maintenance immunosuppressive therapy.

What is the prognosis of autoimmune hepatitis?

The overall survival, including patients with cirrhosis, is >90%.

Wilson's Disease

What is Wilson's disease?

An autosomal recessive disorder of chromosome 13 resulting in progressive copper accumulation affecting the brain, liver, eyes, heart, kidneys, and hematopoietic cells. Normal hepatocyte elimination of copper into the bile is impaired.

What are hepatic manifestations of Wilson's disease?

There are several different manifestations, ranging from asymptomatic liver enzyme abnormalities to cirrhosis or even fulminant hepatic failure. Common biopsy features include macrosteatosis, chronic hepatitis, and fibrosis or cirrhosis.

What are some ophthalmologic manifestations of Wilson's disease?

Kaiser-Fleischer rings (slit lamp) and sunflower cataracts, which are especially prevelant in patients with neuropsychiatric manifestations

What are some renal manifestations of Wilson's disease?

Fanconi syndrome, renal tubular acidosis, kidney stones, and proteinuria

How is the diagnosis of Wilson's disease made?

Elevated serum copper, low serum ceruloplasmin (<20 mg/dL), elevated 24-hour urinary copper (>100 g/day), and elevated quantitative measurement of copper in a liver biopsy specimen

Hereditary Hemochromatosis

What are the genetics of hereditary hemochromatosis?

Most cases are inherited in an autosomal recessive fashion. The most commonly identified *HFE* mutations are the C282Y and H63D mutations. Although uncommon, African American people do develop hemochromatosis, and current gene testing is often unrevealing, suggesting that mutations in other, yet unidentified loci exist. People who are compound heterozygotes (e.g., one C282Y mutation and one H63D mutation) may develop some degree of hemochromatosis.

What tests may be used in attempting to diagnose hereditary hemochromatosis?

Elevated fasting serum transferrin saturation (>50% to 55%), ferritin (may be >1000 ng/mL), and iron. *HFE* gene testing. Imaging studies, particularly MRI, are not diagnostic but may suggest the existence of hepatic iron overload.

What is the hepatic iron index?

The hepatic iron content of a dry liver biopsy specimen is divided by the person's age (in years). Most normal subjects have a hepatic iron index of <1.0. An index >1.9 supports the diagnosis of iron overload. Note: Up to 15% of hemochromatotic patients will have an index <1.9, particularly if they are asymptomatic.

Is a liver biopsy required in all patients with hereditary hemochromatosis?

Not necessarily. Some clinicians defer liver biopsies in people thought to be at lower risk.

What are potential life-threatening complications of hereditary hemochromatosis?

HCC: 20- to 30-fold increased risk (even patients without cirrhosis are at increased risk)

Increased risk of certain infections, such as *Listeria, Yersinia enterocolitica,* and *Vibrio vulnificus* (thus patients should avoid processed meats, high-risk dairy products, and undercooked seafood)

Nonalcoholic Fatty Liver Disease

Who is affected by nonalcoholic steatohepatitis?

Classic risk factors include female gender, obesity, diabetes, and hyperlipidemia. However, it may be seen in patients who have few or none of these characteristics. Children may also be affected.

What are symptoms and signs of steatohepatitis?

Most patients are asymptomatic, although they may have fatigue or right-upper-quadrant discomfort. Hepatomegaly is often seen.

What are laboratory findings of steatohepatitis?

There are no specific diagnostic laboratory tests. Modest transaminitis (two to three times normal) is common. Alkaline phosphatase and bilirubin elevation may occur (in <50% and 10% to 15% of cases, respectively).

How is the diagnosis of steatohepatitis made?

Presence of typical liver enzyme abnormalities, without another explanation despite reasonable evaluation for other causes. Imaging studies may suggest fatty infiltration but cannot differentiate between simple fatty liver versus steatohepatitis. Liver biopsy, although not always absolutely required, is the gold standard.

What is the natural history of nonalcoholic steatohepatitis?

Although this is usually an indolent disease, some patients develop progressive fibrosis with eventual cirrhosis and portal hypertension.

Cirrhosis

What is the Child-Turcotte-Pugh classification?

A scoring system that predicts prognosis and helps in pretransplantation risk stratification.

Table 5–3. Modified Child-Turcotte-Pugh Classification

	1 Point	2 Points	3 Points
Albumin	>3.5	2.8–3.5	<2.8
Bilirubin	<2.0	2.0–3.0	>3.0
Encephalopathy	None	Grade I or II	Grade III or IV
Ascites	None	Mild	Difficult to control
PT (sec/control)	<4	4–6	>6

What is the Child-Turcotte scoring criteria?

Child's class A = score 5 to 6

Child's class B = score 7 to 9

Child's class C = score 10 to 15

What are the 1- and 3-year survivals for a Child-Turcotte:

Class A?

85%, 60%

Class B?

60%, 35%

Class C?

40%, 25%

What other classification systems are available to prognosticate patients with cirrhosis?

In 2002 the United Network for Organ Sharing (UNOS) adopted the Model for End-stage Liver Disease (MELD) Score for determination of organ allocation. The MELD score provides an accurate assessment of 3-month survival and is superior to the Child classification.

What are the components of the MELD score?

It incorporates bilirubin, creatinine, and INR into a log scale.

VARICES

When do varices form?

Varices form when the pressure gradient between the portal and hepatic system reaches >12 mm Hg (normal <5 mm Hg).

What is the risk of developing varices?

Greater than one third of compensated cirrhotics will develop varices. The risk is higher with cirrhosis from alcohol, higher Child classification, and evidence of thrombocytopenia.

What is the prognosis for varices?

Risk of bleeding is increased with variceal size and characteristics (red wale marking) as well as worsening liver function. Overall mortality from bleeding varices is 30%.

What is the acute treatment for esophageal varices?

Acute treatment is aimed at stabilizing the patient with IV fluid, blood transfusion as needed, and an octreotide drip. The patient can then be taken for endoscopic band ligation. Studies have shown that antibiotic coverage during hospitalization for an acute hemorrhage (usually ciprofloxacin) decreases infection and mortality.

What is a final option if bleeding cannot be controlled?

A Sengstaken-Blakemore tube can be used to control bleeding until the patient is stabilized and definitive therapy can be provided. Blakemore tubes pose a high risk of esophageal perforation and infarction.

What is the chronic therapy for esophageal varices to reduce the rebleeding risk in patients who have had prior bleeding?

Prophylaxis is based on directly treating visible esophageal varices with banding along with medical management aimed at decreasing portal hypertension. Portal pressure should be reduced with propranolol, with a target dose based on a 25% reduction in heart rate (or a goal of resting HR 50 to 60) with the addition of a long-acting nitrate if tolerated. TIPS may be necessary for continued variceal bleeding episodes with optimal management.

What is the treatment of bleeding caused by gastric varices?

As opposed to esophageal varices, gastric varices do not respond as well to band ligation or sclerotherapy. TIPS or transplantation have been used in this setting. Studies are being performed to evaluate the efficacy of obliterating gastric varices by injecting them with rapidly polymerizing glue-like compounds.

Table 5–4.   Serum to Ascites Albumin Gradient

SAAG ≥1.1	SAAG <1.1
Pre-liver portal hypertension: PVT, SVT, schistosomiasis	Inflammation: tuberculous peritonitis, secondary peritonitis, pancreatitis, bowel infarct
Liver portal hypertension: cirrhosis, acute liver failure, massive hepatic malignancy	Low oncotic pressure: nephrotic syndrome, protein-losing enteropathy
Post-liver portal hypertension: Budd-Chiari, congestive hepatopathy, tricuspid regurgitation	Malignancy: peritoneal carcinomatosis, Meig's syndrome

ASCITES

How is the serum-to-ascites albumin gradient (SAAG) useful?	A gradient of >1.1 implies that the ascites is a result of portal hypertension (with 97% accuracy). Most commonly this implicates cirrhosis. Preliver causes of an elevated SAAG include portal vein thrombosis and splenic vein thrombosis, while postliver causes include CHF and Budd-Chiari.

SPONTANEOUS BACTERIAL PERITONITIS

What is the pathogenesis of SBP?	Translocation of bacteria through the gut wall into lymphatics or bloodstream, with subsequent seeding of the ascitic fluid. Decreased opsonizing activity within the ascitic fluid also contributes.
What are the most common organisms involved in SBP?	Most commonly aerobic gut flora (e.g., *E. coli, Klebsiella,* and less commonly *Streptococcus* and *Staphylococcus* species). Anaerobic infections are rare.
Why is Gram's staining of ascitic fluid usually a low-yield procedure?	Since organisms average one per milliliter of ascitic fluid, Gram's staining of fluid is almost always negative for organisms.

Therefore, inoculation of blood culture bottles, instead of sending a sample in a syringe or empty tube, can increase the culture-positivity rate from 50% to 80% in patients with >250 polymorphonuclear cells per cubic millimeter in the ascitic fluid.

What if multiple organisms are cultured?

Consider secondary peritonitis (e.g., bowel perforation, abscess)

What ascitic fluid characteristics can help differentiate SBP from secondary peritonitis?

Ascitic fluid glucose <50 mg/dL, total protein >1 g/dL, lactate dehydrogenase greater than the upper normal limit for serum lactate dehydrogenase, and elevated amylase are suggestive of secondary bacterial peritonitis.

What are risk factors for SBP?

Ascitic fluid total protein <1 g/dL

Prior history of SBP

Serum bilirubin >2.5 mg/dL

Variceal hemorrhage

What is the treatment for SBP?

Intravenous cefotaxime should be used for hospitalized patients, while an oral fluoroquinolone can be used as an outpatient therapy for uncomplicated cases. Recent data suggest that intravenous albumin on hospital days 1 and 3 may decrease the incidence of renal failure (which occurs in 30% to 40% of patients with SBP) and decrease overall mortality.

What is the prognosis for patients with SBP?

The incidence of death owing to infectious complications (e.g., shock) has decreased dramatically as a result of early detection and treatment of SBP. In-hospital mortality from other causes approaches 20% to 40%; 1- and 2-year mortality rates remain high (70% and 80%, respectively). Future risk is reduced with appropriate antibiotic prophylaxis and proper diuresis.

HEPATORENAL SYNDROME

What are the clinical manifestations of HRS?	Type 1—the more acute and severe form, manifest by a precipitous decline in renal function (usually to glomerular filtration rate <20 mL/min) within a 2-week period, often with oliguria or anuria
	Type 2—a more insidious, gradual decline in renal function, without other etiologies (e.g., nephrotoxic medications, dehydration), in a patient with advanced liver disease (often with diuretic refractory ascites)
How is the diagnosis of HRS made?	Progressive azotemia with creatinine >2.5 mg/dL, over days to weeks, in patients with acute or chronic liver failure
	Urine volume <500 mL/day
	Urine sodium <10 meq/L (off diuretics) and urine osmolarity greater than serum
	Benign-appearing urinalysis
	Failure to respond to a fluid challenge to exclude prerenal azotemia and exclusion of other causes of renal failure
What is the prognosis of HRS?	>90% mortality Type I—Mean survival 2 weeks Type II—Mean survival 6 months

PORTOSYSTEMIC ENCEPHALOPATHY

What is the mortality of patients diagnosed with PSE?	One-year survival is only 40%.
What are the laboratory findings in PSE?	Increased ammonia level is a marker of PSE (elevated in up to 90% of cases). However, the degree of elevation does not correlate with stage of PSE.
Once PSE is diagnosed, should ammonia levels be followed?	Once a patient is determined to have PSE, there is little benefit from measuring serial ammonia levels.

What are the dietary changes needed to minimize PSE?

Ingestion of animal-derived proteins should be sharply minimized in the acute setting but only modest restriction should be utilized for chronic therapy.

What are the other general treatments for PSE?

Correction of precipitating causes and use of medications to reduce the load of nitrogenous products absorbed from the GI tract are the mainstays of treatment.

What are the main types of medical therapies for PSE, and how do they work?

Lactulose—a nonabsorbable disaccharide, which is metabolized by gut bacteria, leading to acidification of the intestinal contents, resulting in conversion of absorbable ammonia (NH_3) into nonabsorbable ammonium (NH_4^+) and a change in gut flora causing a decrease in NH_3 producing organisms.

Antibiotics (e.g., neomycin, metronidazole)—decrease the numbers of ammonia-producing gut flora.

Zinc supplementation—increases the conversion of NH_3 to NH_4 and can be useful in refractory cases.

HEPATOPULMONARY SYNDROME

What is HPS?

Hypoxemia and frequently platypnea (dyspnea upon standing) and orthodeoxia (oxygen desaturation with upright position) caused by pulmonary vascular dilation and arterial–venous shunts

What else may cause dyspnea and hypoxia in patients with chronic liver disease?

Portopulmonary syndrome and ventilation–perfusion mismatch (caused by diaphragmatic elevation from ascites, resulting in atelectasis)

How is the diagnosis of HPS made?

Contrast echocardiogram (e.g., "bubble" studies) is the initial study of choice.

How is contrast echocardiography useful in HPS?

A contrast material (e.g., bubbles within agitated saline) is injected into a peripheral vein. Bubbles normally appear in the right heart but are filtered by the pulmonary capillaries, so they never reach the left heart. When a right-to-left shunt exists, bubbles are seen in the left heart. If the shunt is an intracardiac shunt, bubbles appear in the left heart within three cardiac cycles, whereas intrapulmonary shunts, such as in HPS, take longer (3 to 7 cardiac cycles).

How is pulmonary angiography used in HPS?

Although not routinely obtained, angiography may reveal abnormalities supporting the diagnosis of HPS, and it helps exclude other causes of hypoxemia, such as pulmonary emboli. Contrast may cause issues, however.

What is the treatment for HPS?

Liver transplantation for patients with significant hypoxia. Case reports suggest benefit from medications such as aspirin and methylene blue.

Why is it important to differentiate HPS from pulmonary hypertension?

Severe pulmonary hypertension is a contraindication to liver transplant.

PORTOPULMONARY HYPERTENSION

What is PPHTN?

Pulmonary hypertension associated with portal hypertension in the absence of secondary causes of pulmonary hypertension

What is the pathophysiology of PPHTN?

Unknown, but may involve humoral mediators from the gut entering the systemic circulation rather than being metabolized by the liver, leading to the pulmonary vasoconstriction, remodeling of the muscle layer within the pulmonary arterial walls, and in situ thrombosis. Genetic factors may play a role.

What are clinical (symptomatic) manifestations of PPHTN?

Symptoms, which may initially be subtle, include dyspnea on exertion, fatigue, chest pain, syncope, orthopnea, or hemoptysis.

What are the physical signs of PPHTN?

Examination may reveal an accentuated P_2, tricuspid regurgitation murmur and edema. Most patients have manifestations of portal hypertension.

How is the diagnosis of PPHTN made?

Echocardiography shows evidence of pulmonary hypertension. Pulmonary angiography is the gold standard. If pulmonary hypertension is identified, tests to exclude other secondary causes should be performed.

What is the treatment for PPHTN?

Like treatments used for primary pulmonary hypertension, including anticoagulants to prevent in situ thrombosis of pulmonary arteries and vasodilators (e.g., epoprostenol, nitrates). Both types of therapy must be used cautiously in patients with chronic liver disease.

Transplantation is considered for mild to moderate PPHTN but may be associated with poor outcomes with severe PPHTN.

What is the prognosis for PPHTN?

Poor, especially without treatment. Major causes of death include right heart failure and infections.

HYPERSPLENISM

Why does hypersplenism occur with cirrhosis?

It results from portal hypertension, causing sequestration and destruction of blood cells.

Should patients with hypersplenism undergo splenectomy?

Surgical splenectomy is not routinely recommended.

TUMORS OF THE LIVER

How are hemangiomas recognized?

They are often found incidentally.

What is the treatment for hepatic adenomas?

Surgical resection

What are the most common malignancies affecting the liver?

Metastases from other sources

Hepatocellular Carcinoma

What is the epidemiology of HCC?

Prevalence varies worldwide, being highest in sub-Saharan Africa, China, Hong Kong, and Taiwan. Although the United States is a low-prevalence region, the incidence has increased during the last two decades.

What are predisposing factors for HCC?

Cirrhosis of any cause. Others include race (e.g., Asian and Eskimo), male gender, environmental carcinogens (e.g., tobacco, aflatoxin, and betel nut chewing), viral infection (especially HBV), hereditary hemochromatosis, and *Clonorchis*.

Does HCC occur in noncirrhotic patients?

Yes. Approximately 20% of cases occur in noncirrhotic livers, whereas 80% occur in the setting of cirrhosis.

What is the annual incidence of HCC in patients with compensated cirrhosis?

Approximately 3% to 4% per year

What are clinical manifestations of HCC?

Many patients do not have symptoms directly attributable to HCC. Manifestations may include abdominal pain, weight loss, early satiety, palpable mass, obstructive jaundice, intraperitoneal bleeding caused by rupture, and bone pain caused by metastases. Rarely, HCC may cause paraneoplastic syndromes, causing hypoglycemia, watery diarrhea, erythrocytosis, or hypercalcemia.

Clinical pearl

HCC should always be considered when a previously stable cirrhotic patient decompensates with worsening encephalopathy or ascites (often as a result of PVT).

What is the concern about liver biopsy for HCC besides bleeding?

Seeding the needle track with tumor cells, resulting in extrahepatic disease

What is the prognosis for HCC?

Most cases are found late in the course of chronic liver disease, resulting in median survivals of 6 to 20 months after diagnosis.

What factors determine prognosis for HCC?

Hepatic function, tumor size, and the presence of metastases. Fibrolamellar HCC occurs more commonly in young patients without underlying liver disease and has a much better prognosis.

For which patients should tumor resection be considered?

Those with adequate liver function reserve, smaller tumors (e.g., >5 cm), and no evidence of metastases.

What factors indicate that liver transplant is a viable option for cure?

Single tumors <5 cm, ≤3 tumor nodules each >3 cm, and absence of metastases or local invasion into blood vessels or lymphatics. In carefully selected patients, 5-year survivals of 70% to 80% may be achieved.

LIVER TRANSPLANTATION

Clinical pearl

Thomas Starzl performed the first human liver transplantation in 1963.

What are the absolute contraindications to liver transplantation?

Advanced cardiopulmonary disease, active sepsis, extrahepatic malignancy, active alcohol or substance abuse, anatomic abnormalities precluding transplantation, and inability of the patient to understand or accept the procedure and subsequent immunosuppressive medications

What are the relative contraindications to liver transplantation?

Advanced age (>65 years), inadequate social or family support, intrahepatic tumor >5 cm, or SBP. In some transplant centers, cholangiocarcinoma and HIV are also contraindications.

What is the usual number of blood transfusions required during cadaveric liver transplantation?

<10 units packed RBCs. No transfusions are needed in up to 30% of cases.

What is the postoperative medical therapy after transplantation?

Immunosuppressive regimens vary but usually include corticosteroids, cyclosporine or tacrolimus, and azathioprine or mycophenolate.

What are the postoperative complications after transplantation at the following times:

    Immediate postoperative period?

Procurement injury (graft dysfunction as a result of inadequate preservation), thrombosis or stenosis of vascular anastomoses, biliary complications in 5% to 10% of cases, and hyperacute rejection (usually as a result of preformed antibodies). The most frequently encountered technical complications result from damage to the biliary tree.

    Early postoperative period?

Acute cellular rejection (usually after the fifth day postoperatively); bacterial, viral, or fungal infection, renal insufficiency

    Late postoperative period?

Chronic rejection (e.g., "vanishing bile duct syndrome") and recurrence of primary disease

When do infections most commonly occur posttransplant?

Patients are at highest risk for bacterial and fungal infections in the first 2 months following transplant. If they are on standard-dose immunosuppressants, their risk of infection approaches that of the normal population at 6 months. The standard use of trimethoprim-sulfamethoxazole and acyclovir, for *Pneumocystis jirovecii* and herpes prophylaxis respectively, has lowered the incidence of these infections.

What is the 1-year survival for patients who undergo liver transplantation in the United States?

Between 85% and 90% for most liver diseases

What is the 3-year survival for patients who undergo liver transplantation in the United States?

>70%. Survivors usually have a good quality of life. Some 85% return to their previous occupation; women have had subsequent normal pregnancies.

What long-term medical problems occur after liver transplantation?

Hypertension as a result of immunosuppressants occurs in 50% of patients. Hyperlipidemia occurs in approximately 25% of patients and is generally treated with statins. Diabetes develops in more than 30% of patients and generally requires insulin for control. Patients are also at increased risk for osteoporosis and skin cancer.

Chapter 6   Hematology

ABBREVIATIONS

ACT	Activated clotting time
APC	Activated protein C
aPPT	Activated partial thromboplastin time
ATIII	Antithrombin III
BMT	Bone marrow transplantation
CKD	Chronic kidney disease
CLL	Chronic lymphocytic leukemia
CML	Chronic myelogenous leukemia
CMML	Chronic myelomonocytic leukemia
CVA	Cerebrovascular accident

DDAVP	1-desamino-8-D-arginine vasopressin (desmopressin acetate)
DIC	Disseminated intravascular coagulation
DTI	Direct thrombin inhibitor
ELISA	Enzyme-linked immunosorbent assay
ET	Essential thrombocytosis
G-CSF	Granulocyte colony-stimulating factor
GFR	Glomerular filtration rate
HELLP syndrome	Hemolysis, elevated liver enzymes, and low platelets
HIT	Heparin-induced thrombocytopenia
HITT	Heparin-induced thrombocytopenia and thrombosis
Hgb	Hemoglobin
HUS	Hemolytic uremic syndrome
ITP	Idiopathic or immune thrombocytopenic purpura
IVF	Intravenous fluid
LAP	Leukocyte alkaline phosphatase
LDH	Lactate dehydrogenase
MCV	Mean cell volume
MDS	Myelodysplastic syndrome(s)
MI	Myocardial infarction
PCR	Polymerase chain reaction
PNH	Paroxysmal nocturnal hemoglobinuria
PT	Prothrombin time
PV	Polycythemia vera
RA	Refractory anemia
RAEB-1	Refractory anemia with excess blasts (<5%)
RAEB-2	Refractory anemia with excess blasts (5–19%)
RARS	Refractory anemia with ringed sideroblasts
RCMD	Refractory cytopenia with multilineage dysplasia
RCMD-RS	Refractory cytopenia with multilineage dysplasia and ringed sideroblasts
RDW	Red cell distribution width
RI	Reticulocyte index
RPI	Reticulocyte production index
MDS-U	Myelodysplastic syndrome, unclassified
MDS 5q-	Myelodysplastic syndrome associated with isolated chromosome 5q deletion
RAEB-T	Refractory anemia with excess blasts in transformation
SLE	Systemic lupus erythematosus
TIBC	Total iron-binding capacity
TSH	Thyroid-stimulating hormone
TTP	Thrombotic thrombocytopenic purpura
VTE	Venous thromboembolism
vWD	von Willebrand's disease
vWF	von Willebrand factor

RED BLOOD CELLS

What is hemoglobin A₂?

Hemoglobin A_2 is a tetramer of two alpha and two delta chains. Hemoglobin A_2 constitutes approximately 2% of normal adult hemoglobin.

When are teardrop cells seen?

In disorders that result in infiltration of the bone marrow space, resulting in crowding out of normal bone marrow components. These disorders are known as myelophthisic disorders.

Give examples of myelophthisic disorders:

Examples include malignant infiltration of the bone marrow; myeloproliferative disorders, especially myeloid metaplasia with myelofibrosis; and infections such as in tuberculosis.

What type of blood smear is commonly associated with myelophthisic disorders?

Myelophthisic disorders are commonly associated with a leukoerythroblastic blood smear.

What is a leukoerythroblastic blood smear?

The presence of nucleated RBCs, early myeloid precursors (metamyelocyte and younger), and giant platelets on the smear

What is an acanthocyte?

An RBC with a few irregular spiny projections unevenly distributed on the membrane of a cell with a reduced volume

When are acanthocytes seen?

In spur cell anemia, severe liver disease, and abetalipoproteinemia

What is a burr cell?

Also called echinocytes, burr cells are characterized by numerous regular scalloped projections that are evenly distributed on the RBC surface.

When are echinocytes seen?

In patients with severe renal disease or liver disease

What is a target cell?

An RBC with a "bull's-eye" appearance, with hemoglobin color in the center and periphery of the cell

What causes the target appearance?	The cells have an increased ratio of surface area to volume; the redundant cell membrane causes the target appearance.
When are target cells seen?	In thalassemia or other hemoglobinopathies, liver disease, or disorders of splenic function
What is a stomatocyte?	An RBC with a slitlike central pale area. These cells are also referred to as fish-mouth cells.
When are stomatocytes seen?	In ethanol abuse and in an inherited disorder called hereditary stomatocytosis

ANEMIAS

How may anemias be categorized?	A useful formulation is to think of anemias as arising from RBC underproduction, destruction or loss, or sequestration.
What tests should be ordered in the initial workup of anemia?	The MCV can be used to categorize the anemia as microcytic, normocytic, or macrocytic. Measuring the reticulocyte count, checking renal function, and reviewing the peripheral smear are also integral parts of the initial workup.
What is a corrected reticulocyte count?	One that is corrected for the baseline hematocrit—i.e., an adequate reticulocyte count in someone with a severe anemia should be higher than that in a nonanemic person.
What is a normal (nonanemic) corrected reticulocyte count?	$\leq 5\%$
What methods can be used to determine the reticulocyte count?	1. The absolute reticulocyte count equals the percentage of reticulocytes multiplied by the RBC count. 2. The corrected reticulocyte count is determined by multiplying the percentage of reticulocytes by the patient's hematocrit and dividing by the normal hematocrit.

What absolute reticulocyte count suggests an adequate marrow response to anemia or blood loss?	An absolute reticulocyte count $>100,000/\mu L$ usually suggests an adequate bone marrow response to blood loss or hemolysis.
What is the reticulocyte index?	A correction factor
How is the reticulocyte production index calculated?	Take the corrected reticulocyte count divided by $(1 + x)$, where $x = 0.5$ for every 10% decrease in Hct.
How is the reticulocyte count useful?	Under conditions of severe anemia, reticulocytes are released from the marrow prematurely and finish their maturation in the peripheral circulation, giving a falsely high estimate of daily RBC production.
What does an elevated reticulocyte count suggest?	An appropriately elevated reticulocyte count suggests that the anemia is secondary to acute blood loss or a hemolytic process.
What does a low reticulocyte count suggest?	An inappropriately low reticulocyte count suggests that the process is at least partly caused by decreased bone marrow production. So a RI <2 for a Hct of 10% to 35% indicates a hypoproliferative anemia. Very frequently, mixed pictures are present.

MICROCYTIC ANEMIAS

What are the causes of microcytic anemia?	Iron deficiency, thalassemias, sideroblastic anemia, and sometimes anemia of chronic disease
In a patient with an elevated reticulocyte count and microcytic anemia, what diagnosis is suggested?	Thalassemia. To confirm this suspicion, the peripheral smear should be reviewed and a hemoglobin electrophoresis ordered.
In a patient with a microcytic anemia and a low reticulocyte count, what test should be ordered?	A serum ferritin level

What does a low ferritin level indicate?

If the ferritin is low, the patient likely suffers from iron deficiency anemia, at least in part.

How sensitive and specific is a low ferritin level with regard to the diagnosis of iron deficiency?

A ferritin <15 ng/mL has a specificity of 99% for iron deficiency anemia but a sensitivity of only 60%. Note: A cause of blood loss must be identified.

If the ferritin is normal with a low reticulocyte count, what test should be ordered next?

Serum creatinine

What does an elevated creatinine and normal ferritin suggest?

If the patient has an elevated creatinine with a normal ferritin, the likely cause of anemia is renal insufficiency.

What other lab test should be considered in patients with mild to moderate renal dysfunction?

In patients with mild-to-moderate abnormalities of renal function, it is useful to check an erythropoietin level for confirmation.

In a patient with a low reticulocyte count, normal ferritin, and normal renal function, what blood test should be done?

TIBC or transferrin

What do low TIBC or transferrin levels indicate?

A low TIBC or transferrin suggests a diagnosis of anemia of inflammation/chronic diseases.

What is the most common cause of significant microcytosis without anemia?

Thalassemia

Iron Deficiency

Does a normal serum ferritin rule out iron deficiency anemia?

No. Inflammatory states and liver disease can elevate the serum ferritin level into the normal range (ferritin is an acute-phase reactant). In these cases, the anemia is usually multifactorial.

What is the "gold standard" for the diagnosis of iron deficiency?

Prussian blue stain for iron stores in a bone marrow aspirate

After making the diagnosis, what is the next critical step?

Finding the reason for the iron deficiency which is commonly blood loss from the GI tract

When should the iron be taken?

Ferrous sulfate is best absorbed away from meals; however, it is better tolerated with food.

Is there anything that can be done to improve the iron absorption?

Simultaneous administration of vitamin C facilitates iron absorption.

What are some of the side effects of oral iron therapy?

Gastrointestinal upset, constipation, and nausea. Stool softeners should always be used with iron therapy.

What is done for patients who do not absorb iron well or cannot tolerate the medication?

IV iron formulations are sometimes needed if the patient cannot tolerate oral iron or does not absorb it.

How long does it take for oral iron to begin to increase the reticulocyte count?

The reticulocyte count peaks in 5 to 10 days. It usually takes 2 to 3 months of continuous iron therapy to reestablish the body's iron stores.

Thalassemias

What is the hemoglobin electrophoresis pattern with alpha thalassemia trait?

Normal. A low MCV with normal ferritin without evidence for beta thalassemia or a hemoglobinopathy are clues to the diagnosis. PCR analysis can now be done to confirm the diagnosis of alpha thalassemia.

What is hydrops fetalis in relation to thalassemia?

Deletion of all four alpha-globin genes. This is incompatible with life and the fetus usually dies in utero.

What is hemoglobin H disease?

Three of the four alpha-globin genes are dysfunctional. Hemoglobin H forms as a result, a tetramer of beta chains. This is the most severe form of alpha-thalassemia that is compatible with life.

How does hemoglobin H disease present?

As significant anemia in early childhood

What are the common consequences of hemoglobin H disease?

Hemolysis, hypersplenism, and anemia. Iron overload (secondary to transfusions) leading to end-organ damage is relatively uncommon.

How is the diagnosis of beta thalassemia minor made?

By demonstration of microcytic anemia with target cells and ovalocytes, moderate poikilocytosis, basophilic stippling, and reticulocytosis. Hemoglobin electrophoresis shows an elevated percentage of hemoglobin A_2.

What is beta thalassemia major?

Abnormalities of both beta-globin genes with markedly reduced-to-absent beta-chain synthesis. This disorder is also referred to as Cooley's anemia.

How does beta thalassemia major present?

With severe anemia within the first 6 months of life resulting in growth retardation unless the patients are transfused

What are the predominant medical problems in patients with beta thalassemia major due to?

Transfusion-related infections and iron overload secondary to massive transfusion requirements.

What is beta thalassemia intermedia?

Both beta-globin genes are abnormal, but one of the genes is partially functional and can still synthesize a small amount of normal beta-globin chain.

What are the signs and symptoms of beta thalassemia intermedia?

Usually, patients do not require transfusions and have mild splenomegaly. However, cardiomegaly and osteoporotic fractures can develop.

Sideroblastic Anemia

What is a sideroblast?

An erythroid precursor with increased iron granules in the cytoplasm

What are ringed sideroblasts?

Erythroid precursors with large iron granules within mitochondria ringing the nucleus. Normal erythroid precursors have a few small punctate iron granules scattered throughout the cytoplasm.

What is the defect that results in the accumulation of iron within the mitochondria in ring sideroblasts?

An enzymatic defect of heme synthesis does not allow iron to be incorporated into the heme molecule. There are both hereditary and acquired causes. When this is a lifelong process, however, it is likely due to hereditary sideroblastic anemia.

What are the acquired causes of sideroblastic anemia?

Idiopathic, MDS, lead poisoning, and drug use (e.g., use of isoniazid, hydralazine, chloramphenicol, and ethanol)

What is the treatment for sideroblastic anemia?

Phlebotomy or chelation. Pyridoxine (vitamin B_6) may lead to an increase in the hematocrit in some patients with the hereditary forms. Removal of offending drugs/toxins is vital for acquired causes. Supportive care is the mainstay in the MDS variety. Some idiopathic forms respond to erythropoietin and G-CSF.

Hemoglobinopathies

How are acute painful episodes (vaso-occlusive crisis) in sickle cell patients managed?

IVF and pain management with opioids. Avoid meperidine (the metabolite accumulates and can cause seizures). Give supplemental oxygen if patient is hypoxic.

What is sickle cell chest syndrome characterized by?

Hypoxia, infiltrate on CXR, pain, and dyspnea

What are the causes of sickle cell chest syndrome?

May be due to infection, thrombosis, or fat emboli

How is sickle cell chest syndrome managed?

Transfusions to decrease the percentage of Hb S

What causes aplastic anemia in sickle cell patients?

Parvovirus B19 infection, which is usually self-limited in immunocompetent patients.

What is hemoglobin SC disease?

A heterozygous condition in which one allele for the beta chain is hemoglobin S and the other allele is hemoglobin C

How is hemoglobin SC disease different from sickle cell anemia?

Patients with hemoglobin SC disease usually have fewer symptoms, but they may be equally affected. Patients with SC disease have a higher frequency of avascular necrosis of the femoral head and proliferative retinopathy.

What is sickle beta thalassemia disease?

One of the beta-chain alleles has hemoglobin S and the other allele has dysfunctional beta-chain synthesis.

How does the course of sickle beta thalassemia disease compare to that of sickle cell anemia?

Even though the disease is usually less severe than sickle cell anemia, the clinical course can be identical. The amount of normal hemoglobin A present usually correlates with the severity of the disease.

NORMOCYTIC ANEMIAS

Anemia of Inflammation

What is seen on bone marrow staining in anemia of inflammation?

Staining the bone marrow reveals normal or increased iron stores, but iron within the erythroblasts is decreased or absent.

How is the diagnosis of anemia of inflammation made?

The diagnosis should be considered in a patient with a systemic illness, a hypoproliferative anemia, and normal iron stores. A low TIBC or transferrin is highly suggestive of anemia of inflammation.

When differentiating iron deficiency anemia from anemia of inflammation, what is seen with regard to:
    The RDW?

In iron deficiency anemia, the RDW is high; in patients with anemia of inflammation, the RDW is normal.

The serum ferritin level?	In iron deficiency anemia, the ferritin is low (unless there is a concomitant inflammatory process, recent blood transfusion, or liver injury). In patients with anemia of inflammation, the serum ferritin level is normal or elevated.
The TIBC and transferring level?	In iron deficiency anemia, the TIBC or transferrin level is elevated. In patients with anemia of inflammation, the TIBC is decreased.
If you still cannot figure it out, what else can be done to differentiate iron deficiency anemia and anemia of chronic disease?	In some situations, an iron stain of the bone marrow is required to differentiate these disorders. Especially in hospitalized patients, both may coexist.
How do you treat anemia of inflammation?	Ideally, the underlying disorder is treated and the anemia resolves. If a patient requires transfusions, alternative causes for the anemia should be considered. If necessary, erythropoietin can increase the hematocrit in many patients.

Anemia of Renal Failure

At what GFR do erythropoietin levels usually drop?	Particularly in patients with a GFR <50 mL/min.
What Hgb level should prompt further evaluation?	Evaluation in patients with CKD should begin when the Hgb is <12 mg/dL in females and <13.5 mg/dL in males.

Hemolytic Anemias

What are the broad categories of hemolytic anemias?	Thalassemias, hemoglobinopathies, autoimmune hemolytic anemia, RBC membrane disorders, microangiopathic hemolytic anemias, and enzyme deficiencies of the hexose monophosphate shunt and the Embden-Meyerhof pathway (i.e., glycolysis)

What is the difference between an extravascular hemolytic anemia and an intravascular hemolytic anemia?

In an extravascular hemolytic anemia, RBCs are removed by the reticuloendothelial system, primarily in the spleen. Intravascular hemolytic anemias result from destruction of RBCs within the vasculature, as happens with the microangiopathies (TTP/HUS, DIC, etc.).

Is the reticulocyte count usually elevated in hemolytic anemia?

Yes, unless the bone marrow is simultaneously affected by a hypoproliferative process such as iron deficiency, vitamin B12 deficiency, anemia of inflammation, or a primary marrow disorder.

What biochemical abnormalities suggest a hemolytic anemia?

Elevated LDH, unconjugated bilirubin, and urine urobilinogen with a decreased haptoglobin or, with severe cases of intravascular hemolysis, hemoglobinuria

What disorders are associated with cold antibody autoimmune hemolytic anemia?

Lymphoproliferative disorders, *Mycoplasma pneumoniae*, infectious mononucleosis, and syphilis

What are cold antibodies?

Antibodies whose affinity for their antigen is increased at relatively low (<37°C) temperatures, usually but not always of the IgM type

What is the treatment of cold antibody autoimmune hemolytic anemia?

Avoidance of cold. Can consider cytotoxic agents particularly if associated with lymphoproliferative disorder. For acute, severe hemolysis, can consider apheresis.

What disorders are associated with warm antibody autoimmune hemolytic anemia?

Idiopathic, autoimmune (SLE), viral, lymphoproliferative disorders (CLL), and numerous drugs

What are the warm antibodies?

IgG antibodies that react with RBC membrane proteins at room temperature

What is the treatment of autoimmune hemolytic anemia?

Steroids are the mainstay to reduce the antibody production. In refractory cases, cytotoxic drugs or splenectomy may be successful. Transfusion of RBCs is imperative in patients with circulatory collapse and symptoms associated with heart disease.

What is the difficulty in transfusing these patients?

Finding compatible blood

What are the RBC membrane disorders associated with hemolysis?

PNH, hereditary spherocytosis, hereditary elliptocytosis, and spur cell anemia of severe liver disease

What are the causes of microangiopathic hemolytic anemia?

Mechanical heart valves, infected heart valves, TTP/HUS, malignant hypertension, DIC, preeclampsia or eclampsia, HELLP syndrome, connective tissue diseases, and malignancy

What is the pathophysiologic process in microangiopathic hemolytic anemia?

Mechanical heart valves may directly shear the RBCs. In other disorders, fibrin strand formation in the microcirculation traps and shears the RBCs.

Macrocytic Anemias

What is megaloblastic anemia?

Macrocytic anemia associated with delayed nuclear maturation and with normal to increased cytoplasmic maturation, producing large erythroid precursors. This type of anemia is caused by disorders affecting DNA or RNA synthesis or repair.

What are the causes of megaloblastic anemia?

Vitamin B12 or folate deficiency, chemotherapy, antiretroviral therapy, and other disorders of DNA synthesis

What should be the first tests ordered for the evaluation of a patient with macrocytic anemia?

Reticulocyte count, serum B12 and folate levels, TSH, and peripheral blood smear

A patient with an elevated reticulocyte count and macrocytic anemia suggests what diagnosis?

Hemolytic anemia

What are the causes of anemia associated with liver disease?

Anemia of inflammation, iron deficiency secondary to gastrointestinal blood loss, vitamin B12 and folate deficiency, hypersplenism, and mild hemolysis

What peripheral smear findings suggest liver disease?

Macrocytosis with target cells. In severe liver disease, markedly abnormal RBC shapes (spur cells) can be seen. These abnormalities appear to be caused by cholesterol synthesis abnormalities in the liver.

What laboratory and peripheral smear findings suggest a MDS?

Cytopenias of two or more lineages (WBC, RBC, platelets) are suspicious. RBCs are usually large, with macro-ovalocytes. Coarse basophilic stippling can be seen. Hypogranulation, nuclear "sticks," and hypo- or hypersegmentation of neutrophil nuclei are highly suggestive.

What test is done to confirm the diagnosis of an MDS?

Examination of the bone marrow aspirate and biopsy are required to make a definitive diagnosis of an MDS. Dysplastic changes of hematopoietic precursors, an increased percentage of blasts, pathologic and ringed sideroblasts, and clonal cytogenetic abnormalities are all suggestive of an MDS.

ERYTHROCYTOSIS

What three mechanisms produce the increased hematocrit seen in cigarette smokers?

1. Decreased plasma volume (unknown mechanism).
2. Underlying lung disease causing hypoxemia.
3. Lower oxygen delivery to tissues. Carbon monoxide from smoke has a higher affinity for hemoglobin than oxygen, resulting in the lower oxygen delivery.

PANCYTOPENIA

What are the causes of pancytopenia?	Disorders involving infiltration of the bone marrow, hypersplenism, vitamin B12 or folate deficiency, myelodysplasia, aplastic anemia, PNH, and medications
What is the characteristic finding on peripheral smear in infiltrative disorders of bone marrow?	Leukoerythroblastosis
What are the disorders of the spleen that result in pancytopenia?	Congestive splenomegaly (e.g., cirrhosis and portal vein thrombosis), lymphomas, Gaucher's disease, Niemann-Pick disease, Letterer-Siwe disease, and infectious diseases (e.g., kala-azar, miliary tuberculosis, and syphilis)

APLASTIC ANEMIA

What is the differential diagnosis of aplastic anemia?	Toxin effects, viral infection, hypoplastic MDS, hypoplastic acute leukemia, PNH, and myelofibrosis
Pure RBC aplasia may be caused by what infectious agent?	Parvovirus B19
What tumor may be associated with pure RBC aplasia?	Thymoma
What are treatment options for aplastic anemia?	Immunosuppression with antithymocyte globulin and/or cyclosporine plus steroids, or allogeneic BMT

LEUKOCYTES

LEUKOPENIA

Below what neutrophil count is the patient at significantly increased risk of serious bacterial infection?	0.5×10^9/L

What are some common drug-related causes of neutropenia?	Clozapine, thioamides, trimethoprim-sulfamethoxazole, phenytoin, chemotherapy, phenothiazine, procainamide, and beta lactams
What are some of the other causes of neutropenia?	Bone marrow disorders (e.g., tumor infiltration, fibrosis, leukemia, aplastic anemia), megaloblastic disorders, sepsis, autoimmune neutropenia, collagen vascular diseases, and hypersplenism
What is seen on the bone marrow examination of patients with agranulocytosis?	No myeloid activity. Patients are at extremely high risk of infection and sepsis.
What is the treatment for agranulocytosis?	Immediate discontinuation of all drugs associated with agranulocytosis and administration of antibiotics for signs or symptoms of infection. Should granulocyte activity not reestablish itself, G-CSF may be started.

LEUKOCYTOSIS

What is a leukemoid reaction?	An increase in the WBC count to $>25 \times 10^9$/L secondary to another condition
What are causes of leukocytosis?	Leukemia and reactive states, such as infection, extreme stress, trauma, and cancer

NEUTROPHILIA

What are toxic granulations?	An increase in intensity of staining and number of myeloperoxidase granules within neutrophils
In whom are toxic granulations seen?	In patients with active infection or bone marrow stress, including that caused by G-CSF
How can a leukemoid reaction be differentiated from CML?	In CML, the spleen is usually enlarged, the LAP level is very low, and there is often basophilia, none of which characterize a leukemoid reaction. If in doubt, the presence of the Philadelphia chromosome is pathognomonic for CML.

LYMPHOCYTOSIS

What are the causes of marked lymphocytosis ($>15 \times 10^9$/L)?	Infectious mononucleosis, pertussis infection, chronic lymphocytic leukemia, and acute lymphocytic leukemia

EOSINOPHILS

What are causes of peripheral eosinophilia?	Think **NAACP:** Neoplasm (acute leukemia or chronic myeloid disorders), allergic reactions, autoimmune, collagen vascular/cortisol insufficiency, and parasitic infections
What is the hypereosinophilic syndrome?	Rare disease with persistent eosinophilia ($>1.5 \times 10^9$/L for more than 6 months) in the absence of an identifiable underlying cause and with organ involvement
What organs are commonly involved in the hypereosinophilic syndrome?	Heart (endomyocardial fibrosis), liver, skin, lungs, and central nervous system
What is the standard first-line therapy for hypereosinophilic syndrome?	Corticosteroids

PLATELETS

What are some of the platelet dense granule contents?	Calcium, serotonin, and adenosine diphosphate
What are some of the platelet alpha granule contents?	Platelet factor 4, alpha-thromboglobulin, factor V, vWF/FVIII, plasminogen activator inhibitor (PAI), FXIII, and transforming growth factor beta

THROMBOCYTOPENIA

At what platelet count is there a significantly increased risk of bleeding from trauma or surgery?	Platelet counts $>50 \times 10^9$/L are usually sufficient to prevent major bleeding from surgical procedures and trauma. The more severe the trauma and the larger the

operation, the greater the risk of bleeding; neurosurgical procedures generally require a platelet count closer to 100×10^9/L, but rigorous studies supporting this requirement have not been performed.

At what platelet count does spontaneous hemorrhage become a risk?

Ecchymoses and petechiae usually do not occur until the platelet count is $<50 \times 10^9$/L.

At what platelet count does spontaneous life-threatening hemorrhage become a distinct possibility?

$<5 \times 10^9$/L for children and $<10 \times 10^9$/L for adults

When should platelets be transfused?

At a platelet count of $<100 \times 10^9$/L when there is life-threatening or clinically significant bleeding. Prophylactic platelet transfusion is routinely given to patients with platelet counts $<10 \times 10^9$/L when they have decreased platelet production ($<20 \times 10^9$/L if there is concomitant infection, fever, uremia, or other additional bleeding risk).

What is the differential diagnosis of decreased platelet production?

Drugs, liver injury, sepsis, myelophthisic disorders, acute leukemia, myelodysplasia, aplastic anemia, viral infections, AIDS, vitamin B12 and folate deficiency, or splenomegaly

What are the causes of increased destruction or consumption?

ITP, TTP/HUS, and DIC

IMMUNE THROMBOCYTOPENIC PURPURA

What diseases are associated with ITP?

Chronic lymphocytic leukemia, Hodgkin's disease, non-Hodgkin's lymphoma, SLE, rheumatoid arthritis, Hepatitis C and HIV

What are some alternative treatments for steroid-refractory patients with ITP?	Intravenous immunoglobulin, which gives a rapid but transient increase in platelet count, anti-D immunoglobulin (for Rh-positive patients), B-cell depletion with rituximab, splenectomy, danazol, and rarely, cytotoxic chemotherapy agents

THROMBOTIC THROMBOCYTOPENIC PURPURA AND HEMOLYTIC UREMIC SYNDROME

What is the pentad of TTP?	Fever, hemolytic anemia with schistocytes, thrombocytopenia, neurologic changes, and renal dysfunction
What two of the five criteria above are sufficient to prompt treatment of TTP?	The presence of microangiopathic hemolytic anemia and thrombocytopenia without apparent cause is sufficient to begin treatment for TTP.
What is HUS?	A triad of thrombocytopenia, hemolytic anemia with schistocytes, and renal failure
What are the differences between TTP and HUS?	HUS is associated with a greater degree of renal failure and, less often, with other end-organ damage (e.g., heart, brain, lungs, gastrointestinal tract, and retinal vessels). Thrombocytopenia and hemolysis are more profound in TTP than in HUS. It is often difficult to distinguish between TTP and HUS owing to clinical overlap, so many consider them as a continuum of disease. HUS as a distinct entity is more frequent in children.
What is the differential diagnosis of TTP/HUS?	DIC, preeclampsia, and eclampsia, HELLP syndrome, malignant hypertension, and severe vasculitis; or multiple simultaneous comorbidities (e.g., sepsis causing renal failure, altered mental status, and DIC) mimicking its clinical picture
What are some inciting factors for TTP/HUS?	Infection, pregnancy, immune disorders, allogeneic BMT, and drugs (including chemotherapy)
Which drugs are associated with TTP and HUS?	Cyclosporine, ticlopidine (Ticlid), clopidogrel (Plavix), and mitomycin C

What is the treatment for TTP?	Daily apheresis of 3 to 4 L leads to improvement in many patients within 1 week. Before the institution of apheresis therapy, TTP was nearly universally fatal. Steroids are sometimes used as an adjunct to plasma exchange. HUS is treated similarly but may respond more poorly.
Should platelets be transfused in patients with TTP or HUS?	In both disorders, platelet transfusions are contraindicated.

THROMBOCYTOSIS

What two laboratory tests may help differentiate reactive thrombocytosis from essential thrombocythemia?	Fibrinogen and C-reactive protein levels, which are often elevated with reactive thrombocytosis because many of the reactive disorders cause elevation of acute-phase reactant protein levels

MYELOPROLIFERATIVE DISORDERS

What are the four myeloproliferative disorders?	PV, essential thrombocythemia, CML, and myelofibrosis with myeloid metaplasia

POLYCYTHEMIA VERA

Is only the hematocrit elevated in PV?	No. The leukocyte count is elevated in two thirds of patients and the platelet count is elevated in 50%.
What are the major criteria making the diagnosis of PV?	Elevated RBC mass (Hgb >18.5 g/dL for men and Hgb >16.5 g/dL for women), oxygen saturation >92%, splenomegaly
What are the minor criteria making the diagnosis of PV?	Leukocytosis, thrombocytosis, elevated LAP, and elevated B12 binding proteins
How is the diagnosis of PV made?	The presence of the three major criteria or the first two major criteria and two of the minor criteria are sufficient to make the diagnosis.

What is key in making the diagnosis of PV?

The key issue is distinguishing PV from other causes of reactive erythrocytosis, which is why the serum erythropoietin level is tested; it is usually markedly decreased in PV.

What is the median survival of patients with PV?

10 years with phlebotomy

What is the major cause of death in PV?

Thrombosis; less often, hemorrhage

Is there an increased risk for development of acute leukemia in PV?

Yes. This risk is not nearly as high as that seen with MDS, and it is often associated with attempts to treat the condition with alkylating agents or radioactive phosphorus.

What is the treatment for PV?

Phlebotomy to a hematocrit of $\leq 42\%$ to 45%. Aspirin is recommended for all patients who do not have a contraindication. Hydroxyurea is indicated if the patient's age is >40 years and there is a history of thrombosis or platelet count >400,000/μL. Anagrelide may be used to decrease the platelet count without the (debated) potential leukemogenic potential of hydroxyurea.

What is the "spent phase" of polycythemia?

The development of myelofibrosis with associated low cell counts and possible transfusion dependence. This state is indistinguishable from agnogenic myeloid metaplasia.

When is the spent phase seen, and how common is it?

The onset averages 10 years from diagnosis and occurs in approximately 15% of patients with PV. Increasing splenomegaly, anemia, and bone marrow fibrosis with associated leukoerythroblastic blood smear marks this phase.

How often is acute leukemia seen in patients in the "spent phase"?

Acute leukemia eventually develops in 25% to 50% of patients with this complication.

ESSENTIAL THROMBOCYTHEMIA

What is essential thrombocythemia?	A myeloproliferative disorder with persistent thrombocytosis (platelet count $>600 \times 10^9$/L) that is not reactive to another disorder and is not caused by another myeloproliferative disorder. Bone marrow biopsy shows megakaryocyte hyperplasia and clustering.
What are some of the common clinical problems in patients with essential thrombocythemia?	Arterial or venous thrombosis and hemorrhage (CVA, MI, digital ulceration, VTE, epistaxis, and gastrointestinal bleeding). Also headache, visual symptoms, and livedo reticularis.
What abnormalities are seen in the peripheral blood in essential thrombocythemia?	Thrombocytosis, often with very large platelets; leukocytosis (30% of cases); leukoerythroblastic blood smear (25% of cases); eosinophilia; and basophilia
What is the differential diagnosis for essential thrombocythemia?	Other myeloproliferative disorders, MDS (e.g., 5q-), and reactive thrombocytosis
What is the typical age of onset of essential thrombocythemia?	It is usually not seen until the sixth or seventh decade of life, but a cohort of young women in the fourth and fifth decades of life occasionally present with the condition.
What is the acute treatment for essential thrombocythemia?	For acute thrombosis: plateletpheresis is followed by administration of platelet-lowering drugs (hydroxyurea or anagrelide). For hemorrhage: platelets, then platelet-lowering drugs.
What defines a high-risk patient with essential thrombocytosis?	Age >60 years or history of thrombosis
What defines a low-risk patient with essential thrombocytosis?	Age <60 years, no history of thrombosis, and platelet count < 1,500,000/μL

What is the chronic treatment for essential thrombocythemia?	It is somewhat controversial for asymptomatic patients. Low-risk patients may not need therapy. In patients at high risk for thrombosis, the platelet count should be lowered into the normal range with hydroxyurea or anagrelide.
How does hydroxyurea work?	Hydroxyurea nonspecifically interferes with DNA synthesis.
How does anagrelide work	Anagrelide specifically blocks platelet production and does not have the (debated) leukemogenic potential of hydroxyurea.
Should aspirin be used in these patients?	Low-dose aspirin is also recommended in symptomatic or high-risk patients.

CHRONIC MYELOGENOUS LEUKEMIA

How is a leukemoid reaction distinguished from early CML?	The LAP is characteristically very low in CML and is markedly elevated in a leukemoid reaction.
What is the usual length of the chronic phase of untreated CML?	3 to 5 years
What is imatinib mesylate (Gleevec)?	A tyrosine kinase inhibitor that specifically targets the ABL tyrosine kinase
What is its effect in chronic phase CML?	It has shown dramatic effectiveness in restoring normal blood counts, causing loss of the Philadelphia chromosome as well as major reductions in *BCR-ABL* transcripts as measured by PCR DNA.
What brings about the progression from the chronic phase to the accelerated phase to the blast phase in CML?	Likely accumulation of additional genetic errors: new nonrandom cytogenetic abnormalities have been found in up to 80% of patients in the blast phase.

What changes occur at the onset of the accelerated phase of CML?

An elevated leukocyte count, persistent thrombocytosis, increase in percent blasts and promyelocytes in blood and bone marrow, increased splenomegaly, development of myelofibrosis and development of chloromas (focal leukemic tumors)

What is the clinical course of the accelerated phase of CML?

Usually, over a period of several months, transformation into the blast phase occurs.

What indicates the onset of the blast phase of CML?

>20% blasts in the peripheral blood or bone marrow

What is the usual phenotype of the CML blasts?

Usually myeloid but occasionally lymphoid. Treatment for each phenotype is different.

What is the treatment of the blast phase of CML?

Same as for de novo acute leukemia. With chemotherapy, some patients can be converted back into the chronic phase. The duration of partial or complete remission is usually short.

MYELOFIBROSIS WITH MYELOID METAPLASIA

What is myelofibrosis with myeloid metaplasia?

A neoplastic hematopoietic stem cell disorder characterized by bone marrow fibrosis, marked splenomegaly, extramedullary hematopoiesis, pancytopenia, and a leukoerythroblastic blood smear

What are some of the findings on peripheral smear in myelofibrosis with myeloid metaplasia?

Teardrop RBCs with nucleated RBCs, early myeloid forms including blasts, and large platelets

What is the differential diagnosis for myelofibrosis with myeloid metaplasia?

Other myeloproliferative disorders, metastatic carcinoma, lymphoma, hairy cell leukemia, MDSs, disseminated tuberculosis, and histoplasmosis

What is the treatment for myelofibrosis with myeloid metaplasia?

Supportive care with transfusions, growth factors, and antibiotics as needed. A trial of thalidomide and steroids may be offered to improve anemia and platelet counts. Hydroxyurea, splenectomy, and radiation therapy can palliate symptomatic splenomegaly.

What are the common causes of death attributable to agnogenic myeloid metaplasia?

MI or heart failure (30%), hemorrhage (25%), acute leukemia (20%), and infection (10%)

MYELODYSPLASTIC SYNDROMES

How does MDS commonly present?

Symptoms are attributable to cytopenias. Anemia results in weakness and congestive heart failure, for example, neutropenia results in infection, and thrombocytopenia results in bleeding.

What is the median survival of patients with MDS?

From approximately 6 years to 4 to 5 months.

What are the causes of death in patients with MDS?

Acute leukemia in 30% and cytopenias in 30%. The remainder die of unrelated comorbid conditions, as MDS is usually a disease of the elderly.

What are the most important prognostic factors for MDS?

Percentage of blasts in the bone marrow, presence of particular chromosomal abnormalities (e.g., deletions of chromosome 7, complex karyotypes), and presence of pancytopenia are the strongest predictors of a poor prognosis.

What clonal cytogenetic abnormality can portend a good prognosis for MDS?

5q-: the 5q-syndrome is classically seen in elderly women with transfusion-dependent anemia, thrombocytosis, and a normal leukocyte count.

What is the treatment of MDS for patients with the 5q- abnormality?

In patients with the 5q- abnormality with or without other chromosomal abnormalities, treatment with the immunomodulator lenalidomide may be offered.

What other chemotherapy may be offered for patients with a good performance status?

Hypomethylating agents such as 5-azacytidine or decitabine

When should BMT be considered?

In young patients requiring frequent transfusions or with excess blasts

What therapies can be offered when the MDS transforms to an acute leukemia?

Induction chemotherapy may be considered, but complete response rates are considerably less than in de novo acute leukemia and the overall prognosis is very poor.

SPLEEN AND LYMPH NODES

If the spleen is palpable, how much bigger than normal is it?

About 2.5 times

What infections commonly cause splenomegaly?

Epstein-Barr virus–mediated mononucleosis, viral hepatitis, malaria, and rickettsial infections

What are the common causes of lymphadenopathy?

Reactive to a systemic process: e.g., viral and certain bacterial infections (Epstein-Barr virus, HIV, syphilis)

Direct infiltration by pathogens: e.g., mycobacterial, fungal, or staphylococcal infections

Neoplasia: e.g., lymphomas, leukemias, and locally advanced or metastatic cancer

Miscellaneous: e.g., sarcoidosis or nonneoplastic lymphoid conditions

TRANSFUSION MEDICINE

Transfusion of 1 unit of packed RBCs should increase the patient's hematocrit by how much?

Approximately 3% per unit transfused, but this relationship may not hold for extremely large or small patients

When after the transfusion do delayed hemolytic transfusion reactions usually occur?

2 to 10 days

What is the cause of delayed hemolytic transfusion reactions?

An anamnestic increase in previously formed antibodies or the formation of new antibodies to minor antigens on the transfused RBCs

What types of antibodies cause delayed hemolytic transfusion reactions?

IgG. These antibodies are directed against blood group antigens other than the A and B antigens. These reactions are predominantly seen in individuals who were previously transfused.

What kind of hemolysis occurs in a delayed transfusion reaction?

Extravascular. The decrement in hematocrit is generally less than in an immediate transfusion reaction mediated by ABO incompatibility, which is intravascular.

What is the importance of the Rh RBC antigen system?

Rh-positive patients have an immunogenic D antigen on their RBCs. After exposure to Rh-positive RBCs, approximately 50% of Rh-negative individuals produce anti-D antibodies with resultant delayed transfusion reaction on subsequent transfusion of Rh-positive (D antigen–positive) blood.

HEMOSTASIS AND THROMBOSIS

Is FXII a necessary enzyme in the cascade?

Not in vivo, but to make blood clot in vitro where tissue factor is not available, FXII is a necessary protein. Patients with FXII deficiency do not bleed spontaneously and are at no higher risk for bleeding during surgical procedures.

APPROACH TO BLEEDING DISORDERS

What are the four broad categories of bleeding disorders?

Disorders arising from platelet dysfunction, clotting factor deficiency or dysfunction, vascular dysfunction (e.g., connective tissue diseases), or hyperfibrinolysis

What is platelet-type bleeding?

Bleeding at mucocutaneous sites, multiple small bruises, and immediate bleeding after trauma or surgery

What disorders are associated with platelet-related bleeding?

Thrombocytopenia, platelet function defects, and vWD

What is clotting factor–type bleeding?

Soft tissue bleeding with occasional large bruises or hematomas and delayed bleeding after trauma or surgery

What are the causes of clotting factor–type bleeding?

Hemophilia A (FVIII deficiency), hemophilia B (FIX deficiency), hemophilia C (FXI deficiency), and other rare deficiencies of FII, FV, FVII, FX, and fibrinogen

What factor deficiency is associated with delayed bleeding and poor wound healing and normal PT and PTT?

FXIII

How is bleeding associated with FXIII deficiency treated?

Cryoprecipitate

What suggests the presence of a true bleeding disorder in patients with easy bruisability?

Spontaneous bruising (i.e., bruising not associated with trauma), bruising located on the trunk or in other areas not typically prone to ordinary trauma, large size of bruises, and long period of time for bruising to resolve

What bleeding disorders may be associated with an isolated prolonged PT?

FVII and vitamin K deficiencies, warfarin use, and liver dysfunction. Deficiencies of FII, FV, FX, and fibrinogen are usually associated with prolongation of both the PT and aPTT.

What bleeding disorders may be associated with an isolated prolongation of the aPTT?

Deficiencies of FVIII, FIX, and FXI, and vWD (due to coexistence of FVIII deficiency)

What bleeding disorders may be associated with a prolongation of the PT and aPTT?

Simultaneous deficiency of multiple factors, as seen with liver disease, vitamin K deficiency, malnutrition, and DIC. Rarer causes include isolated deficiencies or acquired inhibitors of factors II, V, and X, or fibrinogen.

What does the ACT assay measure?

The clotting time of whole blood in the presence of an activating substance. This allows for a quick bedside assessment of anticoagulant (typically heparin) adequacy.

What are some disorders that can prolong the bleeding time?

vWD, platelet function defects (e.g., Bernard-Soulier syndrome), essential thrombocythemia, paraproteinemias, microangiopathic hemolytic anemias, uremia, and dysfibrinogenemia

What is cryoprecipitate?

A concentrate of plasma enriched in vWF/FVIII, FXIII, and fibrinogen

What is the treatment for acute bleeding in a patient with FXI deficiency?

Fresh-frozen plasma; FXI concentrates are available in some other countries.

What are the common causes of bleeding in patients with cirrhosis?

Thrombocytopenia, coagulation factor deficiencies (both from impaired synthetic function and vitamin K deficiency), platelet dysfunction, low-grade DIC, and increased fibrinolysis

von Willebrand's Disease

What is the function of vWF?

vWF mediates adhesion of platelets to the vessel wall basement membrane after vascular injury, and is the carrier protein for FVIII.

What laboratory tests are used in testing for vWD?

vWF and FVIII antigen levels, ristocetin cofactor activity, and vWF multimer testing

What does the ristocetin cofactor activity measure?

It is an approximation of vWF function.

What are the 4 types of vWD?

Type 1
Type 2
Type 3
Platelet type

Describe the abnormality with type 1 vWD:

Quantitative decrease in levels of functionally normal vWF

How common is type 1 vWD?

This subtype is the most common, comprising 70% to 80% of cases.

Describe the abnormality of type 2 vWD:

Qualitative abnormalities of vWF

How common is type 2 vWD?

This subtype comprises 15% to 30% of vWD cases. There are several subtypes of type 2.

Describe the abnormality of type 3 vWD:

Absence of vWF

How common is type 3 vWD?

This is a rare form and may be associated with profound bleeding problems.

Describe the abnormality of platelet type vWD:

The platelet receptor for vWF (glycoprotein Ib) has increased affinity for vWF, resulting in increased clearance of plasma vWF.

Why is it important to distinguish type 2B vWD and platelet type vWD from all other types of vWD?

Because administration of DDAVP can cause thrombocytopenia in patients with these subtypes

How is vWD inherited?

Usually autosomal dominant, but patients with type 3 may be autosomal recessive or doubly heterozygous. In contrast, hemophilia A and B are X-linked.

What is the treatment of bleeding in patients with type 1 vWD?

Desmopressin (DDAVP)

How is bleeding treated in patients who cannot receive or do not respond to DDAVP?

FVIII concentrates. For major operations or life-threatening hemorrhage, these concentrates should be given to all subtypes.

When should cryoprecipitate be used to treat vWD?

In an emergency when DDAVP is not appropriate and when no virally inactivated intermediate-purity factor VIII product is available

What are the adverse effects of DDAVP?

DDAVP may be contraindicated in certain subtypes of vWD. DDAVP can cause hyponatremia, facial flushing, minor alterations in blood pressure, nausea, and headache.

What is the most common cause of aPTT prolongation in severe vWD?

FVIII deficiency. FVIII circulates attached to vWF. In the absence of vWF, the half-life of FVIII is shortened.

THROMBOTIC DISORDERS

Under what circumstances should a hypercoagulable state be suspected?

Thrombosis without a precipitating risk factor, thrombosis at a young age, recurrent thromboses, thrombosis in an unusual location (e.g., upper extremity, portal vein, mesenteric vein, cerebral vein), a family history of thrombosis, and resistance to anticoagulation with heparin or warfarin

What are the known common inherited hypercoagulable states?	APC resistance (FV Leiden mutation), prothrombin (FII) gene mutation, protein C deficiency, protein S deficiency, AT III deficiency, dysfibrinogenemia, and hyperhomocysteinemia. More than 30% of patients who clinically appear to have an inherited hypercoagulable state currently have no identifiable abnormality.
What are the two most common inherited disorders associated with an increased risk of venous thrombosis?	APC resistance (FV Leiden mutation), and prothrombin (FII) gene mutation
How is APC resistance diagnosed?	Patient plasma demonstrates decreased prolongation of the aPTT compared with that of normal subjects after the addition of APC. Alternately, genetic studies can be ordered to screen for the FV Leiden mutation.
What acquired conditions are associated with a hypercoagulable state?	Malignancy, myeloproliferative disorders, PNH, connective tissue diseases (e.g., SLE, rheumatoid arthritis, etc.) and other inflammatory conditions, antiphospholipid antibody syndrome, hyperviscosity states (e.g., paraproteinemia and untreated PV), HITT, TTP/HUS, DIC
How is protein C activated?	After binding to endothelial cell thrombomodulin, thrombin cleaves protein C, generating APC.
What does protein S do?	Protein S is a cofactor to APC.

Antiphospholipid Antibody Syndrome

What is the antiphospholipid antibody syndrome?	A disorder where the patient has a history of thromboembolic events or pregnancy mishaps—e.g., recurrent spontaneous abortions—as well as autoantibodies to complexes of phospholipids and plasma proteins

What is lupus anticoagulant?

Autoantibodies against phospholipid-protein complexes. Their presence is inferred from abnormalities in various phospholipid-dependent clotting tests (e.g., aPTT).

What are anticardiolipin or beta-2-glycoprotein-1 antibodies?

Antibodies measured in serum with specificities toward a specific phospholipid, cardiolipin, or to beta-2-glycoprotein-1.

When are antiphospholipid antibodies clinically meaningful?

In the setting of a thromboembolic event or recurrent miscarriage, they are suggestive of a hypercoagulable state; if the antiphospholipid antibody persists, long-term anticoagulation should be considered.

How do you diagnose antiphospholipid syndrome?

The American College of Rheumatology classification involves one clinical (vascular thrombosis or frequent miscarriages) and one lab criterion listed above.

Disseminated Intravascular Coagulation

What is DIC?

DIC is a syndrome in which diffuse activation of coagulation factors overwhelm the body's normal anticoagulant regulatory systems, leading to excessive fibrin formation and platelet activation, followed by depletion of clotting factors and platelets.

What is the clinical result of DIC?

Diffuse microvascular clot formation with organ damage and dysfunction, followed by clinical hemorrhage. Sequentially, the fibrinolytic system becomes activated, lysing thrombi and exacerbating hemorrhage.

What are the common causes of DIC?

Sepsis, head trauma, cancer, abruptio placentae, amniotic fluid embolism, fat embolism, eclampsia, snake bites, viral and rickettsial infections, and collagen vascular diseases

How is the diagnosis of DIC made?

In the appropriate clinical setting, prolongation of the PT, elevation of the D-dimer titer with thrombocytopenia, and hypofibrinogenemia. Serial measurements of the variables listed are usually helpful.

ANTICOAGULATION

What are the most commonly used anticoagulants in the United States?

Heparin, low-molecular-weight heparins (enoxaparin, dalteparin, tinzaparin), and warfarin. In the inpatient setting, direct thrombin inhibitors (argatroban, lepirudin, bivalirudin) are commonly used. The pentasaccharide fondaparinux is becoming more commonly used, and oral DTIs are in development.

How is low-molecular-weight heparin different from standard heparin?

Smaller fragments of heparin interact with ATIII to have greater inhibition of FXa and lesser inhibition of thrombin. Their pharmacokinetics are more predictable than that of unfractionated heparin.

How are the effects of low-molecular-weight heparins or fondaparinux monitored?

They are dosed in a weight-based fashion and normally do not need monitoring. If necessary, inhibition of FXa may be assayed.

Why should the platelet count be monitored if a patient is receiving heparin or low-molecular-weight heparins?

To monitor for the development of HITT

What platelet counts should signal the consideration of HIT/T?

A platelet count drop of >50% from baseline

Why is HITT such an important illness to diagnose?

This is a disorder in which limb- or life-threatening thrombosis can occur. If HIT/T is suspected then all heparin and/or low molecular weight heparin must be stopped

In patients with HITT, how is anticoagulation handled?

The patient must be covered with a DTI until the platelet count begins to rise. After the acute risk of thrombosis has passed, the DTI may be transitioned to warfarin.

What is the risk of thrombosis in patients with HITT?

30% or higher

How long should patients remain on warfarin once diagnosed with HITT?

At least 4 weeks even if no thrombosis is evident

What laboratory tests can be done to confirm the diagnosis of HITT?

^{14}C-serotonin release assay has a positive predictive value near 100%, but a negative predictive value of only 20%. The use of ELISA assays for antiplatelet factor 4 (PF4) antibodies has a positive predictive value of 93% for a definitive diagnosis and a negative predictive value of 95%.

How can the effect of warfarin be reversed?

Administration of vitamin K orally or intravenously. For bleeding, plasma or a concentrate of vitamin K–dependent clotting factors may be given. Recombinant FVIIa can be given, which in pharmacologic doses directly activates factor X to bypass the need for clotting factors higher in the cascade.

How do the direct thrombin inhibitors differ from heparin?

ATIII is not a necessary cofactor: thrombin inhibitors inactivate thrombin and only thrombin.

How are the direct thrombin inhibitors monitored?

By aPTT or ACT

How are the effects of direct thrombin inhibitors reversed?

None of the currently available thrombin inhibitors are reversible. If a patient is bleeding he or she must be supported with fluids and/or blood products until the drugs have been cleared from the body.

Infectious Disease

ABBREVIATIONS

AIDS	Acquired immune deficiency syndrome
ALT	Alanine aminotransferase
APH	Acute pulmonary histoplasmosis
AST	Aspartate aminotransferase
BSI	Bloodstream infection
CAP	Community-acquired pneumonia
CBC	Complete blood count
CMV	Cytomegalovirus
CNS	Central nervous system
CoNS	Coagulase-negative staphylococcus aureus
CPH	Chronic pulmonary histoplasmosis
CPK	Creatine phosphokinase
CSF	Cerebrospinal fluid
CT	Computed tomography
DEET	Diethyltoluamide
EBV	Epstein-Barr virus
ELISA	Enzyme-linked immunosorbent assay
ESR	Erythrocyte sedimentation rate
FTA-ABS	Fluorescent treponemal antibody, absorbed
FUO	Fever of unknown origin
GC	Gonococcus
GU	Gonococcal urethritis
HIV	Human immunodeficiency virus
HPF	High-power field
HSV	Herpes simplex virus
Ig	Immunoglobulin
INH	Isoniazid
IVDAs	Intravenous drug abusers
KOH	Potassium hydroxide
LFT	Liver function test
MAC	*Mycobacterium avium* complex
MHA-TP	Microhemagglutination–*Treponema pallidum*
MRI	Magnetic resonance imaging
MRSA	Methicillin-resistant *Staphylococcus aureus*
NGU	Nongonococcal urethritis
NK	Natural killer
PCP	*Pneumocystis jiroveci* pneumonia
PCR	Polymerase chain reaction
PDH	Progressive disseminated histoplasmosis
PET	Positron emission tomography
PID	Pelvic inflammatory disease
PMN	Polymorphonuclear neutrophil
PZA	Pyrazinamide
RMSF	Rocky Mountain spotted fever

RPR	Rapid plasma reagin
SBP	Spontaneous bacterial peritonitis
SIRS	Systemic inflammatory response syndrome
SLE	Systemic lupus erythematosus
STD	Sexually transmitted disease
TSS	Toxic shock syndrome
UTI	Urinary tract infection
VDRL	Venereal Disease Research Laboratory
VRE	Vancomycin-resistant enterococcus
VZV	Varicella zoster virus
WBC	White blood cell

DIAGNOSTIC METHODS

What is PCR?
Polymerase chain reaction. It uses the enzyme DNA polymerase to increase (amplify) the number of copies of DNA or RNA in a sample. PCR is very sensitive because only a few copies of genetic material (and not whole organisms) need to be present. It is useful for organisms that are difficult to culture (including HIV).

What is serologic testing used for?
To diagnose infection when the pathogen cannot be cultured. It measures acute and convalescent sera to detect a fourfold increase in titer (synonymous with recent infection). Diagnosis can be made only retrospectively.

ANTIMICROBIAL THERAPY

GENERAL PRINCIPLES

In which diseases is bactericidal therapy mandatory?
Meningitis, endocarditis, brain abscess, osteomyelitis, and neutropenia

What are reasons for antimicrobial treatment failure?
Development of resistance in vivo, superinfection, decreased activity at the site of infection (e.g., necrotic tissue, foreign body, and lack of penetration into abscess), impaired immune host defenses, improper dosing, and altered pharmacokinetics secondary to drug interactions

What is pharmacodynamics?

Pharmacodynamics describes the biochemical and physiologic effects of the drug and its mechanism of action.

What makes an antimicrobial agent *bacteriostatic?*

It is bacteriostatic if it inhibits growth and replication.

What makes an antimicrobial agent *bacteriocidal?*

It is bacteriocidal if it causes bacterial cell death.

What determines whether a drug is bacteriostatic or bacteriocidal?

The antimicrobial concentration at the site of action

What is the MIC_{90}?

The minimum concentration of an antimicrobial that is inhibitory for 90% of all isolates of a bacterial species

What is concentration-dependent killing of bacteria?

Antibiotics that develop high concentrations at the bacteria binding site have concentration-dependent killing where peak/MIC ratio is critical.

What are the concentration-dependent killing agents?

Fluoroquinolones, aminoglycosides, macrolides, azalides, ketolides, and metronidazole

What is time-dependent (concentration-independent) killing of bacteria?

Antibiotics that spend an extensive amount of time bond to a bacteria. Therefore, the time the antibiotic is bound to the bacteria at greater than MIC is critical.

What are the time-dependent killing agents?

Penicillins, cephalosporins, aztreonam, vancomycin, carbapenams, linezolid, and clindamycin

ANTIBACTERIAL AGENTS

Note: General statements regarding antimicrobial susceptibilities are difficult owing to changing resistance patterns. Consideration of individual organism and local resistance patterns is needed in selecting appropriate antimicrobial therapy.

What is the mechanism of action of penicillins and other beta lactams?

Inhibition of bacterial cell wall synthesis

What are the other beta-lactam antimicrobials?

Cephalosporins, carbapenems, and monobactams

What is the only monobactam?

Aztreonam

What is the most common method of resistance to penicillins and other beta lactams?

Beta-lactamase production

How do beta lactamases work?

They covalently react with the beta lactam ring and hydrolyze it, causing destruction of the activity of the drug.

What are the three beta-lactamase inhibitors?

Clavulanate, sulbactam, and tazobactam

What are the combination beta-lactam/beta-lactamase inhibitor antimicrobials?

Amoxicillin-clavulanate (Augmentin), ticarcillin-clavulanate (Timentin), ampicillin-sulbactam (Unasyn), pipercillin-tazobactam (Zosyn)

What is the incidence of hypersensitivity reactions with penicillins?

Allergic reactions from penicillins occur with a frequency of 7 to 40 of every 1000 penicillin treatment courses.

Name the four types of penicillin hypersensitivity reactions.

Type 1 (IgE)—urticaria, angioedema, anaphylaxis. Occurs in 4 to 15 of every 100,000 penicillin treatment courses; fatality occurs once in every 32,000 to 100,000 treatment courses.

Type 2 (IgG, cytotoxic antibodies)—hemolytic anemia

Type 3 (immune complexes)—serum sickness

Type 4 (cell-mediated)—contact dermatitis, idiopathic maculopapular rash, interstitial nephritis, drug fever, eosinophilia, exfoliative dermatitis, Stevens-Johnson syndrome

Through what routes is vancomycin absorbed?

Vancomycin is effective in systemic infections only if given intravenously. The oral form does not have significant systemic absorption; it is effective only against *Clostridium difficile,* since the site of action is in the GI tract.

What is the antimicrobial activity of daptomycin?

A lipopeptide antibiotic with broad gram-positive activity including MRSA and VRE. Currently approved for skin infections, bacteremia, and endocarditis.

What is the antimicrobial activity of tigecycline?

It is a glycylcycline antibiotic (related to the tetracyclines) with activity against gram positives (including MRSA and VRE), enteric pathogens, and anaerobes. It is bacterostatic and not active against *Pseudomonas.*

ANTIMYCOBACTERIAL AGENTS

What is the management of antimycobacterial drug induced hepatotoxicity?

If transaminase levels increase to more than five times upper limits of normal, INH, rifampin, and PZA should be discontinued in favor of an alternative regimen. Possible hepatotoxic drugs are reintroduced one at a time to identify the offending agent.

ANTIFUNGAL AGENTS

What toxicities are associated with amphotericin B?

Dose-dependent decrease in glomerular filtration rate, potassium and bicarbonate wasting (renal tubular acidosis), decreased erythropoietin production, nausea, vomiting, phlebitis, and acute reactions

What acute reactions are associated with amphotericin B infusions?

Chills, fever, tachypnea, hypoxemia, and hypotension may occur 30 minutes after beginning infusion.

What premedication regimen may reduce these side effects?

Premedication with acetaminophen, hydrocortisone, or meperidine may diminish reactions.

What is the antimicrobial spectrum of fluconazole?

Most *Candida* species, *C. neoformans,* and coccidioidomycoses

What is the antimicrobial spectrum of itraconazole?

Blastomycosis and histoplasmosis. Itraconazole may have a role for *Aspergillus* infections when amphotericin B fails or cannot be administered.

What is the antimicrobial spectrum of ketoconazole?

Histoplasmosis and blastomycosis. Ketoconazole is not used commonly because of its side effects. Itraconazole is equally or more effective and less toxic. Newer triazoles with activity against *Aspergillus* sp. are in development.

What is the indication for echinocandin caspofungin?

Refractory invasive *Aspergillus* infection. It also has significant activity against *Candida* sp.

What is the antimicrobial spectrum of voriconazole?

In vitro and in vivo activity has been shown against *Aspergillus* spp. as well as other molds; also active against most *Candida* spp.

What are the indications for the echinocandins (caspofungin, micafungin, and anidulafungin)?

In general, candidemia and esophageal candidiasis. Caspofungin also indicated for febrile neutropenia and refractory invasive *Aspergillus.*

ANTIVIRAL AGENTS

What are the indications for ganciclovir?

Treatment and chronic suppression of invasive CMV disease (e.g., retinitis, pneumonia, and gastroenteritis) in immunocompromised patients

What are the indications for foscarnet?

Progressive CMV disease caused by ganciclovir-resistant strains. It is used most often in AIDS patients with refractory CMV retinitis.

What are the indications for cidofovir?

Refractory CMV retinitis. Its role in the treatment of other CMV diseases and other viral infections is being evaluated.

What is the indication for valganciclovir?

CMV retinitis is currently the only indication.

PATHOGENS

BACTERIA

What are the two main superantigens asscociated with staphylococcal toxic shock syndrome?	Toxic shock syndrome toxin-1 (TSST-1) and staphylococcal enterotoxins
What are the clinical signs and symptoms associated with staphylococcal toxic shock syndrome?	Fever, hypotension, diffuse macular rash that subsequently desquamates, with three of the following organ involvements: liver, blood, renal, mucous membranes, GI, muscular, central nervous system
What is the treatment for staph TSS?	Antibiotics, usually nafcillin or vancomycin if MRSA; IVIg (to help neutralize the superantigen activity of the staphylococcal toxins), intravenous fluids and vasopressors if needed
What groups of patients are at increased risk for *S. aureus* infections?	Hemodialysis, peritoneal dialysis, HIV-infected, IVDAs, diabetics, and alcoholics
What is the pyogenic staph infection of the apocrine sweat glands?	Hidradenitis suppurativa
S. aureus accounts for what percentage of infective endocarditis?	*S. aureus* is responsible for approximately 30% of native valve endocarditis; 70% of endocarditis in IVDAs, and about 20% of those with early or late prosthetic valve endocarditis.
What percentage of CAP or hospital-associated pneumonias are due to _S. aureus_?	*S. aureus* is responsible for less than 10% of CAP but accounts for around 30% of hospital-associated pneumonias.
What percentage of osteomyelitis is caused by _S. aureus_?	Osteomyelitis due to *S. aureus* accounts for 50% to 70% of cases.

What are some of the major infections caused by coagulase-negative staph?	Bacteremia, osteomyelitis, native valve endocarditis, infections of indwelling foreign devices such as prosthetic valve endocarditis and central venous catheters
What drug is most commonly used to treat CoNS infections?	Because CoNS is usually resitant to multiple antibiotics, vancomycin is the drug of choice
What species of *Streptococcus* is Lancefield group A?	*Strep. pyogenes*
What is the hemolytic reaction associated with group A strep?	Beta hemolysis
***Strep. pyogenes* is associated with what major clinical syndromes?**	Pharyngitis, skin/soft tissue and respiratory infections
What species of *Streptococcus* is Lancefield group B?	*Strep. agalactiae*
What is the hemolytic reaction(s) associated with group B strep?	Beta and gamma hemolysis
***Strep agalactiae* is associated with what major clinical syndromes?**	Chorioamnionitis, puerperal sepsis, bloodstream infections in nonpregnant adults
What species are included in the viridans streptococcal group?	This includes the *anginosus*, *bovis*, *mutans*, *salivarius*, and *mitis* species groups.
***Streptococcus pneumoniae* is associated commonly with what clinical syndromes?**	Otitis media, sinusitis, meningitis, community-acquired pneumonia
***Enterococcus* species often have what effect on blood agar?**	Nonhemolysis (or gamma hemolysis)

Enterococci are commonly found where in humans?

As a part of the normal gut flora

What are some common clinical syndromes associated with *Enterococcus* species?

Urinary tract infections (most common), bacteremia and endocarditis, intra-abdominal/pelvic infections, and rarely, wound and tissue infections, meningitis, or respiratory tract infections

Infection with *Listeria monocytogenes* occurs most commonly how?

Ingestion of organisms in a contaminated food source

Why are pregnant women at increased risk for *Listeria* bacteremia?

Because of to a mild impairment of cell-mediated immunity that occurs during pregnancy

During which trimester are they most at risk?

The third trimester

What clinical syndromes other than bacteremia are associated with *Listeria*?

Meningitis, brain abscess, and endocarditis

What is the most common cause of UTI?

Escherichia coli

What are the *E. coli* pathogens that cause diarrhea?

ETEC (enterotoxigenic *E. coli*), EPEC (enteropathogenic *E. coli*), EHEC (enterohemorrhagic *E. coli*), EAEC (enteroaggregative *E. coli*), EIEC (enteroinvasive *E. coli*), DAEC (diffuse adhering *E. coli*)

What are zoonoses?

Infections caused in humans by a variety of pathogens that usually infect nonhuman animals

What zoonosis is commonly transmitted from ingestion of unpatsteurized dairy products?

Brucellosis

What pathogen is commonly isolated from humans bitten by cats or dogs?

Pasteurella

What is the etiologic agent of the plague?	*Yersinia pestis*
What are some of the common animal reservoirs for *Yersinia*?	Rats, ground squirrels, prairie dogs, and field mice
What disease is characterized by the development of a primary cutaneous papule or pustule at the site of inoculation along with regional ipsilateral lymphadenopathy?	Cat scratch disease
What is the causative agent of cat scratch disease?	*Bartonella henselae*
What is the etiologic agent of Lyme disease?	*Borrelia burgdorferi*
What is the time of onset to the three stages of Lyme disease after the initial exposure?	Stage I (early): up to a month Stage II (disseminated): weeks to months Stage III (late): years
What is the classic skin finding in localized stage I Lyme disease?	Erythema migrans
What are the classic findings in stage II Lyme disease?	Cardiac (myocarditis, heart block), neurologic (aseptic meningitis, Bell's palsy, encephalitis), and dermatologic (many annular skin lesions)
What are the classic findings in stage III Lyme disease?	Arthritis and neuroborreliosis
Approximately how long must a tick be attached to a human in order to cause an infection?	Tick attachement for greater than 24 to 36 hours is usually needed to cause infection.

How is Lyme disease diagnosed?

The combination of clinical picture, exposure history in an endemic area, and positive antibody response to *B. burgdorferi* (ELISA and if positive, checking a confirmatory Western blot)

What are the two types of human ehrlichisosis infections?

Human monocytic ehrlichiosis (*Ehrlichia chaffenesis* infects monocytes)

Human granulocytic ehrlichiosis (*Anaplasma phagocytophilum* infects granulocytes)

Human ehrlichiosis is transmitted by what tick?

The Lone Star tick (human monocytic ehrlichiosis caused by *E. chaffeensis*)

The tick *Ixodes scapularis* (human granulocytic ehrlichiosis caused by *A. phagocytophilum*)

What is seen on peripheral blood smear in 1% to 2% of circulating leukocytes in those with human ehrlichiosis?

Morulae (cytoplasmic vacuoles containing *Ehrlichia* organisms)

What is the causative agent of Rocky Mountain spotted fever (RMSF)?

Rickettsia rickettsii

What are the prominent clinical symptoms of RMSF?

Fever, headache, rash

Where on the body does the rash associated with RMSF usually appear?

It usually begins around the wrists and ankles.

When does the rash usually appear with RMSF?

3 to 5 days after the onset of fever

How is the diagnosis of RMSF made?

Treatment decisions are based on clinical grounds and history consistent with possible tick exposure in an endemic area. Serologic testing can check for acute and convalescent antibody titers.

What is a vector-borne disease found in New England that is screened for in blood donor samples from endemic areas?	Babesiosis
What is babesiosis caused by?	*Babesia microti*
How is babesiosis treated?	Clindamycin plus quinine or atovaquone plus azithromycin
What bacilli commonly stain "acid fast"?	Mycobacterial species and *Nocardia*
What is the most common mode of transmission of *Mycobacterium tuberculosis*?	Airborne droplets
The tubercle bacilli transmitted in airborne droplets begin multiplication where in the lungs?	Terminal air spaces
The initial pulmonary focus or tuberculosis is where?	The initial focus is unsually solitary and found in the subpleura and in the midlung zone (lower upper lobe or upper/lower/middle lobes)
How are the types of tuberculosis infections classified?	Primary Superinfection Reactivation
How does the primary infection present?	Occurs as part of the initial infection (when the mycobacteria are not contained by the host's defense mechanisms) and presents as pneumonia or miliary disease.
What is the TB superinection?	Occurs when a patient is already infected with TB but is reexposed to a high quantity of mycobacteria. Pulmonary cavitary disease is seen.

What is TB reactivation?

Occurs years after the initial infection when there is a decline in cell-mediated immunity (as seen with normal aging, malignancy, and HIV)

How long from exposure does the tuberculin skin test turn positive?

3 to 8 weeks

What treatment regimen should be started for TB infection?

An initial four-drug regimen including isoniazid, rifampin, pyrazinamide, and ethambutol or streptomycin. Once the resistance pattern of the TB isolate is known, the therapy can be tailored more specifically.

What is the most common atypical mycobacterial lung infection in the United States?

Mycobacterium avium complex (MAC)

VIRUSES

Herpesviruses

Name the herpesviruses.

HSV-1 and 2, VZV, CMV, EBV, human herpesviruses 6, 7, and 8, and herpesvirus simiae

What are the clinical syndromes associated with HSV 1 and HSV 2?

Mucocutaneous infections (oral-facial and genital), CNS infection, and rarely, visceral organ involvement

What are the clinical manifestations of HSV encephalitis?

HSV encephalitis (typically HSV-1) is characterized by the acute onset of fever and focal neurologic (esp. temporal lobe) symptoms.

What is herpetic whitlow?

HSV infection of the finger

Varicella Zoster Virus

What diseases are associated with VZV?

Primary infection—varicella (chickenpox)

Recurrent infection—herpes zoster (shingles)

Cytomegalovirus

What are the clinical manifestations of congenital CMV infection?

Congenital infection—three fourths of patients are asymptomatic. Symptoms include jaundice, hepatosplenomegaly, petechiae, and CNS involvement.

What are the clinical manifestations of CMV mononucleosis?

CMV mononucleosis—like EBV-related mononucleosis, with fever, mild lymphadenopathy, lymphocytosis, increased liver enzymes, and splenomegaly

What are the potential complications of CMV infection?

Interstitial pneumonitis, hepatitis, Guillain-Barré syndrome, meningoencephalitis, myocarditis, thrombocytopenia and hemolysis, retinitis, and gastrointestinal disease

Papillomaviruses

What are routes of transmission for papillomaviruses?

Close personal contact; anogenital warts are the most common STDs.

Influenza

What are the clinical manifestations of influenza virus infection?

In uncomplicated influenza, incubation is 1 to 2 days followed by abrupt onset of fever, chills, headache, myalgias, malaise, dry cough, and anorexia.

What are the two primary pulmonary complications of influenza?

Primary influenza pneumonia

Secondary bacterial pneumonia

Rapid diagnostic tests for influenza are based on what?

Immunologic detection of viral antigens on respiratory secretions including nasal/throat swab specimens or from a nasal wash

What other complications of influenza can occur?

Other pulmonary processes, myositis, TSS, Guillain-Barré syndrome, and Reye's syndrome

What is the treatment for influenza?

For uncomplicated influenza A, amantadine or rimantadine. Oseltamivir and zanamivir are available for treatment of influenza A and B.

Who should receive the influenza vaccine?

Persons at increased risk of complications from influenza, including persons above 50 years of age, residents of chronic care facilities, and persons with underlying chronic pulmonary or cardiovascular disease, significant metabolic disorders, hemoglobinopathies, renal dysfunction, or immunosuppression. Health-care workers and other persons who provide care to individuals at risk should also be immunized.

Enteroviruses

Name the enteroviruses.

Coxsackieviruses, echoviruses, and enteroviruses

Hepatitis Viruses

Hepatitis A

What type of virus is associated with hepatitis A infection?

RNA picornavirus

How is hepatitis A transmitted?

Fecal–oral route, person-to-person contact, and contaminated food or water

How can hepatitis A infection be prevented?

Avoiding contaminated food/water.

Vaccination is effective if given 2 weeks before travel, otherwise, if possible exposure is anticipated in less than 2 weeks, serum immune globulin can be given to prevent infection.

Hepatitis B

How is hepatitis B transmitted?

Parenterally (IVDAs, blood transfusions), sexual contact, and perinatally. It is not transmitted by the fecal–oral route.

What is the incubation period after exposure to hepatitis B?	1 to 4 months
Which transaminase is usually higher in acute hep B: AST or ALT?	ALT
What is the best indicator of prognosis in those with acute hep B?	PT (prothrombin time)
Acute hep B is diagnosed by evidence of elevation of what viral markers?	The detection of HBsAg, anti-HB$_c$ IgM, HB$_e$Ag (hepatitis B e antigen), and HBV DNA
What viral markers indicate past infection with hepatitis B (immunity through infection)?	Presence of anti-HBsAg, and anti-HB$_c$Ag IgG
What viral markers indicate immunity through vaccination?	Anti-HBsAg
What defines chronic hepatitis B?	The presence of HBsAg for more than 6 months
What is the seroconversion rate for healthy adults and children to the hepatitis B vaccine?	Greater than 90%

Hepatitis C

What are the hepatitis C genotypes?	1b, 1a, 3a, 2b, 2a, 3, 4a, 2, 2c, 4, 1, 5a, other (in order of decreasing frequency)
What are the most common genotypes of hepatitis C in the United States?	60% to 70% of genotypes are of types 1a or 1b
What is the average incubation period for acute hepatitis C?	7 weeks

What are the ways hepatitis C is transmitted?

By IVDAs, sexual contact, and perinatal transmission

What percentage of those with acute hepatitis C develop chronic infection?

50% to 85%

How is the diagnosis of hepatitis C infection made?

Enzyme immunoassay measuring antibodies to recombinant HCV polypeptides, HC viral load to evaluate for persistent infection

How are genotypes used in the treatment of hepatitis C?

As a predictor to response to therapy

Hepatitis D

What is the mode of transmission of hepatitis D?

Primarily the parenteral route, less often by sexual contact, and rarely perinatally

FUNGI

Candida

What are the major *Candida* species?

Candida albicans, glabrata, and *parapsilosis* are the three main pathogens for both bloodstream and mucosal infections.

Aspergillus

Who is most at risk for infections with *Aspergillus* species?

Neutropenic patients, recipients of organ or bone marrow transplantation, those with chronic immunosuppression and acquired or congenital immunodeficiency syndromes

Infection or colonization with *Aspergillus* species may result in what types of diseases?

Allergic bronchopulmonary aspergillosis (allergic response to the *Aspergillus* colonization of airways in patients with asthma or cystic fibrosis), pulmonary aspergilloma, and invasive aspergillosis

Cryptococcus

What types of cryptococcal infections affect immunocompromised patients (in particular AIDS patients or solid organ transplant recipients)?

Invasive fungal infection due to *Cryptococcus neoformans,* which most commonly causes meningoencephalitis or pneumonia. However, cryptococcal infections have been reported in most organ systems.

In addition to starting antifungal therapy for AIDS patients with cryptococcal meningoencephalitis, what else should be done?

Monitoring the opening pressure recorded on the lumbar puncture. It is often elevated in cryptococcal meningoencephalitis. The goal opening pressure should be less than 200 mm water. Daily lumbar punctures may be needed and can be discontinued once the opening pressure is within the normal range for several days.

Histoplasma

Name the three clinically important histoplasmosis syndromes.

APH (acute pulmonary histoplasmosis), CPH (chronic pulmonary histoplasmosis), and PDH (progressive disseminated histoplasmosis)

What are the clinical features of acute pulmonary histoplasmosis?

Patients are asymptomatic in 90% of cases. Symptoms include fever, headache, malaise, and nonproductive cough after a 3- to 21-day incubation period.

What are the symptoms of CPH?

Persistent cough, weight loss, malaise, low-grade fevers, and night sweats over several weeks. Symptoms may mimic those of tuberculosis.

What are the clinical manifestations of PDH?

Severity of PDH ranges from acute illness to more chronic disease lasting for months to years. Manifestations may include hepatosplenomegaly with abnormal LFTs, gastrointestinal mucosal ulcerations, oropharyngeal ulcers, adrenal insufficiency, anemia, interstitial pneumonitis, and renal involvement. More rarely, CNS disease, lytic bone lesions, and lymphadenopathy occur.

Blastomyces

What are the pulmonary manifestations of the following:

    Acute pulmonary blastomycosis? — Typically influenza-like with fevers, arthralgias, myalgias, and cough

    What are the radiographic findings of acute pulmonary blastomycosis? — Chest radiograph is nonspecific, often with localized consolidation; hilar adenopathy is rare.

    Chronic pulmonary blastomycosis? — Cough, sputum production, weight loss, hemoptysis, dyspnea, pleuritic chest pain

    What are the radiographic findings of chronic pulmonary blastomycosis? — Nonspecific radiographic findings

How is the diagnosis of blastomycosis made? — Culture of fungus. A presumptive diagnosis can be made from some histopathologic specimens based on morphology and staining characteristics.

Sporothrix

What are the clinical manifestations of sporotrichosis? — Primarily cutaneous. A papule, chancre, or subcutaneous nodule develops at the site of a traumatic inoculation. Secondary nodules, which often ulcerate and drain, develop along regional lymphatics. Osteoarticular involvement is the most common extracutaneous manifestation.

What hobbies and occupations put individuals at risk for sporotrichosis? — Gardening and farming

HOST DEFENSES

HUMORAL IMMUNITY

What are the consequences of antibody deficiencies? — Increased risk of respiratory infections with *Streptococcus pneumoniae,*

H. influenzae, Neisseria meningitidis (encapsulated pathogens), and mycoplasma, and increased incidence of sinusitis, otitis, and gastrointestinal infections

COMPLEMENT

How is complement activated?

Antigens and antibodies activate the classic pathway; polysaccharides, lipopolysaccharides, and teichoic acid activate the alternative pathway.

What is the result of complement deficiency?

The result depends on which component is deficient and whether that component is absent or reduced. The most common pathogen seen is meningococcus, which is responsible for 80% of infections.

PHAGOCYTOSIS

What pathogens occur in neutropenic patients?

Staphylococci, gram-negative bacilli, and fungi (*Candida, Aspergillus, Mucor*)

CELL-MEDIATED IMMUNITY

What is cell-mediated immunity?

Part of the immune response that is carried out by T lymphocytes, NK cells, and mononuclear phagocytes

What are cytokines?

Proteins or glycoproteins secreted by cells that act as signals between cells of the immune system and mediators of response to infection

What are NK cells?

Closely related to T lymphocytes, NK cells can lyse target cells without major histocompatibility complex restriction or presensitization.

What are mononuclear phagocytes?

Bone marrow progenitors, circulating monocytes, and tissue macrophages

What are the kinds of defects in cell-mediated immunity?	Primary—genetic
	Secondary—drug therapy (immunosuppressive medications including corticosteroids), radiation therapy, organ transplantation, lymphoreticular malignancies, malnutrition, and infections (viral, most notably HIV infection)
What are the pathogens that result from defects in cell-mediated immunity?	Think intracellular organisms including mycobacteria, *Legionella, Salmonella, Chlamydia, Brucella, Yersinia, Nocardia, Rickettsia, Listeria,* fungi (*Histoplasma, Candida, Cryptococcus*) protozoa, and viruses.

MAJOR CLINICAL SYNDROMES

FEVER OF UNKNOWN ORIGIN

What are criteria for defining classic FUO?	A temperature >38°C for >3 weeks, or >2 visits or 3 days in the hospital with evaluation of the cause.
What are the major causes of FUO?	Infection (30% to 40% of cases), neoplasms (20% to 30% of cases), collagen vascular diseases (10% to 15% of cases), and miscellaneous (10% to 20% of cases)
What is included in the initial diagnostic evaluation for FUO?	History (including travel), repeated physical exams, CBC with differential, UA, CXR, blood cultures, ESR, rheumatoid factor, ANA, HIV, tuberculosis skin test
What additional diagnostic tests should be ordered for FUO?	CT of chest, abdomen, and pelvis if initial workup negative. If negative, PET scan may be useful.
What invasive tests should be ordered for FUO?	Always attempt symptom-directed workups. Biopsy of bone marrow, liver, and involved organs should be considered in all patients with FUO.

FEVER AND RASH

What history questions are important to ask in a patient with fever and rash?	Drug ingestion, travel history, occupational or sun exposure, recent immunizations, STD/HIV exposure, exposure to another with similar symptoms/signs, pets and hobbies
What are the common organisms that can cause fever and rash?	HIV, CMV, varicella zoster, RMSF, Lyme, *Ehrlichia, Neiserria meningitidis*

COMMUNITY-ACQUIRED PNEUMONIA

What laboratory abnormality is associated with a poorer prognosis?	Leukopenia
What is the most common bacterial pathogen in CAP?	*Streptococcus pneumoniae*
What are some of the other "typical" bacterial pathogens in CAP?	*Staphylococcus aureus, Haemophilus influenzae, Legionella*
What are some of the "atypical" bacterial pathogen in CAP?	*Mycoplasma pneumoniae, Chlamydophilia pneumoniae*, and *Legionella pneumophila*
What diagnostic tests should be perfomed?	Blood cultures, sputum culture, CXR
What is the empiric therapy for CAP in a non-ICU hospitalized patient?	A respiratory flouroquinolone alone or an advanced macrolide plus a beta lactam
What is the duration of therapy?	The literature on the optimum duration of therapy for CAP is still evolving. On average the treatment course is 7 to 14 days.

PLEURAL EFFUSION AND EMPYEMA

What are the three most common causes of pleural space infections?	Pneumonia, thoracotomy, and trauma

URINARY TRACT INFECTIONS

What are the classic symptoms of lower UTI?	Dysuria, frequency/urgency, hematuria
What are the classic symptoms of upper UTI?	Fever (with occasional chills), flank pain, along with lower tract symptoms
What constitutes pyuria?	Presence of leukocytes at least 10/mm^3 of midstream urine specimen
What are the accepted methods for urine collection?	Midstream clean catch, catheterization, and suprapubic aspiration
What should the initial evaluation include in a hospitalized patient with cystitis/pyelonephritis?	Urinalysis, urine culture, blood cultures, CBC with differential, and a basic chemistry panel
What pathogens are associated with uncomplicated cystitis?	*E. coli, S. saprophyticus, K. pneumoniae, P. mirabilis*
What are the empiric therapy choices for treatment of UTIs?	Trimethoprim-sulfamethoxazole (where local area resistance rates are less than 10% to 15%) or a fluoroquinolone
Generally, what is the duration of therapy for uncomplicated cystitis?	3 days
What is the most common risk factor for *Candida* UTIs?	An indwelling Foley catheter

SEPSIS

What is SIRS?	Systemic inflammatory response syndrome defined as two or more of the following:
	Temperature >38°C or <36°C, Heart rate >90
	Respiratory rate >20, WBC count >12 or <4 or >10% bands

What is sepsis?	The systemic response to infection (SIRS associated with suspected or proven infection)
What is severe sepsis?	Sepsis associated with organ dysfunction away from the site of infection, hypoperfusion, or hypotension
What is in the differential for sepsis?	Trauma, burns, adrenal insufficiency, pacreatitis, pulmonary embolus, myocardial infarction, dissecting or ruptured aortic aneurysm
What antimicrobials should be used for empiric therapy for sepsis?	A broad-spectrum, intravenous regimen that will cover most gram-positive and gram-negative bacteria
What are some choices for empiric antimicrobial therapy for sepsis?	Depending on the suspected source of infection, possibilities include a carbapenem or cefepime plus vancomycin or a beta-lactam/beta-lactamase inhibitor combination agent such as pipercillin-tazobactam.

INTRAPERITONEAL INFECTIONS

What is primary peritonitis?	Also known as SBP (spontaneous bacterial peritonitis), it is an infection of the peritoneal cavity without an evident source.
What population of patients is SBP most commonly seen?	Patients with cirrhosis and ascites
What microbes are usually seen in SBP?	Enteric organisms such as *E.coli* (most common), *K. pneumoniae, S. pneumoniae;* anaerobes are reported infrequently.
What are the clinical manifestations of SBP?	An acute febrile illness with abdominal pain, nausea, vomiting, and diarrhea. However, some cirrhotic patients with SBP will present only with encephalopathy or vague abdominal pain and malaise.

How is the diagnosis of SBP made?	By evaluation of the ascitic fluid obtained by paracentesis. This should be sent for Gram's stain, aerobic/anerobic culture, cell count with differential, protein and albumin. A PML count $>250/mm^3$ is diagnositic (even in the absence of positive Gram's stain and culture).
What drugs are commonly used for empiric therapy for SBP?	A third-generation cephalosporin or a fluoroquinolone
What potential complication of SBP should be evaluated for in those not responding to therapy?	Intraperitonel abscess

INFECTIONS OF THE LIVER AND BILIARY SYSTEM

What are the two main categories of liver abscess?	Amebic and pyogenic
What is the cause of amebic liver abscess?	*Entamoeba histolytica*
In what group is amebic liver abscess most commonly seen in the United States?	Travelers returning from endemic areas
What are the clinical manifestations of amebic liver abscess?	Fever and a dull, aching right-upper-quadrant pain; usually without jaundice. Only up to one third of patients have concurrent gastrointestinal symptoms.
What is the therapy for amebic liver abscess?	Medical management alone is usually successful; treatment with metornidazole 750 mg three times a day for 7 to 10 days.
What are the common etiologies of pyogenic liver abscess?	*E. coli*, *Klebsiella* spp., *Enterococcus* spp., *Streptococcus anginosus* group, *Bacteroides* spp.

What is the most common route of infection in pyogenic liver abscess?	Infection of the biliary tree
What is the classical triad seen in pyogenic liver abscess?	Fever, jaundice, and right-upper-quadrant pain (seen in only 1 in 10)
What is the most frequently abnormal liver function test in pyogenic liver abscess?	An elevated alkaline phosphatase
What is the usual empiric regimen for suspected pyogenic liver abscess?	Ceftriaxone plus metronidazole
What is the mainstay of treatment of pyogenic liver abscess in addition to antibiotics?	Ultrasound or CT-guided drainage of lesion
What infections are associated with the biliary tract?	Cholecystitis, acalculous cholecystitis, and cholangitis
What is the typical presentation of biliary tract disease?	Right-upper-quadrant pain; possibly a Murphy's sign (inhibition of inspiration by pain when the area of the gallbladder fossa is palpated); fever, tachycardia; with cholangitis, Charcot's triad of fever, right-upper-quadrant pain, and jaundice may be seen.

INFECTIVE ENDOCARDITIS

What is infective endocarditis (IE)?	Infection of the endocardial surface of the heart with the physical presensce of microorganisms in the lesion
What is the approximate incidence of IE?	1 case per 1000 hospital admissions
Which heart valve is involved in IE, from the most common to the least?	Mitral (30% to 45%), aortic (5% to 35%), mitral and aortic (0% to 35%), tricuspid (0% to 5%), pulmonary (<1%)

What is the approximate percentage of those with IE who have a murmur?	85%, but it may be absent in right-sided disease. The classic "changing murmur" or new regurgitant murmur occurs only 5% to 10% and 3% to 5%, respectively.
What are some of the common clinical manifestations of IE?	Fever, heart murmur, skin manifestations (such as petechiae), embolic phenomenon
What are some of the common laboratory findings in IE?	Anemia, elevated ESR, abnormal UA (proteinuria, microscopic hematuria), leukocytosis
How should blood cultures be collected in suspected cases of IE?	Three sets of blood cultures from different sites should be collected in the first 24 hours.
What other diagnostic measure is important in the diagnosis of IE?	Transthoracic and sometimes transesophogeal echocardiography
What are the most common bacterial pathogens associated with IE?	*Streptococcus, Staphylococcus, Viridans streptococci, Enterococcus*
What is the empiric therapy for native valve IE?	Vancomycin plus gentamicin
What is the duration of therapy for left-sided IE?	Approximately 6 weeks of intravenous therapy

See Chapter 5 ("Cardiology") for more discussion of endocarditis.

ACUTE MENINGITIS

What are the leading causes of viral or aseptic meningitis?	Enteroviruses, herpesviruses, HIV
What does evaluation of the CSF show in viral meningitis?	A pleocytosis, with the WBC count 100 to 1000/mm^3 (predominately leukocytes), mildly elevated or normal protein, normal or mildly decreased glucose

What is the treatment for most cases of viral meningitis?

Supportive care

What is the specific therapy for herpes meningitis?

Treatment with intravenous acyclovir benefits patients with HSV meningitis and focal neurologic findings.

What are the three most common pathogens associated with bacterial meningitis?

H. influenzae, N. meningitides, S. pneumoniae

What are the symptoms and signs of bacterial meningitis?

Headache, fever, meningismus, altered sensorium

What does the CSF show in bacterial meningitis?

Pleocytosis with WBC 1000 to 5000/mm^3 (neutrophil predominant), glucose $\leq$40, elevated protein (100 to 500 mg/dL), positive Gram's stain 60% to 90%, positive culture of CSF (70% to 85%)

When should a CT scan be performed before a lumbar puncture?

With focal neurological deficits on exam (including altered consciousness), in the immunocompromised, history of CNS disease, new-onset seizures, or papilledema. Blood cultures and antibiotics should be started while awaiting imaging.

What is the role of steroids in the treatment of bacterial meningitis?

Dexamethasone reduces the inflammation in the subarachnoid space following the antibiotic-mediated lysis of bacteria. A meta-analysis evaluated the role of adjunctive dexamethasone given before or at the time of antibiotics and found improved outcomes (most clearly seen for children with pneumococcal meningitis).

What is the empiric antimicrobial therapy for bacterial meningitis?

Vancomycin and a third-generation cephalosporin. Depending on the clinical situation, acyclovir and/or ampicillin can be started as well to treat for HSV and *Listeria* respectively.

EPIDURAL ABSCESS

What is an epidural abscess?	An epidural abscess is a localized collection of pus between the dura mater and the overlying skull or vertebral column.
What are the two main ways epidural abscesses are formed?	Hemotogenous spread from a different foci of infection or by direct extension from vertebral osteomyelitis
What is the most common organism isolated from those with an epidural abscess?	*S. aureus*
What are the four clinical stages associated with thoses presenting with an epidural abscess?	1. Backache and focal vertebral pain 2. Nerve root pain, manifest by radiculopathy or paresthesias 3. Spinal cord dysfunction, manifest by defects in motor, sensory, or sphincter function 4. Complete paralysis
What is the treatment for spinal epidural abscess?	A combined medical/surgical approach. Emperic antimicrobials should be given while the patient is planned for surgical decompression and drainage.
What is the empiric therapy for spinal epidural abscess?	A regimen that contains coverage for *S. aureus*, including resistant organisms and for aerobic gram negative bacilli

GASTROENTERITIS

What is the empiric treatment for inflammatory diarrhea?	Oral rehydration therapy. Therapy with a fluoroquinolone (e.g., ciprofloxacin) may shorten the duration of symptoms if *C. difficile* and *E. histolytica* are not suspected.
What is the treatment for *C. difficile* diarrhea?	Discontinuation of the offending antibiotic if possible Therapy with oral metronidazole or oral vancomycin if patient is refratory or intolerant to metronidazole

What are the causes of noninflammatory diarrhea?	Rotavirus, Norwalk virus, *Giardia, Cryptosporidium, S. aureus, Bacillus cereus, Clostridium perfringens, Vibrio cholerae,* and enterotoxigenic *E. coli*

GENITOURINARY INFECTIONS

Vulvovaginal Candidiasis

What organisms are most commonly associated with vulvovaginal candidiasis?	*Candida albicans* (80% to 90%). *Candida tropicalis,* and *Candida glabrata* also cause vaginitis.
What is the sensitivity of the KOH prep in vulvovaginal candidiasis?	Approximately 50% to 75%

Trichomoniasis

What risk factor is associated with trichomoniasis?	Having an increased number of sexual partners
What is the sensitivity of the wet mount in trichomoniasis?	60% to 80% in symptomatic women

Bacterial Vaginosis

What is seen on wet mount in bacterial vaginosis?	Clue cells and the absence of leukocytes, trichomonads, and the normal flora of rods
What are clue cells?	Squamous epithelial cells with ragged borders and stippling caused by colonization with bacteria

Mucopurulent Cervicitis

What are the etiologic agents of mucopurulent cervicitis?	*Chlamydia trachomatis* and *N. gonorrhoeae*
What are complications of mucopurulent cervicitis?	PID; in pregnant women, preterm delivery and premature rupture of membranes

Pelvic Inflammatory Disease

What are the sequelae of PID?	Infertility, ectopic pregnancy, chronic pelvic pain, and recurrent episodes of PID
What is the differential diagnosis for PID?	Ectopic pregnancy, acute appendicitis, ruptured ovarian cyst, endometriosis, and ovarian torsion

Urethritis

What other pathogens should be treated empirically in patients with gonorrhea?	Chlamydiae
What is the incidence of *Chlamydia* coinfection with GC?	10% to 30% in heterosexual men; 40% to 60% in women

Herpes Genitalis

What is the role of suppressive therapy in herpes infection?	Frequent recurrences may be controlled with daily suppressive therapy, but this does not prevent viral shedding.

Syphilis

What are the stages of syphilis?	Primary—chancre
	Secondary—disseminated (mean of 6 weeks after contact)
	Latent—diagnosed only by serologic testing; early and late stages
	Tertiary—may or may not be clinically apparent; develops in 30% of untreated patients and involves the aorta and CNS
What are the manifestations of primary syphilis?	One or more chancres (ulcerated lesions with heaped-up margins), which are minimally painful, and nontender regional adenopathy
What are the features of secondary syphilis?	Maculopapular, symmetric, generalized rash primarily involving the oral mucous membranes and genitalia but often with involvement of palms and soles; generalized lymphadenopathy; sometimes alopecia

What are the major manifestations of tertiary syphilis?

Lymphocytic meningitis, dementia, tabes dorsalis (posterior spinal column and ganglion disease), aortic disease, or destructive lesions of skin and bone

What are the causes of false-positive nontreponemal tests?

Acute viral illnesses, collagen-vascular diseases, pregnancy, intravenous drug use, and leprosy, among others

SOFT TISSUE, BONES, AND JOINTS

CELLULITIS

What is the presumptive therapy for cellulitis in penicillin nonallergic patients?

Because it is difficult to distinguish clinically between staphylococcal and streptococcal skin infections, initial therapy should adequately cover both organisms. Penicillinase-resistant penicillins or first-generation cephalosporins are antibiotics of choice.

What is the presumptive therapy for cellulitis in penicillin-allergic patients?

Erythromycin, clindamycin, and vancomycin are alternatives for mild and severe infections, respectively, in penicillin-allergic patients.

What is the therapy for suppurative cellulitis?

There has been an increased prevalence of community-acquired MRSA skin infection in patients presenting with suppurative cellulitis. These infections can be treated with clindamycin, trimethoprim-sulfamethoxazole, or rifampin.

What is the therapy for necrotizing fasciitis?

Surgical debridement and antibiotics, which are ultimately guided by bacteriologic data. Depending on clinical circumstances, presumptive therapy may include combinations of the following:

Ampicillin, gentamicin, and clindamycin

Ampicillin, gentamicin, and metronidazole

Ampicillin-sulbactam and gentamicin

What are the principal agents that cause gas gangrene?	*Clostridium perfringens* type A and other *Clostridium* sp.
What is the treatment for gas gangrene?	Emergent surgical debridement Penicillin and additional agents to cover possible anaerobic and Gram-negative copathogens

OSTEOMYELITIS

How can the diagnosis of osteomyelitis definitively be made?	Early bone biopsy for culture and histopathology not only establishes the diagnosis but also often provides the etiologic agent.
What is the role of radiologic studies in diagnosing osteomyelitis?	Plain films are insensitive for diagnosing osteomyelitis. MRI is a very sensitive (98%) and specific (93%) tool for diagnosing vertebral osteomyelitis and diskitis.
What other imaging studies are useful in osteomyelitis?	CT with contrast Radionuclide studies (bone scan or indium labeled WBC scan) can also be performed although there may be false positives with the radionuclide scans due to inflammation.
Are cultures of sinus tracts useful in osteomyelitis?	These cultures reflect colonization of the tract and do not correlate with the underlying bone infection. However, if *S. aureus* is isolated from an open sinus tract, the likelihood is high (>80%) that *S. aureus* is also present in bone.
What is the treatment for osteomyelitis?	1. Debridement of necrotic, avascular infected bone 2. Removal of all foreign objects 3. Pathogen-specific antimicrobial therapy
What is the duration of therapy for osteomyelitis?	Acute—4 to 6 weeks intravenous therapy Chronic—6 weeks intravenous therapy, then several months of oral therapy

INFECTIOUS ARTHRITIS

What is included in the differential for pyogenic arthritis?	Gout, pseudogout, rheumatoid arthritis, SLE, Reiter's syndrome, other infectious but nonbacterial causes
How is the diagnosis of infectious arthritis made?	Identification of bacteria from synovial fluid obtained through arthrocentesis
What are the clinical symptoms and signs of infectious arthritis?	A swollen, painful, erythemetous joint, usually with a visible effusion; usually accompanied by moderated fevers, chills
What does the laboratory findings in infectious arthritis?	Mild leukocytosis, elevated ESR, synovial fluid usually contains an elevated number of WBC/mm^3 (as high as 50,000 to 100,000 in gonoccocal arthritis), a neutrophil predominance

ACQUIRED IMMUNODEFICIENCY SYNDROME

What is HIV?	Retrovirus that causes progressive dysfunction of the immune system
What is AIDS?	Acquired immunodeficiency syndrome is caused by infection with HIV.
What is the definition of advanced immunodeficiency in AIDS?	CD4 cell count of less than 200/mm^3, a percentage of CD4 cells below 14%, or 1 or more of 26 different opportunistic diseases (occurring when at least moderate suppression of cell-mediated immunity is present).
What is the prevalence of HIV infection?	More than 40 million people worldwide; the number of newly infected in 2005 estimated at 4.9 million.
What is the prevalence of AIDS?	In 2007, the number of people living with HIV/AIDS worldwide was 33.2 million. As of 12/2005, an estimated 1.1 million persons in the United States were living with HIV/AIDS, with 25% of those undiagnosed or unaware.
	Currently more than 2.5 million new infections occur yearly, with more than 2.1 million deaths, making HIV/AIDS the leading cause of death as a result of infection.

What is acute HIV seroconversion?

The time right after infection before there is an immune response.

What are the symptoms of acute seroconversion?

An acute mononucleosis-like illness (fever, headache, arthralgias, myalgias, malaise, oral ulcers, weight loss, pharyngitis, rash, gastrointestinal symptoms, and, occasionally, aseptic meningitis) develops. Almost all patients have anti-HIV antibodies by 6 months.

When should combination antiretroviral treatment be initiated in HIV infection?

CD4 count $<200/\mu$L

AIDS-defining illness

HIV-related constitutional symptoms

Asymptomatic patients with CD4 count between 200 to $350/\mu$L; depends on the viral load

What are the most common opportunistic infections in HIV infected persons?

Candidal esophagitis, PCP, MAC, CMV, toxoplasmosis, cryptococcal meningitis, and *M. tuberculosis*

What is MAC?

Mycobacterium avium complex is an atypical mycobacterium that produces disseminated disease in patients with advanced AIDS—the CD4 cell count is usually <50/mm^3. Patients have fever (to $40°$C), night sweats, and weight loss, and they may have abdominal pain or diarrhea. Diagnosis is made by blood culture. Treatment is clarithromycin plus ethambutol.

What is the most common cause of retinitis in AIDS patients?

CMV; it develops late, when CD4 cell counts are <100/mm^3.

How does CMV retinitis present?

Initially, patients may be asymptomatic (disease begins peripherally), but progressive visual loss develops. CMV retinitis has the appearance on funduscopy of "cottage cheese and ketchup."

How is CMV retinitis treated?	Patients with CMV retinitis require therapy with ganciclovir or foscarnet.
What is the most common malignancy in AIDS?	Kaposi's sarcoma
What is the most common cause of a focal CNS lesion in AIDS?	Toxoplasmosis
What are the most common causes of pneumonia in AIDS?	PCP, bacterial pneumonia, tuberculosis, fungi (*Cryptococcus, Histoplasma*)

NOSOCOMIAL INFECTIONS

What is the incidence of nosocomial infection?	Occurs in more than 5% of patients admitted to acute care hospitals

Nosocomial Bloodstream Infection

What are the risk factors for nosocomial BSI?	Indwelling venous catheters, extremes of age, underlying disease, malnutrition, increased length of hospital stay, invasive procedures, ICU stay
What pathogens are associated with nosocomial BSI?	Coagulase-negative staphylococci, *S. aureus*, enterococci, *Candida*, *E. coli*, *Enterobacter*, *Proteus*, *Klebsiella*, and other bacteria (less commonly)

Nosocomial Pneumonia

What is the incidence of nosocomial pneumonia?	More than 250,000 episodes per year. It is the second leading cause of nosocomial infection and the number one cause of death as a result of nosocomial infection in the United States.
How long does a patient need to be hospitalized to be at risk for hospital acquired pneumonia?	48 hours, assuming that he or she was not incubating a pneumonia prior to admission
What are the main pathogens in hospital-acquired or health care–associated pneumonia?	*S. aureus*, *Pseudomonas aeruginosa*, and mutidrug-resistant pathogens in addition to the regular CAP etiologies

What are the risk factors for health care–associated pneumonia?	Hospitalized for at least 2 days within the past 90 days, long-term-care facility resident, has received intravenous antibiotics or chemotherapy within the past 30 days, or has regular visits to an outpatient clinic

Nosocomial Urinary Tract Infection

What is the incidence of nosocomial UTI?	400,000 to 1 million infections per year; 40% of all nosocomial infections

Surgical Wound Infection

What is the treatment for surgical wound infection?	Because skin pathogens are most common, consider nafcillin or vancomycin. Cover gram-negative anaerobes if there is deep wound infection or if the patient is at risk. Surgery is often needed for deep infection.

Nosocomial Gastrointestinal Infections

What pathogens are associated with nosocomial diarrhea?	Bacteria cause more than 90% of episodes, and *C. difficile* causes 90% of episodes in which a pathogen is identified. Rotavirus is the second most common pathogen and is seen in 1 of 20 infections.
What is the treatment for nosocomial diarrhea?	Hydration, supportive care, and, if possible, stop antibiotics. Treat with metronidazole (oral route is preferred to intravenous therapy if the pathogen is *C. difficile*).

Traveler's Syndromes

In what percentage of persons traveling to underdeveloped countries does traveler's diarrhea develop?	30% to 50%
What is the predominant microbial pathogen in traveler's diarrhea?	Enterotoxigenic *E. coli*

What are the contraindications for antimotility agents in traveler's diarrhea?

High fever, bloody stools, or other evidence of an inflammatory colitis or dysentery

Why are antimotility agents avoided with these symptoms?

Toxic megacolon has been reported with the use of antimotility agents with inflammatory diarrhea.

What are the most common causes of febrile illness in returning travelers?

Malaria, enteric fever, hepatitis, and amebic liver abscess

What are the major causes of eosinophilia in travelers?

Helminthic, including filariasis, schistosomiasis, and strongyloidiasis

ABBREVIATIONS

ACE	Angiotensin-converting enzyme
ACEI	Angiotensin-converting enzyme inhibitor
ADPKD	Autosomal dominant polycystic kidney disease
AG	Anion gap
AIN	Acute interstitial nephritis
AKI	Acute kidney injury
ANA	Antinuclear antibody
ANCA	Antineutrophil cytoplasmic antibody
APA	Antiphospholipid antibody syndrome
ARB	Angiotensin receptor blocker
ARF	Acute renal failure
ATN	Acute tubular necrosis
AVP	Arginine vasopressin
BP	Blood pressure
BUN	Blood urea nitrogen
CBC	Complete blood count
C3, C4	Complement components 3 and 4
CHF	Congestive heart failure
CIN	Chronic interstitial nephritis
CK	Creatine kinase
CKD	Chronic kidney disease
CLL	Chronic lymphocytic leukemia
CMV	Cytomegalovirus
CNS	Central nervous system
CrCl	Creatinine clearance
CRI	Chronic renal insufficiency
CSW	Cerebral salt wasting syndrome
CT	Computed tomography
CVA	Cerebrovascular accident
CXR	Chest x-ray
DI	Diabetes insipidus
DKA	Diabetic ketoacidosis
DM	Diabetes mellitus
DNA	Deoxyribonucleic acid
dsDNA	Double-stranded DNA
ECF	Extracellular fluid
EM	Electron microscopy
ESR	Erythrocyte sedimentation rate
ESRD	End-stage renal disease
FE_{Na}	Fractional excretion of sodium
FMD	Fibromuscular dysplasia
FSGS	Focal segmental glomerulosclerosis
GBM	Glomerular basement membrane
GFR	Glomerular filtration rate

GI	Gastrointestinal
GN	Glomerulonephritis
HCO$_3$$^-$	Bicarbonate
HD	Hemodialysis
HELLP	Hemolysis, elevated liver enzymes, low platelet count
HF	Heart failure
HIV	Human immunodeficiency virus
HLA	Human leukocyte antigens
HSP	Henoch-Schönlein purpura
HRS	Hepatorenal syndrome
HTN	Hypertension
HUS	Hemolytic–uremic syndrome
IF	Immunofluorescence
IgA, G, M	Immunoglobulin A, G, M
IV	Intravenous(ly)
IVP	Intravenous pyelogram
LM	Light microscopy
MARS	Molecular absorbent recirculating system
MCD	Minimal change disease
MDRD	Modification of diet in renal disease (study)
MIDD	Monoclonal immunoglobulin deposition disease
MM	Multiple myeloma
MMF	Mycophenolate mofetil
MPGN	Membranoproliferative glomerulonephritis
MRI	Magnetic resonance imaging
MRA	Magnetic resonance arteriography
NDL	Nephrogenic diabetes lusipidus
NKF	National Kidney Foundation
NSAIDs	Nonsteroidal anti-inflammatory drugs
PAN	Polyarteritis nodosa
PAS	Periodic acid–Schiff
PCP	Pneumocystic carinii pneumonia
PCT	Proximal convoluted tubule
P$_{Cr}$	Plasma creatinine
P$_K$	Plasma potassium
PKD	Polycystic kidney disease
P$_{Na}$	Plasma sodium
P$_{osm}$	Plasma osmolality
PT	Proximal tubule
PTH	Parathyroid hormone
PTRA	Percutaneous renal angioplasty
PVD	Peripheral vascular disease
RAS	Renal artery stenosis
RBC	Red blood cell
RBF	Renal blood flow
RF	Rheumatoid factor

RPGN	Rapidly progressive glomerulonephritis
RPN	Renal papillary necrosis
RTA	Renal tubular acidosis
RTC	Renal tubular cell
SIADH	Syndrome of inappropriate antidiuretic hormone
SLE	Systemic lupus erythematosus
SPEP	Serum protein electrophoresis
TB	Tuberculosis
Tc	Technetium
TIPS	Transjugular intrahepatic portosystemic shunt
TTKG	Transtubular potassium gradient
TTP	Thrombotic thrombocytopenic purpura
UAG	Urine anion gap
U_{Cr}	Urine creatinine
U_K	Urine potassium
U_{Na}	Urine sodium
U_{osm}	Urine osmolality
UPEP	Urine protein electrophoresis
UTI	Urinary tract infection
VUR	Vesicourethral junction
WBC	White blood cell

EVALUATION OF KIDNEY FUNCTION

What is the best measurement of kidney function?

GFR

How is GFR estimated?

GFR is not measured directly. Urinary clearance of inulin (a substance that appears in the urine only by filtration) is the "gold standard" for measuring filtration. However, the test is difficult to do. The best estimate of GFR is to use the equation of the MDRD study:

$GFR = 186 \times (Pcr)^{-1.154} \times (age)^{0.203} \times (0.742 \text{ if female}) \times (1.210 \text{ if black})$

How is creatinine clearance assessed?

1. Based on a 24-hour urine collection:
   $CrCl = [U_{cr} \text{ (mg/mL)} \times U_{vol} \text{ (mL/24hr)}] / [Pcr \text{ (mg/mL)} \times 1440 \text{ (min)}]$
2. Estimation using Cockcroft and Gault:
   $\{[140 - age \text{ (yr)}] \times wt \text{ (kg)}] / [Pcr \text{ (mg/dL)} \times 72]\} \times (0.85 \text{ in women})$

Why is GFR a better measure of kidney function than creatinine clearance?

1. Creatinine clearance overestimates GFR because creatinine is secreted by the proximal tubule.
2. Secretion of creatinine can be affected by medications (both trimethoprim and cimetidine decrease secretion).
3. The generation of serum creatinine also varies with age, race, gender, diet, amputation.

What are some factors that can increase the serum creatinine but not affect clearance?

1. Ketotic states and hyperglycemia (if the Jaffe method of determination of creatinine is utilized)
2. Cephalosporins (Jaffe method)
3. Flucytosine (enzymatic method of determination of creatinine)
4. Cimetidine, trimethoprim (inhibit secretion of creatinine)
5. Vigorous exercise
6. Ingestion of cooked meat

What are some of the causes of interpatient variability in GFR?

Gender: GFR approximately 8% higher in males

Body size: GFR conventionally factored by 1.73 m^2

Ethnicity

Age: age-related decline in GFR, 0.75 to 1.0 mL/min/1.73 m^2 (0.01 to 0.02 mL/s/1.73 m^2) per year

Pregnancy: GFR elevated as much as 50% in first trimester and onward; returns toward normal by 4 to 8 weeks postpartum

Protein intake: GFR higher in patients on high-protein diet

Diurnal variation: values tend to be about 10% higher in afternoon than at night

Antihypertensive therapy: secondary to lowering of blood pressure; variable effect not directly predictable

States associated with hyperfiltration: diabetes, obesity, acromegaly

For which patient populations has the MDRD-estimated GFR not been validated?

Age <18 and >70 years, pregnant women, ethnic subgroups other than African Americans and Caucasians

What is the major drawback for the use of the MDRD equation?

Failure to calibrate creatinine assay to the laboratory that developed the estimating equation can introduce error in estimating GFR, especially at higher GFR values.

What is a normal GFR?

Normal GFR has a wide variation. Ages 13 to 21 years (males) 140 ± 30; (females) 126 ± 22.

How does GFR change with aging?

Declines by 1 mL/min/1.73 m^2 per year approximately after 20 to 30 years

Why is urea not a good marker of GFR?

1. It is freely filtered but reabsorbed in the proximal and distal nephron.
2. Urea production is highly variable and greatly influenced by diet and hydration status.

What is cystatin C?

1. Cysteine protease inhibitor produced at a constant rate by all nucleated cells.
2. Freely filtered and then completely reabsorbed by the tubules.
3. Most studies demonstrate that serum levels of cystatin C are a better marker of GFR than creatinine.

What urine findings are markers for kidney disease?

1. Urinalysis with + protein + blood
2. Microscopy with oval fat bodies, fatty casts (nephrotic syndrome); WBCs, WBC casts, tubular casts, granular casts (tubulointestinal process), dysmorphic RBCs, RBC casts (glomerular process)

Why is measurement of proteinuria important?

1. It is a marker of CKD if it persists ≥3 months
2. It is associated with accelerated progression of cardiovascular and kidney disease.
3. It is usually a sign of significant glomerular or tubular damage.

What is the normal rate of protein excretion?

Urine albumin is 10 mg protein per day
Urine total protein is 50 mg protein per day

On a urine collection, what defines proteinuria?

Proteinuria: >300 mg/day on 24-hour collection or >200 mg/g on urine spot

On a urine collection, what defines microalbuminuria?

Microalbuminuria: 30 to 300 mg/day on 24-hour collection or 30 mg/g on urine spot

On a urine collection, what defines albuminuria?

Albuminuria: >300 mg/day on 24-hour collection or >300 mg/g on urine spot

What is the recommended protein to assess for proteinuria?

Albumin

Does proteinuria aid in determining the etiology of CKD?

Yes. Higher levels of proteinuria are associated with glomerular disease and diabetic kidney disease.

What are common causes of false-positive proteinuria?

Hematuria, UTI, exercise, dehydration

Can a single spot urine be used to quantitate proteinuria?

Yes, the ratio of protein or albumin to creatinine in a single early-morning specimen is acceptable.

What proteins are detected by the urine dipstick analysis?

Only albumin. Thus this method is useful only as a screening test and will not detect light chains or nonalbumin proteins in the urine.

What is the first step in evaluating hematuria?

Rule out pigmenturia.

How do you rule out pigmenturia?

By centrifuging the urine sample. If the sediment is red, there is hematuria. If the supernatant is red, there is pigmenturia.

What are common causes of pigmenturia?

Myoglobinuria, hemoglobinuria, beeturia, porphyria

Once hematuria is determined, how is the site of disease localized?

Glomerular hematuria: >70% dysmorphic cells, erythrocyte casts, other cellular casts, proteinuria >1 g/day

Nonglomerular: <30% dysmorphic cells, no casts, absent or minimal proteinuria

ACID–BASE DISORDERS

What is the typical response of the body to an acid load or acid generation?

Initial blood buffering of newly formed acid by bicarbonate and creation of CO_2

Less efficient buffering of acid by hemoglobin in RBCs and by Ca^{2+} exchange in bones

Renal handling of acid load

What is involved with the renal handling of the acid load?

H+ excretion by PT into lumen leads to reclamation of bicarbonate.

H+ also combines with HPO_4^{-2} or HSO_4 (titratable acids) or NH_3 in tubular lumen.

Kidney varies NH_3 production to allow for more acid excretion.

What are the causes of metabolic acidosis?

Increased acid load
  Lactic acidosis

  Ketoacidosis (starvation, diabetic, alcoholic)

  Ingestions: salicylates, methanol, ethylene glycol, toluene, metformin, ammonium chloride, hyperalimentation fluids)

Extrarenal acidosis
  Bicarbonate loss through GI tract: diarrhea, intestinal fistula, ureterosigmoidostomy

Renal acidosis
  Defect in bicarbonate reclamation: type 2 RTA

  Defect in bicarbonate regeneration:
    Diminished NH_4^+ production (type IV RTA)

    Diminished H^+ secretion (type I RTA)

What is the expected respiratory compensation with a metabolic acidosis?

Winter's formula:

$Pco_2 = (1.5 \times bicarbonate) + 8\ (\pm 2)$

How do you calculate the anion gap?

$AG = (Na^+) - [(Cl^-) + (HCO_3^-)]$: normal 8 to 11 meq/L

What is the utility of the plasma anion gap?

Buffering of HA (proton-anion) by bicarbonate in setting of increased acid load leads to increased unmeasured anions (A-) and increased anion gap.

What are the determinants of the normal anion gap?

Unmeasured anions in the plasma, with the major constituent being albumin. Thus the normal anion gap varies directly with the serum albumin level. A correction equation to use with estimating the normal anion gap in the setting of hypoalbuminemia is 3 times serum albumin.

What are the typical causes of an increased anion gap?

Methanol

Uremia/renal failure

Ketoacidosis (starvation, diabetic, alcoholic)

Ethylene glycol

Lactic acidosis

Toluene

Salicylates

Metformin (lactic acidosis)

Tylenol (pyroglutamic acid)

How is ethylene glycol or methanol ingestions treated?

Competitive inhibition of alcohol dehydrogenase with either ethanol or fomepizole decreases production of toxic by-products and hemodialysis.

What are some causes of an increased anion gap not associated with a metabolic acidosis?

Volume depletion (hyperalbuminemia)

Metabolic or respiratory alkalosis

Severe hyperphosphatemia

Presence of anionic paraprotein (often IgA)

What are some causes of an abnormally low or even negative anion gap?

Hypoalbuminemia (most common)

Hypermagnesemia

Hypercalcemia

Lithium intoxication

IgG paraprotein or polyclonal gammopathy

Bromide intoxication

How do you calculate the urine anion gap?

$UAG = [(Na^+) + (K^+)] - (Cl^-)$

What is the utility of the urine anion gap?

In the setting of metabolic acidosis with a normal AG, UAG is helpful to determine extra-renal versus renal acidosis. With normal renal compensation, NH_4+ production increases in response to the acidosis and the UAG becomes more negative (higher Cl^- concentration).

How is the UAG interpreted?

UAG >0 suggests failure to produce NH_4+ and thus a renal (RTA) cause.

UAG <0 suggests normal renal response and extrarenal bicarbonate loss (usually diarrhea).

What is a type I RTA?

Defect in H^+ secretion in the distal tubule
  Defect in H^+-ATPase pump which secretes acid (Sjögren's syndrome)
    Back diffusion of H^+ due to increased tubular permeability to H^+ (amphotericin B)

Decreased distal delivery of Na^+ (volume depletion)
  Decreased cortical reabsorption of Na^+ with net increase in luminal charge and inhibition of H^+ and K^+ secretion (hyperkalemic type I) (urinary tract obstruction and sickle cell disease)

What are the diagnostic features of a type I RTA?

Urine pH >5.3
Plasma K^+ usually low or normal
Plasma bicarbonate low (<14 meq/L)
Nephrocalcinosis

How is a type I RTA treated?

Bicarbonate supplementation (in the form of potassium or sodium/potassium citrate)

What is a type II RTA?

Decreased ability to reabsorb bicarbonate in the PT—new absorptive threshold
  Injury to Na+/H+ antiporter or basolateral Na-K-ATPase (myeloma, Fanconi's syndrome, ifosfamide)

Deficient/inhibited carbonic anhydrase (cystinosis, acetazolamide)

What are the diagnostic features of a type II RTA?

Urine pH >5.3 is serum bicarbonate level above reabsorptive threshold; in steady state usually <5.3.

Plasma K^+ usually low

Bicarbonate low (14 to 20 meq/L)

Often associated with other PT defects (glycosuria, amino aciduria, phosphaturia)

How is a type II RTA treated?

Bicarbonate supplementation (nearly impossible to completely correct serum level). Can add a thiazide diuretic which induces mild volume depletion, causing increased proximal Na+ and bicarbonate resorption.

What is a type IV RTA?

Due to decreased activity of the renin-angiotensin-aldosterone system at any level. The acidosis is worsened by hyperkalemia which inhibits renal ammoniagenesis.

What are some of the causes of type IV RTA?

Diabetes, adrenal insufficiency, heparin, ACEI, ARB, potassium sparing diuretics, HIV infection, and primary adrenal insufficiency

What are the diagnostic features of a type IV RTA?

Urine pH <5.3

Elevated plasma K

Bicarbonate low (14 to 20 meq/L)

How is a type IV RTA treated?

Remove offending medications; often acidosis improves if hyperkalemia is treated; bicarbonate supplementation and steroid replacement if primary adrenal insufficiency

At what GFR does renal ammonia production begin to fall?

At GFR less than 40 mL/min, total ammonium excretion begins to fall and a non-gap acidosis may appear. Generally, the bicarbonate is stabilized at a level from 12 to 20 meq/L through bone buffering of acid.

What are the common causes of a metabolic alkalosis?

Factors that generate a metabolic alkalosis include:

Gastric suction

Vomiting

Antacid therapy

Chloride-losing diarrhea

Diuretics

Mineralocorticoid excess

Hypercalcemia/milk-alkali syndrome

Low chloride intake

Hypokalemia (shift of H+ into cells)

Refeeding (shift of H+ into cells)

Massive blood transfusions

Bicarbonate administration

What are the factors that permit maintenance of metabolic alkalosis?

Normally, the kidney can efficiently excrete bicarbonate and rapidly correct a metabolic alkalosis. Thus the following factors must occur to maintain a metabolic alkalosis:

> Decreased GFR (volume depletion or renal failure)

> Increased tubular reabsorption of bicarbonate (hypokalemia, hyperaldosteronism, chloride depletion)

In the diagnosis of metabolic alkalosis, what are the diagnostic possibilities if the urine chloride is:
  <10 meq/L?

Vomiting or nasogastric suction; diuretics

  >10 meq/L with hypertension?

Cushing's syndrome, hyperaldosteronism, hypokalemia, conditions of apparent mineralocorticoid excess

  >10 meq/L and normal or low blood pressure?

Bartter's or Gitelman's syndrome

How is a metabolic alkalosis treated:
  With a low urine chloride?

Normal saline

  With a high urine chloride?

Treatment of underlying disorder

What are common causes of a respiratory acidosis?

Inhibition of respiratory drive (drugs, sleep apnea, CNS lesions)

Disorders of respiratory muscles (myasthenia, spinal cord injury)

Upper airway obstruction (aspiration, sleep apnea)

Lung disease (pneumonia, asthma, etc.)

What is the renal compensation for a respiratory acidosis:
    If it develops acutely?

Bicarbonate increases by about 1 for every 10 mm Hg rise in $PaCO_2$.

    If it is a chronic problem?

Bicarbonate increases by about 4 for each 10 mm Hg rise in $PaCO_2$.

Should bicarbonate be given to patients with a respiratory acidosis?

Perhaps beneficial in severely acidemic patient. Use with extreme caution.

What are the common causes of a respiratory alkalosis?

Associated with hypoxemia (pulmonary diseases, HF, anemia)

Stimulation of medullary respiratory center (sepsis, liver disease, salicylates, CNS diseases)

Mechanical ventilation

What is the renal compensation for a respiratory alkalosis:
    If it develops acutely?

Bicarbonate decreases by about 1 for every 10 mm Hg rise in $PaCO_2$.

    If it is a chronic condition?

Bicarbonate decreases by about 4 for each 10 mm Hg rise in $PaCO_2$.

What are the most common mixed acid–base disorders?

Mixed respiratory acidosis and metabolic alkalosis (COPD and diuretic therapy)

Mixed metabolic acidosis and metabolic alkalosis (ketoacidosis and vomiting)

Mixed respiratory alkalosis and metabolic acidosis (salicylate intoxication)

What is the Δ anion gap?	ΔAG = measured AG − normal AG
How is it used?	Used to determine if a mixed acid–base disturbance is present
	Most useful to distinguish concomitant metabolic alkalosis and AG metabolic acidosis
What if the ΔAG is +?	Then next look at the measured bicarbonate. Add the ΔAG to the measured bicarbonate.
What if the ΔAG + measured bicarbonate is in the normal range for bicarbonate?	There is no concomitant metabolic alkalosis.
What if the sum of the ΔAG + measured bicarbonate is greater than the normal range for bicarbonate?	There is a concomitant metabolic alkalosis.

WATER BALANCE DISORDERS

HYPONATREMIA

What are the factors that control the serum sodium concentration?	This is due to the finely controlled excretion or retention of water by the kidneys and control of thirst. Thus, disorders of sodium concentration are disorders of water balance.
What are the factors that control renal water excretion?	1. GFR 2. Delivery of filtrate to the diluting segments of the kidney 3. A hypertonic medullary interstitium 4. AVP
What are the symptoms of acute hyponatremia?	Usually related to the CNS: lethargy, obtundation, confusion, seizures, coma, nausea, vomiting
What is the pathogenesis of the symptoms of acute hyponatremia?	They are due to cerebral edema.

What is pseudohyponatremia?

Normal plasmal osmolality with an artificially low measured serum sodium

When does pseudohyponatremia occur?

In states of hyperproteinemia or hyperlipidemia when there is an increase in the mass of the nonaqueous components of serum and when sodium is measured using flame photometry

What are some substances that can increase osmolality without changing the serum sodium (ineffective osmoles)?

Urea, ethanol, ethylene glycol, isopropyl alcohol, methanol. These substances are lipophilic and partition in all body compartments.

What is cerebral salt wasting syndrome (CSW)?

In patients with acute CNS injury (such as subarachnoid bleeds), there is excessive renal loss of sodium (mechanisms unknown), leading to volume depletion and thus a secondary baroreceptor-mediated stimulation of AVP secretion.

How can CSW be differentiated from SIADH?

Patients with SIADH are euvolemic while patients with CSW are hypovolemic.

How is CSW treated?

Vigorous repletion of salt and volume

How do thiazide diuretics cause hyponatremia?

They lead to mild volume depletion with secondary AVP secretion; they also cause potassium depletion, which leads to intracellular movement of sodium. Furthering this is the possibility that thiazides may also increase thirst.

What is the correct therapy of acute symptomatic hyponatremia?

Initial rapid correction of serum sodium at a rate of 1.5 to 2 meq/L/hr until the patient is asymptomatic. Often requires the use of hypertonic (3%) saline. The serum sodium should not be increased more than 8 to 10 meq/L in the first 24 hours.

How can you estimate the change in serum sodium with the infusion of an IV fluid?

Change in serum sodium (per L infused) = [Infusate (Na^+) – Serum (Na^+)]/[Total body water + 1 (liter infused)]

How does potassium influence the correction of hyponatremia?

Since potassium and sodium can exchange across cell membranes, infusion of potassium can lead to an increase in serum sodium; thus, if potassium is given, it should be included in the above equation.

What are the symptoms of chronic hyponatremia?

Given that there is time for adaptation of the brain, cerebral edema is minimized and most patients are minimally impaired with slight confusion, gait difficulties, or no discernible symptoms.

What is the definition of the syndrome of inappropriate ADH (AVP) secretion (SIADH)?

Inappropriately elevated urine osmolality in the setting of a low serum osmolality. Urine osm >100 mOsm/L

Clinical euvolemia

Decreased extracellular osmolality

Normal renal, pituitary, adrenal, cardiac, and hepatic function

What is the most common drug that causes SIADH?

Selective serotonin receptor uptake inhibitors (SSRIs)

What other diseases are associated with SIADH?

HIV, carcinomas, pulmonary disorders, CNS disorders

How is SIADH treated?

1. Removal of all possible causes
2. Water restriction
3. Diuretics to decrease urinary concentrating ability
4. Demeclocycline
5. Vasopressin receptor antagonists

What are vasopressin receptor antagonists?

Oral (tolvaptan) or IV (conivaptan) agents that selectively antagonize the action of ADH at the collecting duct and thus lead to an increase in free water excretion by the kidney

What is the proper therapy for chronic hyponatremia?

If symptoms are acute, some immediate correction is needed, generally not more than a 10% correction in the first 24 hours.

Frequent measurement of urine and serum electrolytes is mandatory. Do not exceed correction rate of 1 to 1.5 meq/L/hr or more than 12 meq/day.

What is the potential risk of correcting chronic hyponatremia too quickly?

Osmotic demyelination syndrome (ODS)

What is the presentation of ODS?

Patients often show initial improvement in mental status with correction of hyponatremia with subsequent development of motor abnormalities, pseudobulbar palsy and mental status changes

How is ODS diagnosed?

Hyperintense lesion on T2-weighted MRI

What is the pathogenesis of exercise-associated hyponatremia?

Excessive water ingestion in the setting of high AVP levels and concomitant salt loss in sweat

HYPERNATREMIA

What are the mechanisms that defend the body against hypernatremia?

The ability of the kidney to excrete a concentrated urine (retain water) and thirst

What is the pathogenesis of hypernatremia?

1. Impaired thirst (elderly, altered level of consciousness, inadequate access to water)
2. Inability of the kidney to retain water (diabetes insipidus)
3. Rarely, sodium gains (hypertonic IV solutions)

What are the signs/symptoms of hypernatremia?

Usually of a neurologic nature due to cellular dehydration: lethargy, hyperreflexia, coma, seizures

What is the mortality associated with acute hypernatremia?

In adults above age 60, the mortality may be as high as 40% and often reflects the severity of the underlying comorbidities.

What is the therapy for hypernatremia?

The primary goal is restoration of serum tonicity. The specific approach depends upon the patient's extracellular volume status. First correct any significant hypovolemia with the best volume expander such as normal (0.9%) saline, then correct the water deficit.

How do you calculate the water deficit?

Water deficit (L) = $0.6 \times$ body wt(kg) $\times$ [(plasma $Na^+/140$) -1]

What is the proper rate of correction?

There is no need to rapidly correct a serum [Na] below 150 meq/L. Generally, in patients with acute hypernatremia, correction of 1 meq/L/hr can be safely achieved. In patients with chronic hypernatremia, the rate should be considerably slower (0.5 meq/L/hr or less).

What is the risk for rapid correction of hypernatremia?

Cerebral edema

What are the forms of diabetes insipidus?

Central and nephrogenic

What are the causes of central diabetes insipidus?

Brain tumors, histiocytosis, trauma, cerebral hemorrhage or infarct, infectious, idiopathic, and metastatic tumors

How is central diabetes insipidus treated?

Desmopressin—a synthetic, long-acting vasopressin analog with minimal vasopressor activity. It can be given intranasally, subcutaneous or IV.

What are the causes of nephrogenic diabetes insipidus (NDI)?

1. X-linked mutations in the vasopressin receptor in the collecting duct
2. Autosomal dominant and recessive mutations in the aquaporin 2 (water channel) gene
3. Acquired causes

What are the common causes of acquired NDI?

Chronic kidney disease, drugs (lithium, colchicine, glyburide, amphotericin, foscarnet), sickle cell disease, amyloidosis, Sjögren's syndrome, sarcoidosis. All associated with impairment in the functioning of the distal tubule and insensitivity to AVP. Also consider hypokalemia and hypercalcemia.

How is NDI treated?

Low-sodium diet, hydrochlorothiazide and/or amiloride, indomethacin (only for short periods of time)

How do these agents work?	They lead to contraction of the extracellular volume and increase proximal tubular fluid reabsorption. This decreases the amount of water that is presented to the distal tubule.

ELECTROLYTE DISORDERS

POTASSIUM

What are the major factors involved in potassium balance?	1. Acid-base status: acidosis leads to shift of potassium out of cells, alkalosis shifts potassium into cells. 2. Insulin: shifts potassium intracellularly. 3. Tonicity: high osmolality shifts potassium out of cells. 4. Beta-2 adrenergic receptor: catecholamines shift potassium intracellularly. 5. Renal excretion (see below). 6. Dietary potassium intake. 7. Small losses in stool.

What are the factors involved in renal excretion of potassium?	The distal tubule is the major site of potassium excretion and regulation, mediated by sodium reabsorption through specific sodium channel in exchange for potassium excretion into tubular lumen. Factors controlling this process are:
	  1. Angiotensin II: increase K^+ excretion
	  2. Aldosterone: increase K^+ excretion
	  3. Distal delivery of sodium and filtrate: more sodium and filtrate delivered to distal tubule, more K^+ that can be excreted

HYPOKALEMIA

What are the common causes of hypokalemia with normal total body potassium (transcellular shift)?	Alkalemia Insulin excess Stress states (acute MI, asthma attacks, etc.) Hypokalemic periodic paralysis Thyrotoxicosis Refeeding syndromes

What are the common causes of hypokalemia with decreased total body potassium?

Decreased intake of K^+ or increased K^+ losses (renal or GI)

What diagnostic tests are useful in determining the cause of hypokalemia?

Determination of urine potassium excretion: either spot urine concentration, transtubular potassium gradient, or 24-hour potassium excretion

In the setting of hypokalemia, what does a low urine K^+ (<20 meq/day) signify?

Extrarenal K^+ losses are more likely, usually from the GI tract

In the setting of hypokalemia, what does a high urine K^+ (>20 meq/day) signify?

Signifies that K^+ losses are derived from the kidney. The next step is to look at the acid–base status and whether the patient is hypertensive to determine the specific etiology.

What are the most common causes of hypokalemia occurring in combination with a metabolic alkalosis?

Most commonly due to diuretics or vomiting. Can be easily determined by measuring the urine chloride, which should be <10 meq/L. However, if the patient is hypertensive, see below.

In a patient with hypertension, hypokalemia and metabolic alkalosis, how do you determine the potential etiologies?

Can be determined by measuring the renin and aldosterone levels. Generally, these patients have either an excess of aldosterone or an aldosterone-like substance that leads to sodium retention and K^+ wasting.

What if it is a high-renin/high-aldosterone state?

RAS, malignant hypertension

What if it is a low-renin/high-aldosterone state?

Primary aldosteronism, glucocorticoid remediable aldosteronism

And the low-renin/low-aldosterone condition?

Liddle's syndrome, Cushing's syndrome, certain forms of congenital adrenal hyperplasia, apparent mineralocorticoid excess syndrome

What is glucocorticoid-remediable aldosteronism (GRA)?

A rare disease where there is a translocation of the promoter (regulatory) elements of the glucocorticoid gene to the aldosterone synthase gene. Thus aldosterone production is now under the control of ACTH and can be shut down with dexamethasone therapy.

What is Liddle's syndrome?

A rare mutation that leads to overactivity of the distal sodium channel, leading to inappropriate sodium retention and K^+-wasting

What is the syndrome of apparent mineralocorticoid excess?

Normally, the aldosterone receptor can be activated by cortisol, but this does not occur owing to the presence of 11-β-OH steroid dehydrogenase, which converts cortisol to the inactive cortisone. In this syndrome, the inactivating enzyme is nonfunctional while the aldosterone receptor responds to both cortisol and aldosterone and is overactive.

What are the causes of hypokalemia, metabolic alkalosis, and an elevated urine chloride with a normal BP?

Bartter's syndrome: a group of mutations affecting the ascending limb of the loop of Henle and leading to impaired $Na^+/K^+/Cl^-$ reabsorption. Similar to the effects of a loop diuretic.

Gitelman's syndrome: a mutation in the distal tubule Na^+/Cl^- cotransporter that impairs Na^+ and Cl^- reabsorption. Effects similar to a thiazide diuretic.

What are the causes of hypokalemia associated with metabolic acidosis?

RTA type I and II (see acid–base section)

What are some causes of hypokalemia associated with a variable pH?

Magnesium deficiency

Anionic drugs, which are delivered to the distal tubule and obligate K^+ losses (such as penicillins)

What is hypokalemic periodic paralysis?

Can occur as either autosomal dominant or associated with thyrotoxicosis.

Rapid intracellular shift of K^+ into cells leading to muscle weakness.

Besides potassium correction, what can help minimize symptoms in periodic paralysis?

Treatment with beta blockers

What are the clinical manifestations of hypokalemia?

Cardiac arrhythmias, digitalis intoxication

Ileus

Skeletal muscle weakness, rhabdomyolysis

Glucose intolerance

AVP resistance (polyuria)

Increased renal ammonia production and metabolic alkalosis

Renal cysts

Chronic renal interstitial fibrosis

What is the therapy for hypokalemia?

If possible, correct the initiating problem.

K^+ deficit can only be approximated.

In general, a reduction in K^+ from 4.0 to 3.0 meq/L requires loss of 200 to 400 meq K^+.

KCl should be the preferred form of replacement except in the presence of an RTA (K^+-citrate).

What is the maximum rate of K^+ IV infusion?

10 to 20 meq/hr

What are the K^+-sparing diuretics?

Amiloride, triamterene, and spironolactone

When should they be used?

Useful to block K^+ excretion in states of aldosterone excess (diuretic therapy, primary hyperaldosteronism)

HYPERKALEMIA

What are the causes of hyperkalemia due to transcellular shifts?	Exercise, especially in the presence of beta blockers
	Metabolic acidosis
	Insulin deficiency
	Tissue breakdown or ischemia (rhabdomyolysis, tumor lysis)
	Succinylcholine
What are causes of spurious hyperkalemia?	Thrombocytosis
	Leukocytosis
	Prolonged tourniquet application (ischemia)
What are the causes of hyperkalemia due to impaired renal K$^+$ excretion?	Low GFR (<20 mL/min)
	Decreased distal sodium delivery (volume depletion)
	Hypoaldosteronism
	Type I RTA, hyperkalemic form
	Drugs that impair K$^+$ secretion (ACEI, ARB, K$^+$-sparing diuretics)
What are some common causes of hypoaldosteronism?	Hyporeninemic hypoaldosteronism (type IV RTA, common in diabetics)
	NSAIDs
	ACEIs, ARBs
	AIDS
	Adrenal insufficiency
	Congenital adrenal hyperplasia (21-OHase deficiency)
	Heparin
	Cyclosporine
What are the common clinical manifestations of hyperkalemia?	Muscle weakness
	Cardiac arrhythmias (especially alterations in T-wave configuration)
	Metabolic acidosis (reduced renal ammonia production)

What is an indirect method of determining the level of aldosterone action on the distal tubule?

Transtubular potassium gradient (TK^+KG):

$[K^+/(Uosm/Posm)]/Pk$

This equation reflects the gradient of K^+ between the distal tubular lumen and the plasma. In the setting of hyperkalemia with adequate mineralocorticoid activity, the value should be high (>7). If low (generally <4), it reflects hypoaldosteronism of some sort.

What should be the first step in deciding the appropriate therapy for hyperkalemia?

Emergent ECG. If there are any T-wave changes, IV calcium should be given immediately. The effect begins within a minute and is short-lived.

What other therapies are available for the treatment of hyperkalemia?

IV insulin and glucose: shifts K^+ into cells

Sodium bicarbonate: shifts K^+ into cells (less effective in patients with advanced CKD)

Beta-2 adrenergic agonists: shifts K^+ into cells

Diuretics: increase renal excretion (takes time and less effective with advanced CKD)

Sodium polystyrene sulfonate (cation-exchange resin): increases GI excretion of K^+

Dialysis: achieves the greatest reduction in K^+ the fastest

What medication can be utilized to treat patients with hyporeninemic hypoaldosteronism (type IV RTA)?

Fludrocortisone, a synthetic mineralocorticoid, can restore K^+ balance, but often at the expenses of Na^+ retention and volume overload

What are potential treatments for chronic hyperkalemia?

Low-potassium diet

Removal of drugs that inhibit K^+ secretion

Loop or thiazide diuretics

Low-dose sodium polystyrene sulfonate

Oral bicarbonate

REGULATION OF CALCIUM AND PHOSPHORUS

What are the major hormones involved in calcium and phosphorus homeostasis?

PTH and 1,25(OH) vitamin D acting on the effector organs: bone, intestine, and kidney

How is PTH secretion regulated?

PTH is released in response to lowering of ionized serum calcium (via Ca^{2+} sensing receptor inactivation). 1,25(OH) vitamin D inhibits PTH secretion. Hyperphosphatemia and hypomagnesemia also stimulate PTH secretion.

What are the activities of PTH?

Increases calcium reabsorption from kidney

Decreases phosphorus reabsorption from kidney

Increases bone resorption with release of calcium and phosphorus

Indirectly increases intestinal absorption of calcium by stimulating conversion of 25(OH) vitamin D to 1,25(OH) vitamin D

How is vitamin D metabolized?

Sources of vitamin D are diet and skin via conversion by UV light to cholecalciferol, which is metabolized by the liver to 25(OH) vitamin D. The active 1,25(OH) vitamin D is formed through the action of a 1-alpha hydroxylase in the kidney.

How is vitamin D synthesis regulated?

1-alpha hydroxylase (rate-limiting step) is increased by low phosphorus, low calcium, and increased PTH. The activity is decreased by 1,25(OH) vitamin D and by kidney failure.

What is the activity of vitamin D?

Acts on intestine to increase calcium and phosphorus absorption

Acts on bone to increase mineralization

Inhibits PTH secretion

CALCIUM

In what ways is calcium stored and transported in the body?	1. 99% stored in bone; 0.9% intracellular, and 0.1% extracellular 2. Extracellular calcium: 50% free (ionized and physiologically active), 10% bound to anions, and 40% bound to albumin
How do you correct total serum calcium for low albumin?	[(Normal albumin concentration – patient's albumin concentration) × 0.8] + patient's calcium concentration
How is calcium handled by the kidney?	60% to 70% absorbed in proximal tubule; 20% to 30% in thick ascending limb of Henle; 10% in distal tubule
What stimulates calcium reabsorption in the kidney?	1. Volume depletion 2. PTH 3. PTH related peptide (PTHrp) 4. Hypocalcemia
What are the signs and symptoms of hypercalcemia?	Nausea, constipation, abdominal pain, decreased mentation, lassitude, thirst, dehydration, reduced urine output, nocturia, polyuria, volume depletion

What are the causes of hypercalcemia?	1. Primary hyperparathyroidism (55%)
	2. Malignancy (35%)
	  a. Humoral due to PTHrp (lung, esophagus, head and neck, renal cell, ovary, bladder)
	  b. Local osteolytic: breast, multiple myeloma
	3. Hematologic malignancy (lymphoma) with ectopic 1,25(OH) vitamin D (also seen in granulomatous diseases)
	4. Misc (10%): drugs (thiazides, lithium, vitamin D); immobilization, pheochromocytoma, thyrotoxicosis, milk-alkali syndrome

What initial diagnostic tests should be obtained in a patient with hypercalcemia?	Calcium, phosphorus, PTH, PTHrp, 25(OH) and 1,25(OH) vitamin D, SPEP, UPEP

What is the acute treatment for hypercalcemia?

1. Volume repletion with IV saline.
2. Once volume is repleted, loop diuretics can be added (must avoid volume depletion to be effective).
3. Bisphosphonates or calcitonin.
4. Corticosteroids if associated with granulomatous disorder.
5. Cinacalcet (calcimimetic) for hyperparathyroidism (binds to calcium receptor to activate it and decreases PTH secretion).

What are the signs and symptoms of hypocalcemia?

Carpal pedal spasm, perioral numbness, tetany, dyspnea, stridor, wheezing, seizures, bone pain, muscle weakness, cataracts (chronic), bone deformities (rickets)

What is Chvostek's sign?

Elicited by tapping on the face just anterior to the ear and just below zygomatic bone. A positive response is twitching of the ipsilateral facial muscles due to neuromuscular irritability.

What is Trousseau's sign?

Elicited by inflating BP cuff over systolic pressure for several minutes. A positive response is flexion of the wrist and metacarpophalangeal joints, hyperextension of the fingers, and flexion of the thumb.

What is the differential diagnosis of hypocalcemia?

1. Low albumin
2. Hypoparathyroidism (surgical, postradiation, congenital, or autoimmune)
3. Vitamin D deficiency (renal failure, poor nutrition, malabsorption)
4. Pancreatitis
5. Pseudohypoparathyroidism
6. Hypomagnesemia
7. Increased phosphorus (binds calcium): rhabdomyolysis, tumor lysis, renal failure
8. Hungry bone syndrome (postparathyroidectomy)

What diagnostic tests should be ordered for the evaluation of hypocalcemia?

Calcium, albumin, ionized calcium, phosphorus, PTH, 25(OH) vitamin D and 1,25(OH) vitamin D

What is the treatment of hypocalcemia?

1. Severe: parenteral calcium (calcium chloride or gluconate)
2. Chronic: oral calcium supplement and vitamin D
3. If magnesium is depleted, it must be replaced as well.

PHOSPHORUS

How is phosphorus stored and transported in the body?

1. 85% in bone, 14% intracellular, 1% extracellular
2. Extracellular phosphorus is bound to albumin and cations, but lab measures only physiologically active form (unlike calcium)

How is phosphorus handled by the kidney?

85% reabsorbed in the proximal tubule through a Na/P cotransporter, remainder taken up in distal segments. Uptake is stimulated by volume contraction, hypophosphatemia. Excretion stimulated by PTH, PTHrp and diuretics.

What are the signs and symptoms of hypophosphatemia?

Muscle weakness, hypoventilation, confusion, seizures, osteomalacia

What are the causes of hypophosphatemia due to decreased intestinal absorption?

Antacids, malabsorption, chronic diarrhea, vitamin D deficiency, starvation, anorexia, alcoholism

What are the causes of hypophosphatemia due to increased urinary loss?

Primary hyperparathyroidism, post–renal transplant, volume expansion, glucosuria, resolving ATN, Fanconi's syndrome, X-linked and vitamin D–dependent rickets, oncogenic osteomalacia

What are the causes of hypophosphatemia due to transcellular shifts?

Respiratory alkalosis, alcohol withdrawal, burns, TPN, refeeding syndrome, leukemic blast crisis

How is hypophosphatemia treated?

Phosphate comes in either Na- or K-salts: choice dictated by other illnesses and electrolyte levels. Oral repletion can also be accomplished with milk. Treat underlying condition.

What are the signs and symptoms of hyperphosphatemia?

Usually asymptomatic unless hypocalcemia occurs due to precipitation of insoluble $CaPO_4$ complexes. Chronic hyperphosphatemia in CKD is associated with vascular calcification and increased mortality.

What are the causes of hyperphosphatemia?

Occurs almost exclusively with decreased GFR. Other rare causes include hypoparathyroidism, acromegaly, thyrotoxicosis, tumor lysis, rhabdomyolysis, vitamin D overdose, phosphate-containing enemas.

What is the acute therapy of hyperphosphatemia?

Dialysis is the most effective, also volume repletion.

What is the chronic therapy of hyperphosphatemia?

Dietary restriction and use of phosphate binders (calcium acetate, calcium carbonate, sevelamer) with meals

MAGNESIUM

How is magnesium stored and transported in the body?

66% in bone, 33% intracellular and 1% extracellular. Serum levels are not reflective of body stores. Extracellular magnesium can be measured as total magnesium, of which 55% is ionized and physiologically active, 15% bound to anions, and 30% bound to albumin.

How is magnesium handled by the kidney?

40% reabsorbed in the proximal tubule, 50% in ascending limb of Henle, 5% reabsorbed actively in distal tubule. Renal tubule reabsorption increased by volume contraction, hypomagnesemia and PTH.

What are the signs and symptoms of hypermagnesemia?

Lethargy, nausea, confusion, hypoventilation, hypotension, arrhythmias, muscle weakness, decreased deep tendon reflexes

What are the causes of hypermagnesemia?

Most often occurs with depressed GFR
1. Increased intake: antacids, laxatives, enemas, treatment of preeclampsia with Mg^{++} salts
2. Decrease renal function
3. Cellular shifts: pheochromocytoma, acidosis

What is the treatment for hypermagnesemia?

If symptomatic, IV calcium salts reverse neuromuscular and cardiac effects. Hemodialysis is the most effective way to remove excess Mg^{++}, especially if GFR decreased.

What are the signs and symptoms of hypomagnesemia?

Tremors, myoclonic jerks, positive Chvostek and Trousseau signs, tetany, generalized muscle weakness (particularly respiratory muscles), vertigo, nystagmus, coma. There is an increased incidence of ventricular arrhythmias, PVCs, ventricular tachycardia, torsades de pointes, ventricular fibrillation. Also increased susceptibility to digitalis-related arrhythmias.

What are the causes of hypomagnesemia?

1. Reduced intake: starvation, alcoholism, prolonged postoperative state
2. Redistribution from extracellular to intracellular fluids: insulin, hungry-bone syndrome, postparathyroidectomy, catecholamine excess, alcohol withdrawal, acute pancreatitis
3. Reduced GI absorption: malabsorption syndromes, post–bowel resection, chronic diarrhea, laxative abuse

What diagnostic tests are useful for hypomagnesemia?

Two available tests to determine total body Mg deficiency:

1. Retention of >75% of Mg^{++} after IV Mg^{++} loading
2. Low urine fractional excretion of Mg^+ is indicative of deficiency

Very low (<1 mg/dL) levels of Mg^{++} in the serum always reflect significant deficiency, as do neuromuscular symptoms.

What is the therapy for hypomagnesemia?

1. Symptomatic or severe: IV magnesium sulfate slowly infused
2. Asymptomatic: oral repletion with magnesium salts: may be limited by diarrhea

ACUTE KIDNEY INJURY

What is the incidence of acute kidney injury (AKI) in the hospital setting?

Approximately 5% of all patients.

Approximately 15% to 20% of intensive care patients. The majority of AKI occurs in the hospital setting.

What is the mortality risk associated with AKI?

Substantial; in one large study, the mortality rate of patients who had a rise in SCr >0.5 mg/dL while hospitalized increased by 6.5-fold.

What are the major causes of acute kidney injury in the hospital setting

Prerenal azotemia and acute tubular necrosis

What are the renal anatomic sites that can be involved in AKI?

Prerenal azotemia: hypoperfusion

Renal artery and vein

Small renal vessels

Glomerular disease

Acute tubular necrosis

Acute interstitial nephritis

Intratubular obstruction

Postrenal obstruction

What are the etiologies of prerenal acute kidney injury?	Intravascular volume depletion
	Distributive shock (early sepsis, third-spacing)
	Low cardiac output
	Renal artery hypoperfusion: NSAIDs, contrast-induced, cyclosporine/tacrolimus, ACEIs/ARBs
What diseases cause acute intrinsic kidney injury?	Renovascular (renal artery or vein thrombosis, atheroembolic disease, large vessel vasculitis)
	Diseases of small vessels and glomeruli (glomerulonephritis, TTP/HUS, malignant hypertension)
	Tubulointerstitial diseases (acute tubular necrosis (ischemic or toxic), acute interstitial nephritis, acute bilateral pyelonephritis)
What are etiologies of postrenal acute kidney injury?	Ureteral obstruction: must be bilateral or unilateral in a patient with single kidney
	Neurogenic bladder
	Cervical/uterine/ovarian cancer
	Prostate disease

ACUTE TUBULAR NECROSIS

What two types of injury can lead to acute tubular necrosis (ATN)?	Ischemic
	Nephrotoxic
What are high-risk clinical settings for ATN?	Sepsis, pancreatitis, burns, post–cardiac surgery, patients with baseline CKD
What are the nonelectrolyte management strategies for the treatment of ATN?	Restoration of kidney perfusion.
	Removal of nephrotoxic agents.
	Treat volume overload with IV diuretics, ultrafiltration if refractory.
	Protein restriction to 0.8 to 1.0g/kg/day, carbohydrate 3 to 5 g/kg/day.
	GI ulcer prophylaxis with histamine antagonist or proton-pump inhibitor.

There are no specific treatments for ATN (controlled trials do not support IV diuretics, dopamine, endothelin-1, atrial naturetic peptide, insulin-like growth factor, mannitol).

What are the electrolyte related management strategies for the treatment of ATN?

Restriction of potassium to <40mmol/day, dialysis if K^+ >6.5 or 5.5 to 6.5 with ECG changes.

Phosphate restriction to <800 mg/day, phosphate binding agents for phosphorus >5.

Dialysis if phosphorus (mg) × calcium (mg) >70.

Sodium bicarbonate to maintain serum levels between 15 and 20 mmol/L and pH>7.2

Hypocalcemia treatment with calcium gluconate

What is the typical time course for the resolution of ATN?

Highly variable and dependent upon the other comorbidities. If a single insult in a relatively healthy patient, should resolve within days to a week.

ACUTE INTERSTITIAL NEPHRITIS

What are the etiologies of AIN?

Drugs

Infections

Systemic disease

Idiopathic

What are the common classes of drugs that cause acute interstitial nephritis (AIN)?

Antimicrobial (penicillin G, ampicillin, methicillin, ciprofloxacin, rifampin, and sulfonamides, including cotrimoxazole)

NSAIDs (aspirin, ibuprofen, fenoprofen, naproxen, indomethacin)

Anticonvulsants (phenytoin)

Diuretics (furosemide)

Antiulcer (omeprazole, cimetidine)

Allopurinol

How does drug-induced AIN present?	In 80% of patients, onset of symptoms is 3 weeks but range is from 1 day to 2 months.
	Clinical findings of flank pain (distension of renal capsule), oliguria, hematuria, pyuria, WBC casts, mild proteinuria, fever, rash, eosinophilia may be present.
What is the average recovery of renal function from drug-induced AIN?	1.5 months
What is the best way to diagnose drug-induced AIN?	Renal biopsy. The presence of urine eosinophils is suggestive, but the finding is very insensitive.
What biopsy findings are consistent with drug-induced AIN?	Interstitial inflammatory infiltrates (T cells, macrophages, plasma cells, eosinophils)
	Interstitial edema
	Tubulitis
	No vascular or glomerular lesions
Are steroids effective in treating drug-induced AIN?	Perhaps. There are no controlled trials but many case reports demonstrating the benefit in select cases. Should be considered in cases that do not have spontaneous improvement in creatinine after 3 to 7 days of withdrawing the offending agent.
What microbes are associated with AIN?	Bacteria: *Staphylococcus, Streptococcus, Escerichia coli, Campylobacter jejuni, Chlamydia, Mycoplasma, Leptospira, Legionella, Mycobacterium tuberculosis, Salmonella, Yersinia*
	Viruses: CMV, EBV, hepatitis B virus HSV, HIV, rickettsia
	Parasites: *Toxoplasma*
What systemic diseases are associated with AIN?	Systemic lupus erythematosus (SLE)
	Sjögren's syndrome
	Sarcoidosis

PIGMENT-INDUCED ACUTE KIDNEY INJURY

In what two clinical settings does heme pigment nephropathy occur?	Rhabdomyolysis and hemolysis
How does rhabdomyolysis lead to acute kidney injury?	1. Fluid sequestration into injured muscle leading to profound volume depletion 2. Cytokine and toxins leading to renal vasoconstriction and tubular injury 3. Myoglobin, freely filtered at the glomerulus, causing tubular cast obstruction and direct tubular injury
What are the clinical features of rhabdomyolysis-induced acute kidney injury?	CK usually >10,000 U/mL Red-brown discoloration of the urine Urine analysis with positive heme but negative RBCs on microscopy Low fractional excretion of sodium
What are the etiologies of rhabdomyolysis?	Muscle injury: burns, trauma, electric shock, seizures, heat exhaustion Drugs: statins, fibrates, neuroleptic malignant syndrome Toxins: alcohol, cocaine, ecstasy, amphetamines Familial: McArdle's disease, malignant hyperthermia
What are the etiologies of hemoglobinuria?	Incompatible blood transfusion, autoimmune hemolytic anemia, paroxysmal nocturnal hemoglobinuria, glucose 6-phosphate dehydrogenase deficiency
What are the management strategies to prevent heme pigment nephropathy?	Aggressive fluid repletion: 1 to 2 L/hr IV normal saline with goal urine output 300 mL/hr. [Less clear role for alkalinization of urine to prevent cast formation with $\frac{1}{2}$ normal saline + 75 meq HCO_3^- titrated to urine pH >6.5. There is no definitive evidence that the alkaline diuresis is more effective than saline diuresis.]

Monitor serum iCa^{++} and serum bicarbonate closely while using bicarbonate.

Consider loop diuretic or mannitol to increase urine output if not at goal.

If acute kidney injury developed, discontinue mannitol and bicarbonate.

CONTRAST NEPHROPATHY

What are the risk factors for developing radiocontrast induced nephropathy (RCIN)?	Renal impairment Rarely seen in patient with normal renal function Creatinine >2.0 mg/dL Diabetes Heart failure Volume depletion, NSAIDs, ACEIs/ARBs
What is the clinical course for RCIN?	Elevation of creatinine 24 to 48 hours postexposure, peak creatinine 4 to 5 days, return to baseline 7 to 10 days If no full recovery, likely concomitant kidney insult (sepsis, hypotension, atheroemboli)

What are the mechanisms for RCIN?	Direct tubular toxicity:
	    Reactive oxygen species causing proximal tubular injury
	
	Kidney vascular hemodynamic changes:
	    Renal vasoconstriction by renin-angiotensin system (RAAS), endothelin, adenosine
	    Osmotic diuresis, thereby increasing NaCl delivery to macula densa and consequent activation of RAAS

How can one minimize the risk for RCIN?	Alternative choice of imaging in high-risk patients Use of low osmolar or iso-osmolar contrast Hydration with NS 1 mL/kg/hr 12 hours before and after contrast exposure

Avoidance of loop diuretics, NSAIDsS, ACEIs prior to contrast

Some studies support N-acetylcysteine 600 q12h × 48 hours prior to procedure

Some studies support bicarbonate or vitamin C prior to procedure

Combination of N-acetylcysteine and bicarbonate with IV fluids may be the best preventive strategy

ATHEROEMBOLIC ACUTE KIDNEY INJURY

When does atheroembolic kidney disease typically occur?

Usually after arterial manipulation: vascular surgery, angioplasty and stenting, arteriography.

It can also occur without manipulation: either spontaneously or after administration of anticoagulants or thrombolytics.

How does acute atheroembolic kidney disease clinically present?

Nonoliguric or oliguric ATN with a high FeNa (intrinsic kidney injury): usually with systemic signs of embolization elsewhere (CNS, confusion; skin, livedo reticularis; feet, ischemic digits)

What is the subacute clinical presentation of atheroembolic kidney disease?

Slow progressive kidney disease with mild proteinuria, hematuria, possible eosinophiluria, labile hypertension. Low-grade fevers may be present.

What laboratory abnormalities may support a diagnosis of atheroembolic disease?

Elevated sedimentation rate, low C3, low C4, elevated liver and muscle enzymes, anemia, eosinophilia, leukocytosis

What is the characteristic kidney biopsy finding of atheroembolic disease?

Cholesterol clefts with giant-cell reaction on light microscopy

What is the therapy for atheroembolic disease?

Generally supportive care. In the setting of AKI, some small case series suggest a role for steroids.

HEPATORENAL SYNDROME

In what patients can hepatorenal syndrome (HRS) occur?

Acute liver disease (severe alcoholic hepatitis)

Chronic liver disease (cirrhosis of any etiology)

Advanced hepatic failure

Portal hypertension

What are the two clinical presentations of HRS?

Type I: Doubling of serum creatinine to >2.5 mg/dL or 50% reduction in creatinine clearance in 2 weeks. Severely jaundiced and coagulopathic

Type II: Slow progressive deterioration in renal function. Less jaundiced and with refractory ascites.

What clinical findings support HRS?

Serum creatinine >1.5 mg/dL, absence of shock and GI fluid losses, persistence of AKI after withdrawal of diuretics and fluid challenge (1.5 L isotonic saline or 100 g albumin in 500 mL saline); oliguria <500 mL, urine sodium <10 mmol/L, urine osmolarity > plasma osmolarity, urine red blood cells <50/hpf, and urinary protein <500mg/L, serum sodium concentration <130 mmol/L, no evidence of obstruction by ultrasound

What is the probability of cirrhotic patients developing HRS?

1-year: 20%

5-year: 40%

What is the prognosis of HRS?

Between 80% and 95%

What is the only established treatment for HRS?

Orthotopic liver transplantation

What pharmacotherapeutic agents are used in the treatment of HRS?

Vasopressin analogs: theoretical reversal of splanchnic vasodilation

Ornipressin 2 IU/hr ×15 days + albumin 1 g/kg first day and then 20 to 40 g daily

Terlipressin + albumin

Splanchnic vasoconstrictors:
Octreotide

Vasoconstrictors: increase mean arterial pressure
Midodrine

Volume expanders:
Albumin

What interventional procedures can be considered for management of HRS?

Paracentesis of 2 L to reduce intra-abdominal pressure

TIPS to reduce portal hypertension

MARS (molecular adsorbent recirculating system) to remove toxic metabolites using an albumin-containing dialysate and charcoal and anion-exchanger columns

Renal replacement therapy

ACUTE KIDNEY INJURY IN THE SETTING OF CANCER

What are common etiologies of acute kidney injury in patients with cancer?

Prerenal: dehydration, hypercalcemia

Vascular: renal vein thrombosis from hypercoagulable state, disseminated intravascular coagulation (acute promyelocytic leukemia), thrombotic microangiopathy

Acute tubular necrosis: sepsis, hypercalcemia, drugs (cisplatin, iphosphamide)

Acute interstitial nephritis: antibiotics, interferon-alpha, IL-2

Malignant infiltration: acute lymphoblastic leukemia, lymphoma

Intraluminal obstruction: tumor lysis syndrome, myeloma cast nephropathy

Postrenal obstruction: ureteral compression from tumor or retroperitoneal fibrosis, bladder cancer

Which patients should be suspected of having tumor lysis syndrome?

Patients with leukemias and lymphomas

Oligoanuric kidney injury

Elevated lactate dehydrogenase levels

Elevated potassium, phosphate, uric acid

What therapies can prevent tumor lysis syndrome?

High dose allopurinol 600 to 900 mg/day prior to chemotherapy

Intravenous fluid loading to have urine output >100 mL/hr

Early continuous dialysis for hyperuricemia and hyperphosphatemia

Urine alkalinization for a pH >7.0 is not recommended because of increased risk of calcium-phosphate precipitation

What are the etiologies of acute reversible kidney injury in patients with myeloma?

Acute kidney injury:

Hypercalcemia

Dehydration

Contrast nephropathy

Cast nephropathy

Infiltration of plasma cells

What is the clinical presentation of direct kidney infiltration by lymphoma or leukemia?

Slow development of nonoliguric acute kidney injury with benign sediment and enlarged kidneys on ultrasound

OBSTRUCTIVE NEPHROPATHY

What are the common causes of intraluminal (tubular) obstruction?

Drugs such as acyclovir, methotrexate, sulfonamides, indinavir, trimethoprim, which can crystallize in the tubules

Uric acid in tumor lysis

Extrarenal intraluminal obstruction can be caused by stones, blood clots, or papillary necrosis

What medications are associated with the development of urinary tract obstruction due to bladder dysfunction?

Any anticholinergic medication and levodopa

What medical conditions are associated with the development of urinary tract obstruction due to bladder dysfunction?

Diabetes mellitus, multiple sclerosis, Parkinson's disease, and strokes can all lead to bladder dysfunction.

What infection can lead to urinary tract obstruction?

Schistosoma haematobium can infect the bladder wall and distal ureter, leading to obstruction.

What are the common causes of extrinsic obstruction of the urinary tract?

Women: gravid uterus, cervical cancer, ovarian cancer or masses, pelvic inflammatory disease

Males: prostatic hypertrophy or cancer

Both genders: retroperitoneal fibrosis, lymphadenopathy, diverticulosis, Crohn's disease, aortic aneurysms

What is the typical clinical presentation of obstructive nephropathy?

Pain

Decreased urinary output or change in character of urinary stream

If bladder outlet obstruction: painful, distended bladder

Urinary tract infections

Uremic symptoms

What are the changes in GFR and tubular function that occur with obstructive nephropathy?

GFR: falls quickly and then resolves as obstruction is relieved. The extent of GFR recovery is dependent on the duration of obstruction.

Tubular function: impaired ability of kidney to concentrate urine (polyuria), development of distal RTA.

What is the test of choice for diagnosing obstructive nephropathy?

Ultrasonography is the quickest and safest method for diagnosis—demonstrates hydronephrosis. Other tests such as CT, MRI, or retrograde pyelography may be useful for localization of the site of obstruction.

What is the treatment of choice for obstructive nephropathy?

Depends upon the cause and site of obstruction. Insertion of nephrostomy tubes is generally the appropriate emergency treatment for upper urinary tract obstruction.

What is a postobstructive diuresis?

Polyuria is common after the relief of obstruction. This is due to salt and water retention during AKI, tubular damage to the kidney preventing urinary concentration, and the buildup of osmotic particles such as urea, which can act like a diuretic. Aggressive attention to volume status and IV hydration is required to avoid volume depletion.

GLOMERULAR DISEASE

What are the clinical presentations of glomerular disease?

Asymptomatic proteinuria (150 mg to 3 g/day), hematuria (>2 RBCs per high-power field or RBC casts), hypoalbuminemia, edema, hypercholesterolemia, lipiduria, oliguria, hypertension, may have signs/symptoms of underlying multisystem disease

What glomerular diseases present as nephrotic syndrome?

Minimal change disease

Focal segmental glomerulosclerosis

Membranous nephropathy

Membranoproliferative glomerulonephritis (MPGN)

Cryoglobulinemic MPGN

Amyloidosis

Diabetic nephropathy

What are the mechanisms for acute renal failure in patients with nephrotic syndrome?

Volume depletion leading to prerenal failure or acute tubular necrosis

Renal vein thrombosis (hypercoagulable state)

Transformation to crescentic type glomerulonephropathy

Acute allergic nephritis from diuretics

Hemodynamic response to ACEI

What are the therapies for treating the complications of nephrotic syndrome?

Nephrotic edema: dietary sodium restriction (60 to 80 mmol/24 hr), oral loop diuretics ± albumin for gradual fluid removal.

Proteinuria: reduction of afferent arteriolar dilation with low-protein diet or dipyridamole. Or blocking efferent arteriolar vasoconstriction with ACEI or ARB.

Hypercoagulability: prophylactic anticoagulation is controversial.

Hyperlipidemia: statin therapy for goal LDL 100 to 129 mg/dL.

Infections: some advocate prophylactic antibiotics, especially for children.

HTN goal: 125/75; first line to consider is ACEI or ARB.

MINIMAL CHANGE DISEASE AND FOCAL SEGMENTAL GLOMERULOSCLEROSIS

What diseases are associated with the development of MCD?

Malignancies: Hodgkin's, mycosis fungoides, CLL.

Drugs: NSAIDs, interferon-alpha, gold.

Allergy: insect stings, pollens.

Most cases are idiopathic.

What are the epidemiologic, clinical, and pathologic features of MCD?

More common in children.

More common in South Asians and Native Americans.

Hypertension at the time of diagnosis is less likely.

Microscopic hematuria is rare.

Light microscopy and immunohistology: normal.

Electron microscopy: podocyte foot process effacement.

Does not progress to renal failure.

What are the epidemiologic, clinical, and pathologic features of primary FSGS?

More common in adults.

More common in African Americans.

Hypertension common at the time of diagnosis.

Microscopic hematuria more common.

Light microscopy: segmental glomerular scarring with adhesions to Bowman's capsule.

Immunohistology: +IgM and C3 deposited in the mesangium.

Electron microscopy: Foot process fusion.

Progresses to renal failure in 50% of patients; degree of proteinuria determines risk.

How is adult MCD treated?

First episode: steroids (prednisone for up to 6 months).

For frequent relapses and steroid-dependent patients, cyclophosphamide can be added.

What is the response rate of MCD to therapy?

Nearly 100% of children and 75% of adults achieve remission. Relapses are common (up to 30% to 40%).

How is primary FSGS treated?

Steroids (prednisone for at least 6 months).

Nonresponders or relapsers: cyclosporine.

Other potential treatments include cyclophosphamide, tacrolimus, mycophenolate.

What is the response rate of FSGS to therapy?

40% of nephrotic patients achieve complete remission and the responders have renal survival >95%.

What factors are associated with secondary FSGS?

Viruses: HIV, hepatitis B, parvovirus

Drugs: pamidronate, heroin

Malignancies: lymphomas

Reduced renal mass: solitary kidney, renal allograft, vesicoureteral reflux

What are the histological variants of FSGS?	Collapsing form Cellular variant Mesangial hypercellularity FSGS with glomerular tip lesions
What is the prognosis for the collapsing form of FSGS?	Severe nephrotic syndrome on presentation, steroid resistance, rapid development of ESRD (median time of 13 months compared with 65 months in other forms of FSGS)
What factors are associated with collapsing FSGS?	Idiopathic, heroin, HIV, pamidronate, parvovirus

HIV-ASSOCIATED NEPHROPATHY

What is HIV-associated nephropathy (HIVAN)?	It is HIV-associated FSGS-variant characterized by a syndrome of massive proteinuria, microhematuria, and azotemia with rapid progression to ESRD. The collapsing form of FSGS is seen on light microscopy.
When does HIVAN occur?	Usually when CD4 cells $<200 \times 10^6$/L. It can also occur during acute HIV infection.
How is HIVAN treated?	No prospective controlled trial has been done. Retroviral therapy may be efficacious. High-dose ACEI/ARB therapy delays the progression of kidney disease. Improvement in renal function correlates with reduction in plasma viral load.

MEMBRANOUS NEPHROPATHY

What is membranous nephropathy?	Glomerular disease as a consequence of IgG deposition on the capillary subepithelial surface. Glomerular permeability is increased, causing nephrotic syndrome. Over time, leads to tubular atrophy and renal failure.
What is the most common cause of membranous nephropathy?	Idiopathic; over 60% of cases have unknown etiology.

What conditions are associated with membranous nephropathy?

Systemic diseases: diabetes mellitus, SLE, solid tumors

Drugs: NSAIDs, penicillamine, gold

Infections: hepatitis B and C

Carcinomas: breast, lung, colon, ovarian, prostate (may be presenting symptom of a carcinoma)

What are the clinical manifestations of membranous nephropathy?

Insidious onset

Women affected > men

Bimodal distribution (ages 30 to 40) and (50 to 60)

Weeks to months of nonnephrotic range proteinuria and then nephrotic range

50% patients with microscopic hematuria

Unusual to have hypertension, red blood cell casts, macroscopic hematuria

What studies should constitute the initial workup for membranous nephropathy?

Assessment of kidney function: serum creatinine and creatinine clearance

Assessment of proteinuria: ratio of urine protein to urine creatinine

Serum albumin, cholesterol, urinalysis

Kidney biopsy to determine exact pathology

Evaluate for associated diseases: hepatitis B surface antigen, hepatitis C antibody or PCR, antinuclear antibody, anti–double-stranded DNA, complements

Consider renal vein angiography depending on probability of renal vein thrombosis (flank pain, hematuria, thromboembolic events)

Age-appropriate cancer screening, particularly if patient's age is >55

What are the outcomes for untreated membranous nephropathy?

30% spontaneous remission

30% partial remission

30% persistent nephrotic range proteinuria with progressive decline in GFR

How is idiopathic membranous nephropathy treated?

Treatment depends on proteinuria and renal function.

If nonnephrotic and normal GFR: treat proteinuria (ACEI and/or ARB), lipid management, blood pressure control.

If proteinuria is 3.5 to 10 g and normal GFR: treatment as above.

If proteinuria is 3.5 to 10 g and reduced GFR: first treat as above. If proteinuria persists on the order of 4 to 8 months, consider cytotoxic agents and steroids.

If urine protein >10 g, regardless of GFR, treat with cytotoxic therapy and steroids.

If patients are on cytotoxic/steroid treatment, what types of prophylaxis is needed?

Antiulcer medications

Bone-stabilizing agents: calcium, vitamin D, bisphosphonates

PCP prophylaxis with trimethoprim/sulfamethoxazole

MEMBRANOPROLIFERATIVE GLOMERULONEPHRITIS

What are the clinical manifestations of MPGN?

Microscopic hematuria

Nonnephrotic-range proteinuria or nephrotic syndrome

Progressive glomerulonephritis

Rapidly progressive glomerulonephritis

What are the etiologies of membranoproliferative glomerulonephritis?

Idiopathic

Secondary: hepatitis C, chronic hepatitis B, HIV, malaria, chronic liver disease, chronic lymphocytic leukemia, lymphoma, thymoma, renal cell carcinoma, SLE, Sjögren's syndrome, hereditary complement deficiency, acquired complement deficiency, bacterial endocarditis

What are the different histological types of MPGN?

MPGN type I (with mixed cryoglobulinemia or without cryoglobulinemia)

MPGN type II (associated with C3 nephritic factor or associated with factor H defect)

MPGN type III (associated with or without terminal complement nephritic factor)

What is the C3 nephritic factor?

An autoantibody formed against the C3 convertase component of the complement cascade. This leads to continuous complement activation and is associated with the development of MPGN.

What types of MPGN are associated with hepatitis C?

MPGN type I with and without cryoglobulinemia

MPGN type III

In which setting is MPGN type I likely to occur?

In conditions with chronic generation of immune complexes (HIV, HCV, HBV, malaria, SLE, chronic lymphocytic leukemia)

In conditions with a patient's inability to clear immune complexes (hereditary complement deficiencies of classic pathway)

In conditions with continuous complement activation (C3 nephritic factor or factor H deficiency)

Where are immune complexes deposited in MPGN type I?

Mesangium and subendothelial space

Where are immune complexes deposited in MPGN type II?

Subendothelial space

Where are immune complexes deposited in MPGN type III?

Mesangium and subendothelial space, but deposition may occur in subepithelial space.

What are findings for MPGN on:

Light microscopy?
Hypercellularity of the glomerulus and prominent lobes of the glomerulus because of mesangial proliferation

Immunofluorescence?
Granular staining of glomerular capillary wall

Electron microscopy?
Subendothelial deposits ± mesangial deposits ± subepithelial deposits with duplicated basement membrane (tram-tracking)

What are cryoglobulins?
Immunoglobulins that are precipitated in the cold

What diseases are cryoglobulins associated with?
Lymphoproliferative disorders, monoclonal gammopathies (myeloma, Waldenström's), HCV, HBV, poststreptococcal glomerulonephritis, endocarditis

SLE

Chronic liver disease

What are the systemic manifestations of cryoglobulinemia?
Artralgias, purpura, Raynaud's phenomenon, digital necrosis, painful skin lesions

How is MPGN treated?
Normal GFR and nonnephrotic: observation

Impaired GFR or nephrotic: steroids

If HCV or cryoglobulin associated and normal GFR: interferon-alpha and ribavirin

If HCV or cryoglobulin associated and reduced GFR: interferon-alpha, ribavirin, steroids

If HCV or cryoglobulin associated and RPGN: methylprednisolone, cyclophosphamide, and cryofiltration (plasmapheresis)

What is the prognosis for MPGN?	Renal replacement therapy needed in >50% at 10 years
Does MPGN recur in kidney transplants?	Yes

NEPHRITIC SYNDROME—GENERAL

What is the nephritic syndrome?	Development of deterioration in GFR associated with:
	Active urine sediment: dysmorphic RBCs, RBC casts, white blood cells, granular casts
	Hypertension
	± Systemic symptoms of the underlying disease (such as SLE)
What glomerular diseases present as nephritic syndrome?	Immune complex: poststreptococcal glomerulonephritis, SLE, endocarditis, IgA nephropathy
	Vasculitis (usually ANCA-positive)
	Associated with anti-GBM antibodies

IgA NEPHROPATHY

What is the most common clinical presentation of IgA nephropathy?	Hematuria during upper respiratory illness (synpharyngitic hematuria) or isolated asymptomatic microscopic hematuria.
	IgA nephropathy is the most common pattern of glomerular disease in the world.
How is Henoch-Schönlein purpura (HSP) differentiated from IgA nephropathy?	The kidney pathology is the same, with diffuse mesangial deposition of IgA. However, in HSP, there are extrarenal manifestations, including vasculitis of the skin, gut, and joints.
What is the pathogenesis of IgA nephropathy?	Likely due to abnormal glycosylation of IgA and formation of circulating IgA, circulating immune complexes that deposit in the mesangium, leading to glomerular injury.

What are the clinical presentations of IgA nephropathy?	Asymptomatic hematuria and proteinuria
	Macroscopic hematuria often with a concomitant upper respiratory tract infection
	Nephrotic syndrome
	Acute kidney injury with crescent formation
	Chronic kidney disease
What are clinical presentations of HSP?	Palpable purpuric rash
	Abdominal pain/bloody diarrhea from intestinal vasculitis
	Polyarthralgias
	Acute renal failure
What is the treatment for IgA nephropathy associated with hematuria and stable kidney function?	Observation
What is the treatment for IgA nephropathy associated with acute kidney injury?	Biopsy to evaluate for crescentic IgA nephropathy. If crescents form, begin prednisone and cyclophosphamide.
What is the treatment for IgA nephropathy associated with proteinuria?	If evidence of minimal change on biopsy, begin prednisone. If proteinuria >1 g/24 hr, use ACEI. For persistent proteinuria on ACEI, consider steroids, azathioprine, or fish oil. Combination of ACEIs and ARBs appears to be particularly beneficial.
What is the role of tonsillectomy in the treatment of IgA nephropathy?	Advocated by some, but the data are inconclusive.
Does IgA nephropathy recur in kidney transplants?	Yes

RAPIDLY PROGRESSIVE GLOMERULONEPHRITIS

What glomerular diseases present as rapidly progressive glomerulonephritis?

Goodpasture's disease

Vasculitis: Wegener's granulomatosis, microscopic polyangiitis, Churg-Strauss

Immune complex: SLE, poststreptococcal glomerulonephritis, IgA/HSP, endocarditis, membranoproliferative glomerulonephritis

What is the diagnostic workup for a patient with RPGN?

Serologic studies: ANA, anti-dsDNA, complement levels (C3, C4), ANCA, anti-GBM antibodies.

Most patients will be biopsied for definitive diagnosis.

GOODPASTURE'S DISEASE

What is the clinical presentation of Goodpasture's disease?

Rapidly progressive glomerulonephritis (RPGN) and hemoptysis. A renal-limited form of the disease is termed anti-GBM disease.

What is the etiology of Goodpasture's disease?

Autoimmunity to a common antigen found on lung and kidney basement membrane

What is the antigen in Goodpasture's disease?

The noncollagenous domain of the alpha-3 chain of type IV collagen: alpha-3(IV)NC1

What precipitating factors may uncover basement membrane epitopes and precipitate the disease?

Cigarette smoking

Hydrocarbon exposure

Infections

Pulmonary edema

What information can be gained by kidney biopsy to determine prognosis?

Degree of necrosis and crescent formation

Degree of tubular loss and chronic scarring

What immunohistologic finding on kidney biopsy is pathognomonic for anti-GBM or Goodpasture's disease?

Linear staining of immunoglobulin along the basement membrane (reacting to the type IV collagen in the basement membrane)

What therapies are available for acute Goodpasture's disease?	Plasma exchange (most effective if initiated early with serum creatinine <6 mg/dL), plus prednisone and cyclophosphamide
What factors predict kidney recovery?	Presenting creatinine <6 mg/dL Nonoliguric
Which patients should be considered for supportive treatment (i.e., no immunosuppression)?	Patients who do not have lung hemorrhage and are dialysis-dependent at onset and with high percentage of crescents, glomerulosclerosis and tubular loss. These patients do not appear to benefit from aggressive immunosuppression.
Does anti-GBM or Goodpasture's disease recur in kidney transplants?	Yes.
What is the optimal timing for kidney transplant in Goodpasture's disease?	Anti-GBM antibodies should be undetectable for at least 6 months to minimize recurrence in transplant.

VASCULITIS

What diseases present with vasculitis involving large vessels?	Giant-cell arteritis Takayasu's arteritis
What diseases present with vasculitis involving medium-sized vessels?	Polyarteritis nodosa Kawasaki's disease
What diseases present with vasculitis involving small vessels?	Wegener's granulomatosis Churg-Strauss syndrome Microscopic polyangiitis Henoch-Schönlein purpura Cryoglobulinemic vasculitis Leukocytoclastic angiitis

What are the clinical manifestations of ANCA-positive (small vessel) vasculitis?

RPGN

Fever, malaise, anorexia, weight loss, myalgias, arthralgias

Palpable purpura

Upper and lower respiratory involvement (most common in Wegener's)

Peripheral neuropathy

What are the two antigens associated with ANCA diseases?

Proteinase 3 (cANCA): Wegener's

Myeloperoxidase (pANCA): microscopic polyangiitis

What is the sensitivity of ANCA for small-vessel vasculitis?

>90%

What is seen pathologically in ANCA diseases?

Focal necrotizing lesions in the glomerulus and vasculature

Crescent formation

Termed pauci-immune secondary to lack of immune deposits and negative immunohistochemistry

How is ANCA-associated RPGN treated?

High-dose methylprednisone IV followed by high-dose oral prednisone

Oral cyclophosphamide daily for 6 to 12 months

Plasma exchange is controversial but likely beneficial if patients have concomitant hemoptysis

What is the percentage of ANCA disease relapse?

25% to 50%

SYSTEMIC LUPUS ERYTHEMATOSUS (SLE)

What are the immunologic findings in patients with SLE nephritis?

Anti-dsDNA and anti-ssDNA antibodies. They also usually have antibodies against C1q and depressed levels of C3 and C4.

For the following features, what percentage of patients have the findings?

Proteinuria	100%
Microscopic hematuria	80%
Tubular abnormalities	60–80%
Nephrotic syndrome	45–65%
Reduced renal function	40–80%
Nephritis	30% to 50%
Granular casts	30%
RPGN	30%
Hypertension	15% to 50%

How is SLE nephritis classified?

By the World Health Organization (WHO) system: based on light microscopy:

WHO class I: normal

WHO class II: mesangial disease

WHO class III: focal proliferative GN

WHO class IV: diffuse proliferative GN

WHO class V: membranous GN

How common are each of the types of SLE nephritis?

Class I: <5%

Class II: 10% to 25%

Class III: 20% to 35%

Class IV: 35% to 60%

Class V: 10% to 15%

What are the different presentations of the SLE nephritis subtypes?

Class I: hematuria, mild proteinuria

Class II: hematuria, proteinuria

Class III: hematuria, proteinuria, HTN, possibly decreased GFR

Class IV: hematuria, proteinuria, HTN, decreased GFR, possibly RPGN

Class V: nephrotic-range proteinuria

How is SLE nephritis treated?

For mild nephritis (WHO class II): prednisone alone

For severe disease (WHO classes III and IV): prednisone plus either cyclophosphamide or mycophenolate

For class V disease: same at classes III and IV or may try cyclosporine as well

What percent of patients with lupus nephritis progress to ESRD?

10% to 15%

COLLAGEN VASCULAR DISEASE

What are the renal manifestations of rheumatoid arthritis?

Membranous nephropathy

Rheumatoid vasculitis

Amyloidosis

Mesangial proliferative GN

What are the renal manifestations of scleroderma?

Mesangial proliferative GN

Scleroderma renal crisis: AKI associated with severe hypertension, renal vasoconstriction, microangiopathic hemolytic anemia. Leads to ischemic injury of the glomerulus and tubules. Treated with high-dose ACEI.

IMMUNOGLOBULIN DEPOSITION DISEASES

What are the two categories of glomerular disease caused by immunoglobulin deposition as seen by electron microscopy?

1. Organized
   Fibrillar (amyloid)
   Microtubular (cryoglobulinemia, immunotactoid glomerulonephritis)
2. Nonorganized (monoclonal immunoglobulin deposition disease)

What is amyloidosis?

Amyloidosis is defined by the ability of a variety of proteins to form beta-pleated sheets and for these proteins to deposit in a variety of organs (kidney, heart, blood vessels, nerves), leading to end-organ dysfunction.

What two types of amyloidosis have kidney involvement?

Primary amyloid (AL, AH)

Secondary amyloid (AA)

How are the two diseases distinguished?

By the precursor proteins:

Both AL and AH amyloid have light-or heavy-chain immunoglobulin deposition.

AA amyloid has SAA apolipoprotein deposition.

What are the main clinical manifestations of AL and AH amyloid?

Nephrotic syndrome

Peripheral neuropathy

Restrictive cardiomyopathy and congestive heart failure

Orthostatic hypotension

What are the light microscopy findings of AL amyloid?

Mesangial expansion, tubular and glomerular basement membrane thickening, and Congo red staining, seen as apple-green birefringence under polarized light

What are the immunofluorescent findings of AL amyloid?

Staining for immunoglobulin molecules

What are the electron microscopy findings of AL amyloid?

Organized fibrils deposited within or alongside capillary basement membrane

What is the median survival for AL amyloid and what is the most significant negative prognostic factor?

Median survival: 16 months

Negative prognostic factor: symptomatic heart failure (median survival 5 months)

What are treatment options for AL amyloid?

Melphalan, prednisone, autologous stem cell transplant

What is monoclonal immunoglobulin deposition disease (MIDD)?

Deposition of monoclonal immunoglobulins in a nonorganized distribution, depicted as granular deposits on electron microscopy. Deposits can be of light chains (LCDD), heavy chains (HCDD), or heavy and light chains (LHCDD)

What is the most common renal presentation of MIDD?

Nephrotic syndrome with progressive decline in GFR

What are the light microscopy findings of MIDD?

Nodular glomerulosclerosis in 30% to 100% of patients, 10% may have positive Congo red staining

What are the immunofluorescent findings of MIDD?

Positive for deposition of immunoglobulin molecules

What are the electron microscopy findings of MIDD?

Dense granular deposits along glomerular basement membrane

What hematologic diseases occur with MIDD?

Multiple myeloma (MM), Waldenström's macroglobulinemia, or chronic lymphocytic leukemia

MULTIPLE MYELOMA

What kidney diseases occur in patients with multiple myeloma?

Prerenal azotemia (volume depletion), often associated with hypercalcemia

ATN

Interstitial nephritis

Myeloma kidney (cast nephropathy)

AL amyloid

LCDD

Plasma cell infiltration

What is the incidence of renal insufficiency in MM?

Over 40% of patients with MM have serum creatinine >1.5 mg/dL. Of these, most cases are caused by cast nephropathy.

What are treatment options for MM and renal failure secondary to myeloma kidney?

Melphalan/dexamethasone or vincristine, doxorubicin (Adriamycin), dexamethasone, and consideration of stem cell transplant and plasmapheresis

Does plasmapheresis lengthen renal survival in patients with myeloma kidney, AL amyloid, or LCDD?

Unknown. To date there is one positive trial and several negative trials regarding the efficacy of plasmapheresis in decreasing death and dialysis and improving renal recovery. The biological limitation is that plasmapheresis can remove only those proteins in the intravascular space. IgGs and light chains are distributed 50% in intravascular and 50% in extravascular space.

THROMBOTIC MICROANGIOPATHY (TMA)

What are clinical presentations of TMA?

Thrombotic thrombocytopenic purpura (TTP)

Hemolytic-uremic syndrome (HUS)

Antiphospholipid antibody syndrome (APA)

What features can distinguish HUS from TTP?

HUS tends to affect children, have higher association with kidney injury and less neurological involvement than TTP. HUS also associated more often with shiga-toxin producing E. coli that leads to bloody diarrhea.

What is the clinical pentad for TTP?

Thrombocytopenia

Microangiopathic hemolytic anemia

Acute kidney injury

Neurologic deficits

Fever

What laboratory values support TTP?

Thrombocytopenia

Hemolytic anemia: high LDH, low haptoglobin, high indirect bilirubin, schistocytes on peripheral smear, negative Coombs' test

Normal coagulation tests

Acute kidney injury

What is in the differential diagnosis for thrombocytopenia, microangiopathic hemolytic anemia, acute kidney injury?	Malignant hypertension, vasculitis, disseminated intravascular coagulation, APA
What are some potential causes of TTP/HUS?	Infections: HIV, Shiga toxin from *E. coli* (0157:H7)
	Drugs: clopidogrel, ticlopidine, rifampin, metronidazole, penicillin, quinine, some antineoplastic drugs or immunosuppressants (cyclosporine, tacrolimus)
	Autoimmune disease: SLE, scleroderma
	Pregnancy: HELLP syndrome, postpartum HUS
	Idiopathic
	Malignancy: metastatic gastric cancer
What is the pathogenesis of idiopathic TTP?	Low levels or activity of a protease (ADAMTS13) that normally cleaves von Willebrand factor multimers
How is HUS secondary to Shiga toxin treated?	Plasma exchange can be considered (adults)
	Supportive care, hydration, electrolyte repletion
	Dialysis for volume or uremic clearance
	No antibiotics for *E. coli* (0157:H7) or antimotility agents
How is idiopathic TTP treated?	Plasma exchange and fresh frozen plasma as replacement fluid
	Cryoprecipitate can be considered for relapsing TTP
	Exchange is done until platelets and LDH normalize
	Other therapies include steroids, vincristine, cyclophosphamide, azathioprine, splenectomy
How is TTP in pregnancy treated?	Plasma exchange and delivery

TUBULOINTERSTITIAL DISEASE

What are the different types of diseases affecting the tubules and interstitium that can lead to chronic interstitial disease?

Collagen vascular diseases (sarcoidosis, SLE, Sjögren syndrome, Behçet's), infectious diseases (EBV, tuberculosis, *Brucella, Toxoplasma,* fungi), drugs (Lithium, tacrolimus, Chinese herbs), VUR, heavy metals, MM, hypokalemia, and hypercalcemia

What are the clinical hallmarks of chronic interstitial kidney disease?

Decrease in GFR, polyuria and nocturia due to incomplete nephrogenic diabetes insipidus, renal tubular acidosis, Fanconi's syndrome due to proximal tubular injury, anemia out of proportion to fall in GFR, proteinuria <1.5 g/day

What percentage of patients with ESRD have CIN as their primary diagnosis?

Varies widely, from ~3% to 8% in the United States to 42% in Scotland, depending on diagnostic precision and geographical factors.

What are the mechanisms by which tubulointerstitial structures are injured?

1. Immune-mediated, involving antibodies directed against tubular epithelial antigens (as in collagen-vascular disease).
2. Direct cytotoxic exposures, as in lead poisoning or analgesic nephropathy.
3. Idiosyncratic reactions, as in cytokine-mediated damage from tacrolimus.
4. The final pathway for all these injuries is interstitial fibrosis, glomerulosclerosis, and tubular atrophy.

What is the histologic appearance of tubulointerstitial nephritis?

Acutely, interstitial edema with a leukocytic (usually lymphocytic) infiltrate; CIN is marked by tubular atrophy and interstitial fibrosis $\pm$ lymphocytic infiltrate. The degree of tubular atrophy and interstitial fibrosis is one of the best predictors of long-term renal outcome.

What are the renal manifestations of sarcoidosis?

Calcitriol is synthesized at a high rate by macrophages in granulomas; this results in hypercalciuria, hypercalcemia, and nephrocalcinosis (the most common cause of CKD in sarcoid). Sarcoid can also cause a granulomatous interstitial nephritis. Rarely, sarcoid can cause GN or retroperitoneal fibrosis causing obstructive uropathy.

What is the treatment of CKD associated with sarcoidosis?

Granulomatous interstitial nephritis often responds well to high-dose corticosteroids; hypercalcemia often responds to a low dose of steroids but is more likely to recur after treatment.

What are the renal manifestations of Sjögren's syndrome?

CIN that predominantly affects the distal tubule, leading to type 1 RTA. Rarely, associated with glomerulonephritis.

What is the treatment of CKD associated with Sjögren's syndrome?

Corticosteroids or cytotoxic drugs; CIN typically responds well, although tubular dysfunction is usually permanent.

What is chronic urate nephropathy?

Interstitial fibrosis secondary to sodium urate crystal deposition in the interstitium of medullary cells; usually seen in patients with tophaceous gout.

Who develops reflux nephropathy?

Children and adults with congenital vesicoureteral (VUR) junction abnormalities that predispose to reflux of urine into the kidney during bladder contraction

What is the pathogenesis of reflux nephropathy?

Recurrent reflux of infected urine is thought to cause renal scarring. Progressive loss of nephron mass leads to glomerular hyperfiltration and in some cases development of FSGS. As VUR is often associated with hypoplastic kidneys, this population may also be more susceptible to any form of kidney damage and CKD.

What are the characteristics of reflux nephropathy?

Recurrent urinary infections, heavy proteinuria (often due to FSGS), slowly progressive decline in GFR

What is xanthogranulomatous pyelonephritis?

A rare complication of chronic urinary inflammation, where granulomatous tissue replaces nearly all renal parenchyma

Aside from reflux nephropathy, what is the role of infectious agents in causing TIN?

Many cases of documented TIN have occurred with infections such as HIV, tuberculosis, leptospirosis, fungi, and others and remitted after treatment. These cases are typically rare. Several investigators have found EBV DNA and antigens in renal biopsies with otherwise unexplained TIN.

What is BK virus nephropathy? Who is at risk and how is it treated?

An acute or chronic interstitial nephritis occurring in post–renal transplant patients caused by BK (or JC) virus. Intranuclear viral inclusions are found on kidney biopsy. Treatment with lowering of immunosuppression or antiviral medications is attempted but often not successful, leading to eventual failure of the kidney transplant.

What is myeloma cast nephropathy?

A form of TIN that occurs more often with kappa-light chain immunoglobulins. Tubular injury and cast formation are caused by light chain precipitation in renal tubules, causing both obstruction and inflammatory damage. Can progress rapidly to ESRD. Hypovolemia plays a prominent role in promoting cast formation.

What are other tubular abnormalities in kidney function caused by MM?

Proximal tubular dysfunction leading to Fanconi's syndrome; urate or calcium stones

Which heavy metals have been implicated in CKD?

Lead, cadmium, and mercury; very rarely, gold, uranium, arsenic, zinc, and others

What are the manifestations of lead nephropathy?

Proximal tubular dysfunction, hyporeninemic hypoaldosteronism, hyperuricemia resulting from decreased uric acid excretion and causing gout, hypertension, progressive renal failure

What is saturnine gout?

Recurring gout, usually tophaceous, that occurs as a result of lead-induced hypouricosuria and resultant hyperuricemia

How is the diagnosis of lead nephropathy made?

As >90% of total body lead is in bone, an EDTA mobilization test is necessary. After administration of EDTA, a 72-hour collection of urine is measured for lead; >600 μg is diagnostic of high lead burden.

How is lead nephropathy treated?

EDTA chelation of lead to decrease progression of CKD

What is renal papillary necrosis (RPN)?

RPN is an uncommon complication of CIN; medullary ischemia caused by a variety of diseases can result in infarction and subsequent necrosis of the renal papillae.

What disorders have been known to cause RPN?

Any cause of CIN; diabetes mellitus, analgesic nephropathy, renal vein thrombosis, pyelonephritis, sickle cell disease, obstructive uropathy, and many others. Transplanted kidneys, especially cadaveric, are more susceptible to RPN.

What is the mechanism by which RPN occurs?

As the renal medulla has a relatively poor blood supply, it is especially vulnerable to hypoperfusion. In most cases of RPN, inflammation of the interstitium results in vasoconstriction and subsequent ischemia leading to infarction. Ischemia may also be due to other causes, such as obstruction of blood flow in sickle cell nephropathy.

How is the diagnosis of RPN made?

Imaging studies such as CT or ultrasound suggest the diagnosis.

What is the significance of RPN?

RPN may result in progressive CKD, tubular defects with electrolyte wasting or concentrating difficulties (polyuria/nocturia); sloughing of necrotic papillae can lead to acute urinary obstruction. Management of RPN is that of the underlying process.

RENOVASCULAR DISEASE

What are the various forms of renal artery stenosis (RAS)?

Fibromuscular dysplasia (FMD)
Atherosclerotic disease

What are the clinical syndromes secondary to atherosclerotic renovascular disease?

Ischemic renal disease (progressive renal failure)
ACEI/ARB-induced AKI
Flash pulmonary edema
Renovascular hypertension
Acute renal infarction
Asymptomatic

What constitutes hemodynamically significant RAS?

>70% stenosis

What are the clinical characteristics of FMD?

Occurs more often in young females and diffusely involves the renal arteries and other arteries as well with a characteristic appearance on angiography ("rosary beading"). Most often presents as isolated hypertension.

What are the clinical characteristics of atherosclerotic renal vascular disease?

Older patients with hypertension, other risk factors for atherosclerotic disease such as smoking, hyperlipidemia, family history. Atherosclerotic disease tends to be restricted to the ostia of the renal arteries. Can present in more varied fashion: hypertension, renal insufficiency, etc.

Can renal artery stenosis be asymptomatic?

Yes, often renal artery lesions are found incidentally and are not functionally significant. In fact, up to 60% of patients age >70 years who die from cardiovascular causes are found to have RAS on autopsy that was not clinically suspected.

What are the characteristics of a bruit due to RAS?

Holosystolic with a short diastolic component heard best in the flank regions or just lateral to the umbilicus

What diagnostic tests have the highest sensitivity and specificity for making the diagnosis of RAS?

MRA

Spiral CT scan with IV contrast

Duplex ultrasonography (highly operator-dependent)

Angiography (the "gold" standard)

What are the complications associated with renal angiography?

Contrast nephropathy

Cholesterol emboli

Renal artery or aortic dissection

Retroperitoneal hematoma

Pseudoaneurysm formation

What is a common problem with all imaging studies for RAS?

The studies detect only the presence of a stenotic lesion; they do not predict functional significance (either in causing progressive renal insufficiency or hypertension).

What is the success rate for percutaneous transluminal renal angioplasty (PTRA)?

Fibromuscular dysplasia: 100% technical success with 50% hypertension cure rate and 50% hypertension improved rate.

Atherosclerotic RAS: >70% technical success with the majority of ostial lesions requiring stent placement. Cure of hypertension is rare (0% to 15%) with improved BP control in 50% to 85% of patients.

What are the clinical clues that suggest a poor outcome from PTRA?	Long-standing hypertension Small (<8 cm) kidneys Creatinine >3 mg/dL Bilateral RAS Diabetes or other causes of progressive kidney disease Poor LV function
Can patients with RAS be managed medically?	Yes. Three randomized clinical trials have looked at this and suggest that a majority of patients can be managed with medical therapy. However, this may be at the expense of additional medications. A larger study (CORAL) is now reinvestigating this question.

GENETIC KIDNEY DISEASES

What is the most common inherited renal disease?	Autosomal dominant polycystic kidney disease (ADPKD); it is the fourth most common cause of ESRD.
What are the various forms of ADPKD?	Types I and II
How do these forms differ?	Type I: accounts for 80% to 90% of cases with ESRD occurring by age 50 to 60 Type II: accounts for 10% to 20% of cases with milder disease and ESRD occurring by age 70
What is the gene involved in ADPKD?	The mutations occur in proteins named polycystins, which are expressed in the renal tubules and are important in cell signaling and proliferation.
What are the renal manifestations of ADPKD?	Hematuria, nocturia (loss of renal concentrating ability), flank pain, nephrolithiasis, cyst rupture, cyst bleeding and cyst infections
What are the extrarenal manifestations of ADPKD?	Liver cysts, pancreatic cysts, cerebral aneurysms, colonic diverticula, mitral valve prolapse

How is ADPKD diagnosed?

Either by ultrasonographic findings of an abnormal number of renal cysts or through genetic testing

What are the features of autosomal recessive PKD?

Early age onset with severe renal abnormalities and early progression to ESRD. May cause neonatal death and associated with progressive hepatic fibrosis.

What are the features of tuberous sclerosis?

Autosomal dominant.

Hamartomas develop in multiple organs.

80% have seizures.

50% have mental retardation.

Skin manifestations are common.

Renal lesions include renal cell carcinoma, cysts, and angiomyolipomas.

What are the features of von Hippel–Lindau disease?

Autosomal dominant

Predisposition for tumors of the eyes, brain, spinal cord, adrenals, and pancreas

Pheochromocytomas in 20%

Associated with renal cysts and development of bilateral renal cell carcinoma

What is Alport's syndrome?

X-linked disease (in a minority of patients, it is an autosomal recessive disorder) characterized by hematuria, progressive renal failure, and hearing difficulties. It is caused by defective production of type IV collagen in the glomerular basement membrane.

What is thin basement membrane disease?

Also a defect in type IV collagen which presents as isolated glomerular hematuria with a very low risk of progressive renal disease.

What are the features of Fabry's disease?

Hereditary deficiency of alpha-galactosidase A

Results in intracellular accumulation of glycosphingolipids

Leads to involvement of the heart, CNS, skin, and kidneys

Leads to proteinuria and progressive renal failure

Treated with human recombinant enzyme

What are the renal manifestations of sickle cell disease?

Impaired renal concentrating ability with nocturia (due to medullary injury)

Hematuria

Papillary necrosis

Distal renal tubular acidosis with hyperkalemia

Focal segmental glomerulosclerosis

Hypertension

ESRD (2% to 5%)

DRUGS AND THE KIDNEY

NSAIDs

What effects do NSAIDs have on the kidney at typical therapeutic doses?

NSAIDs inhibit renal prostaglandin synthesis (PGE_2 and PGI_2), leading to afferent arteriolar constriction.

Which patients are most at risk for NSAID-induced nephrotoxic effects?

Patients with preexisting CKD, AKI, hypovolemia, HF, liver disease

How do NSAIDs cause:
    Prerenal azotemia?

PGI_2 inhibition causing vasoconstriction of afferent arteriole. NSAIDs may also precipitate HRS via a similar mechanism.

    Edema and hypertension?

PGE_2 inhibition causes sodium retention via local and ADH-mediated mechanisms.

    ATN?

PGI_2 keeps renal blood flow constant in ischemic conditions; its inhibition can increase the risk of ATN.

    Type 4 RTA?

Prostaglandin-mediated reduction in renin secretion

AIN?	Typically seen with chronic use
Acute papillary necrosis?	Vasoconstriction, often with hypovolemia
Nephrotic syndrome?	Minimal change disease; less commonly, membranous nephropathy

ACEIS AND ARBS

What is the mechanism of ACEI-induced decrease in GFR?	Reduced levels of angiotensin II, reducing vasoconstriction of the efferent arteriole and reducing vasodilation of the afferent arteriole, thereby decreasing glomerular capillary pressure and filtration
In which conditions have ACEIs been shown beneficial for retardation of kidney damage?	All causes of CKD (except for bilateral renal artery stenosis)
How do ACEIs reduce progression to ESRD and proteinuria?	Reduction of intraglomerular (as well as systemic) pressure, decreasing glomerular permeability and glomerulosclerosis. Reduction of proteinuria has the added benefit of decreasing protein-dependent inflammation and damage.
Are ACEIs equivalent to ARBs in treatment of chronic kidney disease?	As of 2007, the NKF considers ACEIs and ARBs to be interchangeable for treatment of CKD.
Are ACEIs and ARBs complementary in treatment of CKD?	Multiple trials, such as COOPERATE, have demonstrated reduced progression to ESRD and reduced proteinuria with combined ACEI–ARB therapy.
How do ACEIs and ARBs cause hyperkalemia?	Aldosterone deficiency, especially with some degree of reduction in GFR
How can ACEIs and ARBs cause AKI?	Synergistically (in the presence of other factors such as nephrotoxins or hypoperfusion) or by excessive efferent arteriolar vasodilation in bilateral renal artery stenosis

TRIMETHOPRIM/SULFAMETHOXAZOLE

What are the adverse effects of trimethoprim (TMP) that affect the kidneys?	Impair secretion of creatinine causing falsely elevated SCr; hyperkalemia, occasional hyponatremia, normal AG metabolic acidosis
What is the mechanism of TMP-induced electrolyte abnormalities?	TMP is structurally similar to amiloride; it inhibits the ENaC ion channel in the CT, decreasing the electrochemical gradient driving K^+ and H^+ transport. This leads to a distal tubular acidosis similar to type 4 RTA, causing hyperkalemia and occasional hyponatremia and metabolic acidosis. This is usually seen in high-dose TMP (e.g., treatment of PCP).
Who are most at risk for TMP-induced electrolyte abnormalities?	Patients with preexisting CKD, type 4 RTA, hyponatremia (e.g., SIADH); any patient receiving high-dose TMP/SMX, critically ill patients
What are the adverse effects of sulfamethoxazole that affect the kidneys?	AIN, crystalluria leading to tubular obstruction; rarely, rhabdomyolysis

LITHIUM

What are the effects of lithium on the kidney?	NDI (by down regulating aquaporin 2), nephrotic syndrome (MCD or FSGS), chronic interstitial nephritis, CKD
How common is NDI in patients receiving lithium chronically?	10% to 20% have at least some degree of concentrating impairment.
What other effects are seen in acute or chronic lithium toxicity?	Nausea, delirium, hypo/hyperthyroidism, hypercalcemia, aplastic anemia, long-QT syndrome, seizures, arrhythmias
Which conditions predispose to a higher risk of lithium toxicity?	Preexisting renal dysfunction, use of ACEIs, chronic lithium use
At what serum lithium levels are these effects seen?	Toxic levels >1.5 meq/L chronically, higher levels in acute intoxication

At what point is dialysis indicated to remove lithium?

Any serum level >4 meq/L, >2.5 meq/L with renal insufficiency or neurologic symptoms, increasing levels after admission, or any level in ESRD with symptoms. Dialysis should be extended to account for tissue redistribution and prevent rebounding levels post-HD.

What other treatments for lithium-induced NDI exist besides dialysis?

Amiloride (blocks lithium reuptake in the collecting tubules); thiazides and NSAIDs

ANTI-INFECTIVE DRUGS

How do various anti-infective agents cause AKI:

    Beta lactams?

AIN; several cephalosporins and carbapenems are toxic to proximal tubular cells and can cause ATN

    Aminoglycosides?

Dose-related proximal tubular toxicity; may cause ATN.

    Vancomycin?

AKI due more to the vehicle vancomycin is suspended in, which is substantially less nephrotoxic than in the past. Vancomycin alone rarely causes AKI these days; AKI is usually seen in combination with other drugs (e.g., aminoglycosides).

    HIV protease inhibitors (adefovir and tenofovir) and cidofovir?

Accumulate in proximal tubular cells (reuptake by organic anion transport channels) leading to proximal tubular toxicity (ATN and Fanconi's syndrome)

    Acyclovir and indinavir?

Crystalluria causing obstructive nephropathy, TIN, ATN

    Foscarnet?

Direct tubulotoxic causing AKI, hypocalcemia, nephrogenic diabetes insipidus (DI)

    Amphotericin B?

Intrarenal vasoconstriction plus direct toxicity to proximal tubular cells

CYTOTOXIC AND IMMUNOSUPPRESSIVE DRUGS

What effects do tacrolimus and cyclosporine have on renal function? Which effects are reversible and which are not?

Both tacrolimus and cyclosporine nephrotoxicity result from calcineurin inhibition. Reversible, dose-dependent reduction in RBF (due to afferent arteriole constriction) is mediated by increased endothelin and angiotensin II activity and decreased nitric oxide activity. Irreversible interstitial fibrosis is thought to be cytokine-mediated and dose-independent.

What is the mechanism of tacrolimus-induced hyperkalemia?

Suppression of mineralocorticoid synthesis

What is the mechanism of cyclosporine-induced hyperkalemia?

Suppression of plasma renin activity and renal tubular aldosterone resistance

Compared to tacrolimus, does sirolimus have similar effects on the kidney?

Sirolimus likely has some nephrotoxicity. However, sirolimus can increase CyA nephrotoxicity by raising tissue CyA levels. Also, both tacrolimus and sirolimus can cause TTP-HUS.

Is mycophenolate mofetil nephrotoxic?

No

How can methotrexate (MTX) cause AKI?

Tubulotoxicity and precipitation of MTX crystals in tubules

What are specific treatments for MTX-induced AKI?

Prevention with hydration and urinary alkalinization has greatly reduced AKI.

What are the nephrotoxic effects of ifosfamide?

Tubular toxicity causing Fanconi's syndrome and occasionally AKI

What effects can cisplatin have on the kidney?

Tubulotoxicity causing progressive renal failure, magnesium wasting; with bleomycin, can cause TTP-HUS

MISCELLANEOUS DRUGS AND HERBS

What is the danger of metformin in patients with reduced GFR?

Severe lactic acidosis in patients with overdose or impaired renal function; unclear mechanism

What are potential adverse effects of opioids in CKD or AKI?

Some opioids (especially meperidine and morphine) have metabolites with significantly prolonged half-lives and/or adverse effects (e.g., seizures with meperidine)

How can bisphosphonates cause AKI?

ATN, collapsing FSGS

How do drugs that expand plasma volume (IV immunoglobulin, hetastarch, mannitol, dextran) cause AKI?

Osmotic nephrosis (uptake of substances into PCT cells leading to swelling and resultant tubular obstruction)

Which herbs and alternative medicines have been implicated in kidney disease?

Aristolochia sp. causes TIN and chronic interstitial fibrosis (Chinese herb nephropathy); licorice (mineralocorticoid activity causes HTN, hypokalemia, Fanconi's syndrome in chronic use); many traditional African herbal therapies cause ATN.

DIABETIC KIDNEY DISEASE

What percentage of patients with type I and type II diabetes develop nephropathy?

Type I: 25% to 30% after 25 to 40 years

Type II: 25% after 20 years

What are the risk factors for the development of diabetic nephropathy?

Ethnicity (African Americans and Mexican Americans at highest risk)

Hypertension

Higher levels of proteinuria

Poor glycemic control

What is the pathologic lesion of diabetic nephropathy?

Nodular glomerular lesions (Kimmelsteil–Wilson) are located in the central regions of the glomerulus and have a hard, eosinophilic appearance. There is also expansion of the mesangium with capillary wall and basement membrane thickening.

What are the stages of diabetic nephropathy?

Stage 1: renal hypertrophy and hyperfiltration

Stage 2: development of pathological changes with normal GFR

Stage 3: development of microalbuminuria (usually 6 to 15 years after development of diabetes)

Stage 4: worsening proteinuria, development of hypertension, decline in GFR begins

Stage 5: ESRD (develops on average 7 years after the development of persistent proteinuria)

What are the screening recommendations for microalbuminuria in diabetics?

Type I: yearly after 5 years of diabetes or over age of 12

Type 2: yearly after diagnosis

Screening can be done with a spot albumin–creatinine ratio. If elevated, three timed overnight urine collections should be obtained to verify.

What is the significance of microalbuminuria?

Evidence of incipient diabetic nephropathy with high risk for both progressive nephropathy as well as CV disease

What other forms of kidney disease are diabetics susceptible to?

Membranous nephropathy

Renal papillary necrosis

Renovascular disease

Obstruction due to autonomic neuropathy of the bladder

Higher risk for UTIs and pyelonephritis

Higher risk for contrast nephropathy

What clinical evaluation should be done in diabetics with proteinuria?

Quantitate proteinuria

Renal ultrasound

Rule out UTI

Urine microscopy

Serology if glomerulonephritis suspected: complements, ANCA, anti-DNA antibodies

Does tight glycemic control prevent diabetic nephropathy?

Yes. Good glycemic control can slow progression of nephropathy, especially in the early stages. In the DCCT (Diabetes Control and Complications Trial), those with lower HgBA1C values had a lower risk for development of microalbuminuria.

In patients with nephropathy, does tight glycemic control slow the progression?

It has been more difficult to show that tight glycemic control slows progressive nephropathy.

What is the goal BP for a diabetic patient?

130/80 in the absence of proteinuria.

The exact goal BP for diabetic patients with proteinuria is not clear, however a goal of 125/75 has been suggested.

What are the preferred antihypertensive drugs for diabetic patients with microalbuminuria?

ACEIs or ARBs. ACEIs have been most studied in type 1 diabetes and ARBs in type 2 diabetes. These drugs have specific antiproteinuric effects and slow renal progression above their antihypertensive effects.

Do ACEIs prevent the development of microalbuminuria?

Yes

What other therapies are important in slowing the progression of diabetic nephropathy?

Statins

Smoking cessation

Low-protein diets

Is there a role for combined use of ACEIs and ARBs in treatment of diabetic nephropathy?

Probably. Small trials have shown a synergistic fall in proteinuria with both drugs, but no long-term outcome studies looking at renal function are available as yet.

What are the complications associated with ACEIs or ARBs in diabetic patients?

Angioedema (ACEIs $\gg$ ARBs)

Cough (ACEIs)

Hyperkalemia

Worsening GFR

Can ACEIs be used in patients with elevated creatinine?

Yes. ACEIs have been safely used in patients with Cr up to 3.0 mg/dL. Need to monitor for hyperkalemia and increase in serum Cr >30% from baseline.

How can you manage hyperkalemia and continue the ACEI or ARB?

Low-potassium diet

Addition of diuretic

Sodium bicarbonate

CHRONIC KIDNEY DISEASE

What is chronic kidney disease (CKD)?

For ≥ 3 months, a GFR <60 mL/min/ 1.73 m^2 or GFR >60 mL/min/1.73 m^2 with a marker of kidney damage (proteinuria, hematuria, HTN related to kidney disease)

What are the stages of CKD?

Stage 1: GFR ≥ 90 mL/min with kidney damage

Stage 2: GFR ≥ 60 to 89 mL/min with kidney damage

Stage 3: ≥ 30 to 59 mL/min

Stage 4: ≥ 15 to 29 mL/min

Stage 5: <15 mL/min

What are the management strategies for:
    Stages 1 and 2 CKD?

Avoidance of nephrotoxic drugs, lifestyle modifications to reduce cardiovascular disease, yearly monitoring of renal function, aggressive treatment of hypertension, hyperlipidemia

Stage 3 CKD?

Interventions as above. Nutrition counseling. Evaluation for secondary hyperparathyroidism and anemia associated with CKD.

Stages 4 and 5?

As above, and preparation for renal replacement therapy. Referral to nephrologist is recommended.

What are the complications of CKD?

Hypertension, normocytic anemia, hyperphosphatemia, hypocalcemia, secondary hyperparathyroidism, increased risk of cardiovascular disease, malnutrition

What is done to slow the progression of CKD?

General measures include antihypertensive therapy, especially with ACEIs or ARBs, hyperlipidemia therapy, smoking cessation, anemia treatment. Specific therapies depend upon the underlying disease.

What is end-stage renal disease (ESRD)?

Medicare ESRD program definition: patients on dialysis or transplant regardless of GFR. Other definitions: all patients with GFR <15 or patients restarting dialysis after failed transplant.

What is the prevalence of ESRD?

According to USRDS data from 2004, the prevalence of ESRD is over 335,000.

What is the annual mortality rate of patients with ESRD?

>20%.

What guidelines are available for management of patients with CKD?

The NKF's K/DOQI: Kidney Disease Outcomes Quality Initiative, found at http://www.kidney.org/

What is uremia?

The constellation of symptoms due to renal failure. These include: fatigue, nausea, vomiting, anorexia, volume overload, encephalopathy, peripheral neuropathy, pericarditis, and in very late stages, coma.

What are the indications to start patients with CKD on dialysis?

Uremic symptoms, which can be very subjective, or GFR <15 mL/min or life-threatening electrolyte imbalances such as hyperkalemia

What is the pathogenesis of anemia due to CKD?

Loss of erythropoietin production by the kidney as GFR falls <60 mL/min

Why is treating anemia in CKD patients important?

Anemia is associated with increased hospitalizations, cognitive and functional impairment, and increased cardiovascular disease, especially left ventricular hypertrophy.

When should anemia workup be initiated?

GFR ≤ 60; Hgb <11 (Hct 33% in premenopausal women); Hgb <12 in postmenopausal women and in men

What is the initial workup?

Hgb/Hct, reticulocytes, RBC indices, serum iron, total iron-binding capacity,% transferrin saturation, fecal occult blood testing, vitamin B12 and folate levels

What therapies are available and what are treatment targets?

Erythropoietin SC for goal of Hgb 11 to 12 g/dL or Hct 33% to 36%

Iron IV or oral for goal of % transferrin saturation >20% and ferritin >100 ng/mL

What is the pathogenesis of secondary hyperparathyroidism?

As GFR falls, hyperphosphatemia and decreased production of 1,25 vitamin D occurs. This leads to hypocalcemia and increased levels of PTH.

How is secondary hyperparathyroidism treated?

1. Control serum phosphorus levels: achieved by using oral phosphate binders (calcium carbonate, calcium acetate, or sevelamer) with meals
2. Low-phosphorus diet
3. Replace active 1,25 vitamin D to suppress PTH production

What are the consequences of untreated secondary hyperparathyroidism?

1. Osteitis fibrosa cystica (increased risk of fractures)
2. Tertiary hyperparathyroidism
3. Increased risk of cardiovascular disease

What are dietary and nutritional goals for patients with CKD?

Low-protein (no more than 0.8 g/kg/day), low-potassium, low-phosphorus diet

What are the daily protein intake goals for patients with CKD?

<0.6 to 0.75 g/kg/day for patients with GFR <25, as reduced protein intake is correlated with slower progression to ESRD.

For patients on dialysis, goal is 1.2 g/kg.

What is the etiology of metabolic acidosis in patients with CKD?

Non-gap acidosis due to reduced ammoniagenesis by tubular cells; anion gap acidosis due to acidic uremic toxins (phosphates, etc.)

Should metabolic acidosis in patients with CKD be treated?

Yes. Correction of acidemia has been associated with reductions in hypoalbuminemia and metabolic bone disease. Goal is [$HCO3-$] of at least 22 meq/L, achieved with oral $NaHCO3$.

What is the leading cause of death in patients with stages 3 to 5 CKD?

Cardiovascular disease

What are the risk factors for cardiovascular disease in this population?

Typical risk factors such as diabetes, hypertension, hyperlipidemia, smoking, family history, age account for only 40% to 50% of attributable risk. Other nontraditional risk factors include inflammation, secondary hyperparathyroidism, vascular calcification, and numerous unidentified risk factors.

What is the typical lipid profile for a patient with stage 4 to 5 CKD?

Low HDL, low to normal LDL, high triglycerides

What is nephrogenic fibrosing dermopathy?

More recently termed nephrogenic systemic fibrosis. A rare fibrosing condition that occurs in patients with advanced CKD (stages 3 to 5). The dominant clinical manifestations involve the skin. Leads to progressive restriction in joint movement and functional incapacity. Associated with the exposure to the MRI contrast agent gadolinium.

HEMODIALYSIS

What are the mechanisms governing the clearance of toxic solutes from the blood during dialysis?

1. Diffusion: solute moves from the side of higher concentration to the side of lower concentration.
2. Ultrafiltration: movement of solvent (water) across a semipermeable membrane from a region of high pressure to one of low pressure.
3. Convection: as solvent moves down a pressure gradient, dissolved solutes are dragged across the membrane.

How are these mechanisms utilized in dialysis?

1. Diffusion: removal of small molecules such as electrolytes and urea
2. Ultrafiltration: removal of body water
3. Convection: removal of larger molecules and protein-bound molecules

What is the dialyzer?

This is the critical part of the dialysis machine where the exchange of molecules and water occurs. It consists of thousands of hollow capillary fibers composed of a biocompatible semipermeable membrane. Blood flows through these fibers, whereas the outer surface is bathed in the dialysate solution.

How is dialysis therapy monitored?

The amount of solute removed is measured in terms of clearance. Clearance reflects the volume of blood or plasma cleared of a given solute in a unit time. Dialysis therapy is prescribed to give each patient a minimum acceptable clearance, and this is closely monitored.

What solute clearances are monitored?

Blood urea nitrogen serves as the marker for clearance.

What are uremic toxins?

These are a group of ill-defined molecules that lead to the symptoms of uremia. These molecules include urea, beta-2 microglobulin, and many others. One goal of dialysis is to remove these toxic substances.

What is KT/V?

This is a measure of dialysis adequacy that incorporates:

1. K: clearance of urea
2. T: time on dialysis
3. V: total body water

A goal KT/V of 1.2 is set for all patients.

What are signs and symptoms of inadequate dialysis?

Malnutrition (low serum albumin), weight loss, anorexia, nausea, vomiting, declining functional status, encephalopathy, peripheral neuropathy, pericarditis, persistent volume overload, KT/V <1.2

Which is the preferred form of AV access?

AV fistula: longest life span and fewest complications. AV grafts typically develop stenotic lesions at the venous anastomosis.

How is an AV fistula created?

A surgeon forms an anastomosis between an artery and vein usually in the forearm of the nondominant arm. Arterial pressure is transmitted to the vein, which dilates, becomes thickened, and then can be used to cannulate for access to the bloodstream.

How is an AV graft created?

A tubular graft (polytetrafluoroethylene) is interposed between an artery and vein and tunneled beneath the skin.

What are the problems associated with central venous dialysis catheters?

Infections, clotting, low blood-flow rates, and poor dialysis clearances

What are the complications associated with a dialysis session?

Hypotension, cardiac arrhythmias, muscle cramps, nausea, vomiting, headaches. Complications due to machine-related issues include air embolism, hemolysis (usually due to exposure of blood to contaminants in the dialysis water), and hypersensitivity reactions to the dialysis membrane.

What is dialysis disequilibrium syndrome?

An uncommon reaction that usually occurs during the first dialysis treatment. Symptoms include headaches, nausea, vomiting, disorientation, seizures, obtundation, or coma.

What is the cause of this syndrome?

It is believed that the rapid removal of extracellular solute leads to movement of water into the CNS and the development of cerebral edema.

What is the mortality associated with chronic hemodialysis?

The life expectancy of ESRD patients is only one-fourth to one-sixth that of the age-matched general population.

What is the leading cause of death in these patients?

Cardiovascular disease

Do statins lower the risk of CV mortality in patients on hemodialysis?

Observational studies suggest decreased CV mortality; however, the one randomized control trial (RCT) failed to show a statistically significant benefit. Further studies are needed.

What is continuous renal replacement therapy (CRRT)?

Modality of hemodialysis utilized in the ICU for critically ill, hemodynamically unstable patients. CRRT uses lower blood flow rates and lower dialysate flow rates along with a slower removal of body fluid to maximize stability of blood pressure. Since the flow rates are lower, CRRT needs to run continuously to ensure removal of toxins.

What do the following terms mean for the various forms of CRRT:
CVVH?

Continuous venovenous hemofiltration. Here there is no dialysate solution and removal of toxins and body water is through ultrafiltration only.

CVVHD?	Continuous venovenous hemodialysis. Here there is a dialysis solution that is used to remove solutes via diffusion.
CVVHDF?	Continuous venovenous hemodiafiltration. This modality combines dialysis and hemofiltration to maximize solute and water removal.
What is SLED?	SLED is slow, low-efficiency dialysis. This is another form of slower dialysis similar to CRRT that runs for 6 to 12 hours during the day and not continuously.
Is there a preferred modality of hemodialysis therapy in the ICU?	No. Clinical trials have not conclusively determined that one modality is superior to another.

PERITONEAL DIALYSIS

How is fluid removed from the body with PD?	A hypertonic solution of dextrose is used as the dialysate. Water from the vascular space enters the peritoneal cavity down the osmotic gradient, and then this excess ultrafiltrate is drained out by the patient.
What are the common complications of PD?	1. Peritonitis 2. Failure of the peritoneal membrane to act as an effective dialyzer 3. Catheter malfunction 4. PD fluid leaks (either internal or external) 5. Hernia development
What are the symptoms/signs of peritonitis?	Abdominal pain, fever, cloudy dialysate
How is peritonitis diagnosed?	Finding of WBCs $>100/mm^3$ in a dialysate sample.
What are the most common organisms associated with peritonitis?	*Staphylococcus aureus, Staphylococcus epidermidis*, enterococci, gram-negative organisms including *Pseudomonas* spp.

What is the correct empiric therapy for PD-associated peritonitis?

First-generation cephalosporin (cefazolin) or vancomycin in combination with either an aminoglycoside or third- or fourth-generation cephalosporin. Generally, antibiotics should be given intraperitoneally to maximize efficacy.

KIDNEY TRANSPLANTATION

How does the cost of a kidney transplant compare with that of hemodialysis?

The average yearly cost of hemodialysis is $50,000. The cost of a kidney transplant is $100,000 for the first year and then approximately $10,000 per year after this. After 4 years, the overall costs of successful kidney transplantation are lower than those of dialysis.

How does the survival of patients receiving a kidney transplant compare with that of those remaining on dialysis?

Overall, after 100 days posttransplant, a mortality advantage is seen in patients receiving a transplant. The magnitude of the survival benefit of transplantation varies according to patient age and comorbidities and is greatest in young diabetics.

What are the events required for T-cell activation?

There are at least two different signals:

1. Binding of the foreign antigen presented by the HLA antigen to the T-cell receptor.
2. Interaction of accessory molecules on T-cells and antigen-presenting cells (such as between CD28 and B7).
3. A third signal is due to elaboration of cytokines (especially IL-2), which leads to T-cell activation, cell division, and clonal expansion.

How are these events utilized to design immunosuppressive therapy?

1. With agents that target signal 1: these include monoclonal (OKT3) and polyclonal (thymoglobulin) agents targeted to the T-cell receptor complex. The drugs tacrolimus and cyclosporine inhibit IL-2 production through blockade of calcineurin.

2. Agents that block this step are in development.
3. The humanized monoclonal antibodies basiliximab and daclizumab are targeted against the IL-2 receptor. Sirolimus acts on the signaling pathway downstream from the cytokine receptor. Mycophenolate mofetil and azathioprine impair de novo nucleotide synthesis and cell division.

What HLA antigens are routinely tested for prior to transplantation?

HLA A (class 1), B (class 1) and DR (class 2). Since we inherit one allele from each parent, six potentially unique antigens can be present in an individual. Blood group antigens are also tested, and while transplants can be undertaken across mismatched ABO blood types, there is an extremely high likelihood of rejection and special protocols are required.

At what GFR can a person be placed on the waiting list for a kidney transplant?

GFR of 20 mL/min

What are the factors that determine the outcome of kidney transplantation?

1. Cadaveric versus live donor: superior outcomes with live donation
2. HLA-matching: superior outcomes with five- or six-antigen matched kidneys.
3. Race: poorer outcomes in blacks
4. Recipient age: worse outcomes in the very young and old
5. Donor age: worse outcome with increasing age
6. Comorbidities: worse outcome in diabetics, hepatitis C-positive
7. Rejection: worse outcome with prior episodes of rejection

What is the typical immunosuppressant protocol utilized posttransplant?

Tacrolimus or cyclosporine plus mycophenolate mofetil (MMF) plus prednisone

What are calcineurin inhibitors?	This class of medications includes tacrolimus and cyclosporine. These drugs block the expression of critical cytokine genes such as IL-2
What are the major side effects of calcineurin inhibitors?	Nephrotoxicity including chronic kidney disease, hypertension, hyperkalemia, hypomagnesemia, hypertrichosis (cyclosporine), alopecia (tacrolimus), gingival hyperplasia (cyclosporine), hyperlipidemia (cyclosporine), glucose intolerance, (tacrolimus), neurotoxicity (taciolimus), infections and malignancy
What is the risk of using a statin with a calcineurin inhibitor?	Increased risk of rhabdomyolysis with all statins (lower likelihood with pravastatin)
What is the mechanism of action of mycophenolate mofetil (MMF)?	MMF inhibits the production of de novo purine synthesis which is required for cell division of lymphocytes.
What are the side effects of MMF?	The major side effects are GI: diarrhea, nausea, vomiting. Other side effects are leukopenia, thrombocytopenia, and increased risk for infections.
What is sirolimus?	Immunosuppressant that blocks the downstream effects of IL-2 to inhibit cytokine-mediated cellular proliferation. It can be exchanged for calcineurin inhibitors when toxicity of these drugs warrants a switch.
What is thymoglobulin?	It is made by immunization of rabbits with human lymphoid tissue and is a polyclonal antibody preparation used at the time of transplantation (induction therapy) to deplete peripheral lymphocytes.
How is acute rejection manifested?	Rise in serum creatinine or rarely, pain over the allograft. Rejection is diagnosed with a biopsy of the allograft.

What do biopsies in acute rejection show?

The biopsy typically reveals an acute inflammatory infiltrate surrounding the renal tubules and occasionally (in more severe cases) involving the vasculature or glomerulus.

How is acute rejection treated?

1. Pulse high-dose corticosteroids
2. If severe, thymoglobulin may also be used
3. Intensification of immunosuppression

What are the advantages of living kidney donation?

1. Better short- and long-term results
2. Lower incidence of delayed graft function
3. Avoidance of long wait for cadaveric transplant
4. Capacity to optimally time transplant procedure

What are the potential risks to the donor?

1. Donor operative mortality (less than 1 in 2000)
2. Operative and post-op morbidity and recovery time
3. Post-op complications
4. Increased risk of long-term hypertension and perhaps proteinuria

What is the evaluation process for a potential donor?

1. Education
2. ABO blood type and cross-match
3. Complete history and physical
4. Comprehensive lab screening (CBC, chemistries, HIV, lipids, hepatitis B, C, CMV, glucose tolerance test)
5. Urine for creatinine clearance, proteinuria
6. CXR, ECG, and possibly stress test
7. CT or MRI of the kidney

What are the exclusion criteria for living donation?

1. Age <18 or >70 years (differs across programs)
2. Hypertension
3. Diabetes
4. Proteinuria
5. Abnormal GFR
6. Hematuria

7. Significant medical illness
8. Obesity
9. Strong family history of renal disease, hypertension, or diabetes
10. Psychiatric contraindications

What are the contraindications for cadaveric transplantation?

1. Chronic kidney disease
2. Age >70 years (relative)
3. Potentially metastasizing malignancy
4. Severe hypertension
5. Sepsis
6. IV drug abuse
7. HIV-positive
8. Hepatitis B surface antigen–positive
9. Oliguric acute kidney injury

Is there a higher incidence of malignancy in renal transplant patients?

Yes, the risk for non-skin malignancies is 3.5-fold higher.

What malignancies are noted?

Lymphomas as well as malignancies related to viral etiologies, such as posttransplant lymphoproliferative disease (EBV) and cervical cancer (HPV)

What is chronic allograft nephropathy?

This is a common cause of late graft failure and is due to both immunological factors (rejection) and nonimmunological factors (diabetes, hypertension, hyperlipidemia).

What is the most common viral infection after transplantation?

CMV; thus prophylaxis with an antiviral agent such as ganciclovir is recommended.

How does CMV infection present?

Most commonly as fever, malaise, leukopenia, and transaminitis. More severe presentations include pneumonitis, gastritis, esophagitis, and hepatitis.

What other prophylactic antimicrobials are given to kidney transplant patients?

TMP/SMX to prevent PCP and oral nystatin to prevent thrush

MAJOR TRIALS IN NEPHROLOGY

1. Prevention of Diabetic Nephropathy: Role of Angiotensin Blockade
   a. Type 1 diabetes: Lewis et al. (*N Engl J Med* 1993;329:1456) demonstrated that the ACEI captopril significantly slowed the progression of renal disease in type I diabetics as compared to a group of patients treated with other agents to an equivalent blood pressure.
   b. Type 2 diabetes: Two studies—RENAAL (*N Engl J Med* 2001;345:861) and IDNT (*N Engl J Med* 2001;345:851)—in type 2 diabetic patients with nephropathy have demonstrated that the ARBs losartan and irbesartan, respectively, significantly slowed the progression of renal disease as measured by either the doubling of serum creatinine or development of ESRD.
2. Prevention of Diabetic Nephropathy: Role of Glycemic Control
   a. The Diabetes Control and Complication Trial demonstrated that intensive glycemic control could lessen the risk of development and slow the progression of diabetic nephropathy. There was no clear threshold value of HgBA1C but progression was slow, with values less than 7.5% (*N Engl J Med* 1993;329:977).
   b. The UKPDS (United Kingdom Prospective Diabetes Study) demonstrated that blood pressure control had a much larger effect on slowing progression of nephropathy than glycemic control (*Br J Med* 1998;317:693).
3. Prevention of Progressive Chronic Kidney Disease
   a. The role of blood pressure control: The Modification of Diet in Renal Disease (MDRD) study evaluated whether lower blood pressure targets gave greater renoprotection. Recommendations based upon a secondary analysis of this trial were that in patients with proteinuria of >1 g/day, blood pressure below 125/75 mm Hg was associated with a slower rate of renal disease progression (*Ann Intern Med* 1995;123:754).
   b. The role of angiotensin blockade: In the REIN study, 352 patients with nondiabetic CKD randomized to either ACE-inhibitor or placebo with equal blood pressure in both groups. The ACE-inhibitor group had a much slower rate of progressive CKD, especially in those patients with urine protein >3 g/day (*Lancet* 1997;349:1857).
   c. The role of dihydropyridine calcium channel blockers: In the African American Study of Kidney Disease (AASK), patients with CKD and hypertension were randomized to either an ACEI, a dihydropyridine calcium channel blocker (amlodipine), or a beta blocker. The amlodipine arm of the trial was stopped early due to more rapid progression of CKD in this arm, especially in those patients with proteinuria >1 g/day (*JAMA* 2001;285:2719).
   d. The role of protein-restricted diets: The MDRD study (above) randomized patients to either 1.3 g/kg/day (usual) or 0.58 g/kg/day (low) protein diets. A second arm of the study added a very low (0.28 g/kg/day)

arm. Primary analysis of the results demonstrated no significant renoprotection associated with the low-protein diet. Secondary analysis revealed benefit from the low-protein diet in those patients with a greater initial decline in renal function, and extrapolation of the trends in decline in GFR predicted a benefit if the trial had been extended in length.

4. Prevention of Contrast Nephropathy
   a. While no trials of deliberate hydration have been tested in a randomized trial versus no therapy, the study by Solomon et al. (*N Engl J Med* 1994; 331:1416) demonstrated that a protocol of IV hydration with 0.45% saline led to a lower incidence of contrast nephropathy (defined as a 0.5 mg/dL or greater rise in serum creatinine within 48 hours of the procedure) as compared with saline plus either mannitol or furosemide.
   b. Aspelin et al. (*N Engl J Med* 2003;348:491) demonstrated that the iso-osmolar contrast agent iodixanol led to fewer instances of contrast nephropathy as compared to low-osmolar contrast agents in patients at high risk for developing AKI.
   c. Tepel et al. (*N Engl J Med* 2000;343:180) demonstrated that oral N-acetylcysteine 600 mg twice a day in addition to 0.45% saline before and after the procedure led to a significant reduction (2% versus 21%) in the development of contrast nephropathy in high-risk patients. Subsequently, Marenzi et al. (*N Engl J Med* 2006;354:2773) demonstrated the superiority of a regimen of N-acetylcysteine (1200-mg IV bolus before angioplasty followed by 1200 mg orally twice daily for 48 hours) over either a 600-mg dose of N-acetylcysteine or IV fluids alone.
   d. Merten et al. (*JAMA* 2004;291:2328) demonstrated in a prospective randomized trial of 119 patients at high risk for the development of contrast nephropathy that IV hydration with an isotonic solution of sodium bicarbonate was superior to that of saline (1.7% versus 13.6% developed contrast nephropathy in each group respectively).

5. Renal Artery Stenosis
   Three randomized controlled trials have investigated the blood pressure outcomes of medical therapy versus percutaneous transluminal renal angioplasty in patients with renal artery stenosis. Webster et al. (*J Hum Hypertens* 1998;12:329) studied 55 patients and showed no difference in blood pressure, renal function, or survival in either group. Plouin et al. (*Hypertension* 1998;31:822) studied 49 patients and showed no difference in blood pressure but slightly fewer antihypertensive medications in the angioplasty group. In the largest study, van Jaarsveld et al. (*N Engl J Med* 2000;342:1007) studied 106 patients and once again showed no difference in blood pressure between the groups at 12 months. However, 44% of the patients in the medical therapy arm crossed over to receive subsequent angioplasty.

6. Hemodialysis
   a. The National Cooperative Dialysis Study (NCDS) (*N Engl J Med* 1981; 305:1176–1181) set the initial guidelines for dosing of hemodialysis and demonstrated that focusing on a minimum amount of urea clearance was important to ensure good outcomes.
   b. The HEMO Study (*N Engl J Med* 2002;347:2010) evaluated the potential benefits of increasing the dialysis dose above currently recommended target levels. There was no significant difference in mortality between the high and standard dialysis dose groups.
7. Continuous Renal Replacement Therapy:
   Mehta et al. (*Kidney Int* 2001;60:1154) conducted the only randomized controlled trial of CRRT (84 patients) versus standard intermittent hemodialysis (82 patients) in patients with acute renal failure in the intensive care unit. Intermittent hemodialysis resulted in a lower mortality (41.5%) than occurred with CRRT (59.5%). However, despite the randomization process, patients allocated to CRRT had more severe illness. Several other trials have not shown a significant benefit of CRRT over conventional intermittent dialysis (*Lancet* 2006;368:379).
8. Hepatorenal Syndrome
   Angeli et al. (*Hepatology* 1999;29:1690) demonstrated significant benefit of combined therapy with IV albumin, octreotide, and midodrine in patients with hepatorenal syndrome. Those patients treated with these drugs demonstrated improved renal function and urine output. This has recently been confirmed in another study with a larger number of subjects (*Dig Dis Sci* 2007;52:742).

ABBREVIATIONS

ACS	American Cancer Society
AFP	Alpha-fetoprotein
AIDS	Acquired immunodeficiency syndrome
ALL	Acute lymphocytic leukemia
AML	Acute myeloid leukemia
CBC	Complete blood count
CLL	Chronic lymphocytic leukemia
CML	Chronic myelogenous leukemia
CNS	Central nervous system

CT	Computed tomography
DCIS	Ductal carcinoma in situ
DIC	Disseminated intravascular coagulation
EBV	Epstein-Barr virus
EGGCT	Extragonadal germ-cell tumor
ERCP	Endoscopic retrograde cholangiopancreatography
5-FU	5-Fluorouracil
GCT	Germ-cell tumor
GRFoma	Gastrin-releasing factor–producing tumor
Beta-HCG	Beta-human chorionic gonadotropin
H&P	History and physical examination
HPV	Human papillomavirus
HTLV 1	Human T-cell lymphotrophic virus type 1
ITP	Idiopathic thrombocytopenic purpura
LCIS	Lobular carcinoma in situ
LGL	Large granular lymphocyte
MGUS	Monoclonal gammopathy of undetermined significance
MRI	Magnetic resonance imaging
NHL	Non-Hodgkin's lymphoma
NK	Natural killer
NSCLC	Non–small cell lung cancer
NSGCT	Nonseminomatous germ-cell tumor
PDA	Poorly differentiated adenocarcinoma
PDC	Poorly differentiated carcinoma
PP	Pancreatic polypeptide
PPoma	Pancreatic polypeptide–producing tumor
PSA	Prostate-specific antigen
PSC	Primary sclerosing cholangitis
PT	Prothrombin time
PTC	Percutaneous transhepatic cholangiogram
PTT	Partial thromboplastin time
RPLN	Retroperitoneal lymph node
RPLND	Retroperitoneal lymph node dissection
RTIO	Radical transinguinal orchiectomy
SCLC	Small cell lung cancer
SLL	Small lymphocytic lymphoma
SMA	Superior mesenteric artery
SVC	Superior vena cava
TNM	Tumor, node, metastasis
VIPoma	Vasoactive intestinal polypeptide–producing tumor
WBC	White blood cell
WDLL	Well-differentiated lymphocytic lymphoma

ONCOLOGIC EMERGENCIES

SPINAL CORD COMPRESSION

What are the most common malignancies involved in spinal cord compression?

Lung, breast, prostate, lymphoma, and multiple myeloma. Other more unusual cancer causes are colorectal, melanoma, sarcoma, and renal cell carcinoma.

In a cancer patient with back pain and no neurologic symptoms, what is the first study that should be done?

Plain radiographs of the affected area.

What should be done if the plain films show metastatic changes?

If the plain films show evidence of metastatic cancer, an MRI should be done on an outpatient basis.

What should be done if the plain films are negative for metastatic changes?

If the plain films are negative, a bone scan should be done.

Can a patient have spinal cord compression with normal plain radiographs?

Yes. Therefore, if neurologic symptoms are present, an MRI of the spine to rule out cord compression should be done.

What is the radiographic study of choice to rule out spinal cord compression?

A CT myelogram is probably the most specific and sensitive study. However, MRI has virtually supplanted the myelogram as the initial study because it is nearly as accurate, noninvasive, and quicker.

What is the prognosis for regaining lost neurologic function?

Poor. Few patients with paraplegia regain neurologic function. Most patients (80%) who are ambulatory at the time of treatment are ambulatory after treatment. As many as one third of patients with mild to moderate neurologic dysfunction have improvement of symptoms with treatment.

Who should receive radiotherapy for the treatment of spinal cord compression?	Patients with a known radiation-sensitive tumor and no spinal instability, those with spinal involvement without spinal instability or neurologic deficit, or for palliation in patients who are poor candidates for surgery
Who should receive surgery followed by radiation in treatment of spinal cord compression?	Patients with a pathologic fracture with spinal instability or compression of the spinal cord by bone, patients with radiation-resistant tumors with neurologic deficits, and patients with an unknown tissue diagnosis
Who should receive surgery alone in treatment of spinal cord compression?	Patients whose tumors relapse or fail to respond to radiation
Who should receive chemotherapy alone in treatment of spinal cord compression?	Pediatric patients with responsive tumors, adults with responsive tumors, and patients whose tumors relapse at a site of radiation and surgery

INCREASED INTRACRANIAL PRESSURE

When is surgery indicated in cases of increased intracranial pressure presumed to be related to cancer?	1. To make a diagnosis 2. If symptoms are refractory or progressive after medical or radiation therapy 3. If the patient has had good performance status with a single metastasis and a long disease-free interval
What are the usual LP results regarding glucose and protein levels?	The glucose level is usually less than 45 mg/dL, the protein level is generally increased.
What is the treatment for carcinomatous meningitis?	Whole brain radiation therapy. Intrathecal chemotherapy is occasionally successful for a short time, depending on the underlying tumor type.
What is the prognosis for patients with carcinomatous meningitis?	Generally poor, with median survival in the 4- to 6-month range

SUPERIOR VENA CAVA SYNDROME

What are the causes of SVC syndrome?	Malignant causes (80% to 90% of cases)—most commonly, lung cancer, lymphoma, thymoma, GCTs, and breast cancer
	Nonmalignant causes (10% to 20% of cases)—histoplasmosis with mediastinal fibrosis, syphilis, tuberculosis, and thrombosis, usually as a result of an indwelling central venous catheter

HYPERCALCEMIA

What is the treatment for hypercalcemia?	Aggressive hydration is the mainstay. Diuretics after aggressive intravenous hydration can enhance kaliuresis but should not be initiated until the patient has been generously hydrated. Bisphosphonates are effective and are commonly used after rehydration.

HYPERURICEMIA

What malignancies are commonly associated with hyperuricemia?	Acute leukemias, high-grade lymphomas, and myeloproliferative disorders (including CML)
What is the management of hyperuricemia?	Prophylactic measures need to be undertaken before cytotoxic chemotherapy. Medications that lead to an elevated serum uric acid or that acidify urine are discontinued. Allopurinol is started, intravenous hydration is begun to maintain good urine output, and urine is alkalinized with sodium bicarbonate to a pH of 7.0 to 7.5.

TUMOR LYSIS SYNDROME

Which labs need to be monitored for tumor lysis syndrome?	Serum uric acid, phosphate and uric acid. These are released from the breakdown of malignant cells.
How is tumor lysis syndrome treated?	Hydration and alkalinization of the urine (the urinary pH is maintained at 7.0 to 7.5)

What prophylactic therapy should be used in patients with a large tumor burden who are at risk for tumor lysis syndrome?

Allopurinol. The dose often needs to be adjusted for renal insufficiency in this setting.

Rasburicase, a recombinant urate oxidase enzyme, is indicated as prophylaxis in pediatric patients at high risk for tumor lysis syndrome. Its use in adults has not been studied in randomized controlled trials.

NEUTROPENIC FEVER

Which patients with neutropenia are at greatest risk for infection?

Those with prolonged neutropenia and those with immunodeficiencies as a result of their primary disease or therapy (e.g., leukemias and lymphomas)

Are there cases where additional coverage should be considered?

Consider additional coverage for gram-positive organisms for severe mucositis or any indwelling catheters.

What should be done if fevers persist despite antibiotics?

If fevers persist after 2 to 5 days, agents that are effective against fungi should be considered.

ACUTE LEUKEMIA

What are urgent clinical findings in acute leukemia?

Neurologic findings including altered mental status, seizures, headache, and cranial nerve palsies or other focal neurologic signs, suggesting leukemic meningitis, leukostasis, or bacterial meningitis

Pulmonary edema secondary to leukostasis

Tumor lysis

Hemorrhage (CNS, visceral, or gastrointestinal)

Infection or fever with or without neutropenia

What are the treatment options for leukostasis with neurologic findings?

Leukophoresis and hydroxyurea acutely, with initiation of induction chemotherapy as soon as possible

How do you manage hemorrhage in acute leukemia?	RBC and platelet transfusion to maintain platelet count >20,000/mm^3 and hematocrit >25 to 30 mg/dL. Check for evidence of DIC with PT, PTT, fibrinogen, and D-dimer.

ACUTE LYMPHOID LEUKEMIA

What cytogenetic groups convey a poor prognosis in adult ALL?	t(9;22), the Philadelphia chromosome; t(4;11); trisomy 8; and hypodiploidy
What is the long-term disease-free survival rate in adults?	30% to 40%. In contrast, nearly 80% of children are long-term disease-free survivors.
What is the standard induction regimen for ALL?	Vincristine, prednisone, l-asparaginase, and an anthracycline. The complete remission rate in adults is 80% to 90%.
What are the good prognostic factors for ALL?	Hyperdiploidy and complete response to induction chemotherapy
What are the bad prognostic factors for ALL?	Adverse cytogenetics, WBC >50,000/mm^3, age older than 60 years, and time to complete response of >4 to 6 weeks

ACUTE MYELOID LEUKEMIA

What is the basis for WHO reclassification of AML?	Cytogenetics, molecular genetics, therapy related AMLs, and biphenotypic leukemias (with features of AML and ALL)
Which subtype of AML is commonly associated with DIC?	Promyelocytic
What vitamin induces a complete remission in 90% of patients with promyelocytic leukemia?	Transretinoic acid

What percent of AML patients achieve complete remission with induction chemotherapy?

50% to 70%

What is the standard induction regimen for AML patients?

Cytarabine (100 mg/m^2) by continuous infusion over 24 hours for 7 days and daunorubicin (45 mg/m^2) intravenously for 3 days (commonly abbreviated as 7 + 3)

How many patients are cured if they go into complete remission?

None. They all need some form of consolidation chemotherapy.

What is the 5-year survival rate in patients who undergo treatment for AML?

Varies dramatically with underlying cytogenetics: 60% for good cytogenetics t(15;17), t(8;21), and inv(16); 40% for normal cytogenetics; 20% or less for poor cytogenetics [such as del(5), del(7) and complex karyotypes]

What are good prognostic factors for AML?

De novo leukemia (i.e., leukemia that is not preceded by a myelodysplastic syndrome), young age, and presence of specific cytogenetic abnormalities, including t(15;17), t(8;21), and inv(16)

What are poor prognostic factors for AML?

Leukemia evolving out of a prior myelodysplastic syndrome or associated with prior alkylating chemotherapy, advanced age, high peripheral WBC count, and the presence of the following cytogenetic abnormalities: –5, 5q–, –7, +8

LYMPHOPROLIFERATIVE DISORDERS

What are the lymphoproliferative disorders?

CLL, hairy cell leukemia, LGL leukemia, lymphoma (e.g., Hodgkin's disease and NHL), and plasma cell dyscrasias (e.g., multiple myeloma and Waldenström's macroglobulinemia)

CHRONIC LYMPHOCYTIC LEUKEMIA

Patients with CLL are susceptible to what types of infections?

Both bacterial and viral infections secondary to hypogammaglobulinemia and defects in cell-mediated immunity

Do patients with CLL have an increased incidence of autoimmune diseases?

Yes. Autoimmune hemolytic anemia occurs in 10% to 25% of cases. ITP and pure red blood cell aplasia are also more common in CLL.

With regard to the diagnosis of CLL, what are the usual physical exam features?

Frequently, there is lymphadenopathy and splenomegaly.

With regard to the diagnosis of CLL, what is seen on peripheral blood smear?

An increase in the absolute number of lymphocytes in the peripheral blood, which, on the peripheral smear, appear morphologically as small, mature lymphocytes

With regard to the diagnosis of CLL, what is seen on flow cytometry?

Flow cytometry shows a monoclonal population that coexpresses CD19 and CD5.

What is the differential diagnosis for CLL?

Lymphoproliferative disorders such as the leukemic phase of follicular lymphoma, monocytoid B-cell lymphoma, mantle cell lymphoma, SLL, LGL syndrome, lymphoplasmacytic lymphoma, Sézary cell lymphoma, hairy cell leukemia, splenic lymphoma with villous lymphocytes, and Waldenström's macroglobulinemia. A few of the nonmalignant causes of lymphocytosis include tuberculosis, mononucleosis, and pertussis infection.

What is the median survival expectation for a person with CLL?

Varies dramatically with stage and cytogenetics. With low-risk cytogenetics (isolated 13q deletion), median survival is >10 years; with high-risk cytogenetics (17p deletion, p53 gene), median survival is 4 to 5 years.

What is the Rai staging system for CLL and survival for each stage?	Stage 0: lymphocytosis alone; 15 years
	Stage I: lymphocytosis with lymphadenopathy; 9 years
	Stage II: lymphocytosis with spleen or liver involvement; 5 years
	Stage III: lymphocytosis with anemia; 2 years
	Stage IV: lymphocytosis with anemia and thrombocytopenia; 2 years
What is the treatment for asymptomatic patients with CLL?	Observation if the patient is asymptomatic
What is the treatment for symptomatic patients with CLL?	Oral alkylating agents or fludarabine are commonly used in symptomatic patients.

HAIRY CELL LEUKEMIA

What is often noted on bone marrow aspiration?	The bone marrow is often difficult to aspirate, resulting in a "dry tap."
How is the diagnosis of hairy cell leukemia made?	By the appropriate clinical scenario and by "hairy cells" seen on peripheral smear or bone marrow examination. A special stain called TRAP (tartrate-resistant acid phosphatase) is confirmatory, as is flow cytometric data.

LARGE GRANULAR LYMPHOCYTE SYNDROME

What is an LGL?	On peripheral smear, an LGL appears as a large lymphocyte with abundant pale cytoplasm with prominent azurophilic granules.
What is the presentation of T-cell LGL?	Chronic, sometimes severe neutropenia with frequent bacterial infections. Infiltration of the spleen, bone marrow, and liver are not uncommon. Interestingly, 25% of cases are associated with rheumatoid arthritis, making it difficult to distinguish from Felty's syndrome.

| **What is the presentation of NK-cell LGL?** | Usually, an acute clinical course involving fever and B symptoms (e.g., fever, drenching night sweats, anorexia, weight loss). Anemia and thrombocytopenia are more common than with T-cell LGL. Massive hepatosplenomegaly, lymph node involvement, and gastrointestinal symptoms are common. |

LYMPHOMA

| **What are B symptoms?** | Fever, drenching night sweats, anorexia, and weight loss |
| **What are typical physical findings in lymphoma?** | Lymphadenopathy and hepatosplenomegaly are the most predominant findings. |

HODGKIN'S DISEASE

| **What are the WHO histologic subtypes of Hodgkin's disease?** | Nodular lymphocyte predominant and classic Hodgkin's lymphoma (classic further divided into nodular sclerosing, mixed cellularity, lymphocyte rich, and lymphocyte-depleted) |
| **What are the stages in the Modified Ann Arbor staging system and the corresponding 5-year survival rates?** | Stage I: involvement of a single lymph node region or single extralymphatic site (IE); 90%

Stage II: involvement of two or more lymph node regions on the same side of the diaphragm or localized extranodal extension plus one or more nodal regions (IIE); 80% to 90%

Stage III: involvement of lymph node regions on both sides of the diaphragm, may be accompanied by localized extralymphatic extension (IIIE) or splenic involvement (IIIS); 60% to 85%

Stage IV: diffuse or disseminated involvement of one or more extralymphatic organs or tissues with or without associated lymph node involvement; 50% to 60% |

What are the dominant factors that determine therapy in Hodgkin's disease?	Stage, presence of extranodal disease, bulk of disease, and the presence of B symptoms. Histologic subtype has little or no bearing on choice of therapy.
How is bulky disease defined?	Bulky disease within the chest is defined as lymphadenopathy greater than one third of the diameter of the chest. Bulky disease elsewhere is defined as lymphadenopathy >10 cm.
What are late complications of treatment of Hodgkin's disease?	Acute leukemia and myelodysplasia as a result of alkylating agent chemotherapy Solid tumors within and adjacent to the radiation port Cardiac disease as a result of radiation and doxorubicin (Adriamycin) exposure Sterility and hypothyroidism

NON-HODGKIN'S LYMPHOMA

What is the staging system for NHL?	The Modified Ann Arbor staging system; see under Hodgkin's disease above
What monoclonal antibody therapy is used in the treatment of NHL?	Rituximab targets the CD20 receptor and is being investigated as initial therapy, in chemotherapy combinations, and as single agent maintenance therapy.

PLASMA CELL DYSCRASIAS

What are the major plasma cell dyscrasias?	MGUS, multiple myeloma, Waldenström's macroglobulinemia, and amyloidosis
What are the diagnostic criteria for an MGUS?	An MGUS must have: Serum M protein <3.5 g/dL (IgG) or <2 g/dL (IgA) <10% plasma cells in the bone marrow Urine light chains <1 g/24 hr No lytic bone lesions

Does an MGUS transform into a plasma cell dyscrasia?

Yes. 1% to 2% per year progression to myeloma. Recently the serum-free light chain has been used to help determine risk of progression in a single patient and is gaining wider use.

MULTIPLE MYELOMA

Do all patients with multiple myeloma have a monoclonal protein in the serum?

No. Only 80% of patients have an M protein in serum; 20% have only light chains, which must be measured in a 24-hour urine collection, or with the new serum light chain assay. Approximately 1% of patients with multiple myeloma are termed nonsecretors and have no identifiable monoclonal protein.

In nonsecretors, where is the immunoglobulin?

On staining of the plasma cells, the protein is shown to be within the cytoplasm, but the plasma cells cannot excrete the immunoglobulin molecule.

What are some of the newer treatments for multiple myeloma?

Thalidomide analogs and bortezomib, a proteasome inhibitor. Allogeneic bone marrow transplantation can cure the disease, but its use is limited because multiple myeloma is a disease of the elderly. Nonmyeloablative transplantation is being investigated. High-dose chemotherapy with peripheral stem cell rescue has been shown to lengthen time to relapse compared with standard therapy; however, long-term disease-free survival is limited.

What is the median survival?

Untreated, 6 months; treated, 2 to 3 years; 5-year survival is <10%

WALDENSTRÖM'S MACROGLOBULINEMIA

What are the differences between Waldenström's macroglobulinemia and

multiple myeloma in respect to the following?

Physical findings	Patients with Waldenström's macroglobulinemia commonly have lymphadenopathy with hepatosplenomegaly and rarely have bone lesions.
Paraproteins	By definition, Waldenström's macroglobulinemia must involve a monoclonal IgM paraprotein, whereas in multiple myeloma, IgG and IgA are the most common immunoglobulins involved.
Neoplastic cells	Waldenström's macroglobulinemia shows lymphoplasmacytic morphology, and the neoplastic cell in multiple myeloma is a plasma cell.
Symptom complex	Hyperviscosity is a more common problem in Waldenström's macroglobulinemia.

What are common presenting symptoms of Waldenström's macroglobulinemia?

Weakness, fatigue, oral and nasal mucocutaneous bleeding, symptoms attributable to splenomegaly, and symptoms attributable to hyperviscosity

What is the median survival for patients with Waldenström's macroglobulinemia?

3 to 5 years, but expected to improve with newer, more effective therapies

HEAD AND NECK CANCER

What percent of patients present with localized disease?

30%, but this amount varies with tumor location

When a patient is first seen, at which anatomic locations is disease more commonly advanced?

Supraglottic larynx, oropharynx, and hypopharynx

What are the staging criteria for head and neck cancer?

Each site has its own specifics. The four general stages are (I) local, (II) locally advanced but resectable, (III) locally advanced but unresectable, and (IV) metastatic.

What is the general treatment approach for head and neck cancer?

Local disease—radiation or surgery with curative intent. Radiation chosen when organ preservation is important, as in laryngeal cancer

Resectable locally advanced disease—surgery followed by radiation with concurrent chemotherapy

Unresectable locally advanced disease—concurrent chemotherapy and radiation

Metastatic disease—palliative chemotherapy and or palliative radiation

What is the surgical procedure for head and neck cancer?

Wide local excision with ipsilateral radical neck dissection. Contralateral radical neck dissection is performed if clinical or radiologic evidence of disease is present within the contralateral neck.

What is the 5-year survival rate for the following:
    Local disease?

60% to 90%

    Locally advanced disease?

30%

    Metastatic disease?

<5%

What is the incidence of new aerodigestive cancers arising in a patient previously rendered disease-free from a head and neck cancer?

Each year, a new cancer of the aerodigestive epithelium develops in 3% to 7% of patients. This effect is referred to as field cancerization.

BREAST CANCER

What inherited genetic abnormalities are associated with breast cancer?

It is estimated that 5% to 10% of all cases of breast cancer in the United States are related to inherited genetic abnormalities.

Genes involved include BRCA1, BRCA2, PTEN (associated with Cowden syndrome), TP53 (associated with Li-Fraumeni syndrome), and STK11 (associated with Peutz-Jegher's syndrome)

What percentage of patients with breast cancer present with metastatic disease?

6%

Is lumpectomy plus radiation equivalent to mastectomy in the primary management of breast cancer?

Yes. This has been confirmed by seven studies. About 25% of women require mastectomy because it is necessary for complete excision or because radiation is contraindicated in the patient.

What is the role of bone marrow transplantation in the management of breast cancer?

Stem cell transplantation had shown initial promise in patients with locally advanced or metastatic disease; however, subsequent randomized controlled trials showed no survival benefit for autologous bone marrow transplantation.

What monoclonal antibody therapy is available to individuals with breast cancer?

Herceptin targets the HER2/neu antigen and is available to individuals with tumors that overexpress HER2/neu. It is most effective when combined with cytotoxic therapy, and its use was recently expanded to the adjuvant setting.

What is the 5-year survival rate for women with breast cancer?

Roughly 80% to 85% for all stages. For women with cancers localized to the breast, the 5-year survival rate is 96%. Women with regional metastases (positive axillary node involvement) have a 75% 5-year survival rate. Those with distant metastases have a 20% 5-year survival rate.

LUNG CANCER

What are the chest radiograph findings for the following histologies?
   Squamous cell carcinoma?

A central lesion with hilar involvement and frequent cavitation

Adenocarcinoma?

A peripheral lesion, which can also cavitate

Bronchoalveolar carcinoma?

Peripheral, sometimes multifocal, "ground-glass opacity"

Large cell carcinoma?

Usually a peripheral lesion, which can cavitate

Small cell carcinoma?

A central lesion with hilar mass and early mediastinal involvement, which does not cavitate

How is SCLC staged?

Limited and extensive.

What is "limited" SCLC disease?

In limited-stage SCLC, all disease is within a single radiation port within the chest and supraclavicular fossa

What is the cure rate for limited SCLC?

There is a 15% to 20% cure rate in limited SCLC with combined radiation and chemotherapy.

What is "extensive" SCLC disease?

Extensive-stage SCLC extends outside a single radiation port within the chest.

What is the treatment of extensive-disease SCLC?

Combination chemotherapy offers a 60% to 90% response rate with a median survival for all patients of 9 to 11 months. In untreated disease, the median survival is 6 weeks.

What is the current chemotherapy standard for SCLC?

Cisplatin or carboplatin and etoposide

What is the staging of NSCLC?

Stage I: negative nodal involvement and an easily resectable tumor

Stage II: resectable tumor with ipsilateral peribronchial or hilar node involvement

Stage IIIA: potentially resectable tumor with positive ipsilateral mediastinal and/or subcarinal lymph node involvement

Stage IIIB: any tumor with contralateral lymph node or supraclavicular lymph node metastases. Any tumor, regardless of lymph node status, that invades the mediastinum, heart, great vessels, trachea, esophagus, vertebral body, or carina, or has a malignant pleural effusion. Not surgically resectable.

Stage IV: distant metastases

What is the treatment of NSCLC?

Stages I and II: surgical resection. Role for adjuvant chemotherapy under investigation. Some trials show benefit for stage II.

Stage IIIA: neoadjuvant chemotherapy ± radiation followed by surgery in resectable patients. Patients who are found to have stage IIIA after surgical resection (microscopic N2 involvement) benefit from adjuvant chemotherapy. Unresectable patients are treated with radiation and concurrent chemotherapy.

Stage IIIB: radiation with concurrent chemotherapy.

Stage IV: combination chemotherapy for patients with good performance status improves survival and quality of life.

What are the commonly used chemotherapy drugs for NSCLC?

Carboplatin, cisplatin, paclitaxel, gemcitabine, navelbine in combination for first-line therapy. Bevacizumab, an antibody against vascular endothelial growth factor (VEGF) in combination with carboplatin and paclitaxel has resulted in the best survival, with median survival reported around 12 months. Docetaxel, pemetrexed, and erlotinib as single agents in the second-line setting.

What is the approximate 5-year survival rate of NSCLC for the following:

    Stage I 50%

    Stage II 30%

Stage IIIA	20%
Stage IIIB	15%
Stage IV	<5%

GASTROINTESTINAL CANCER

ESOPHAGEAL CANCER

What are the most common histologies of esophageal cancer?	Squamous cell and adenocarcinoma
What has occurred with the histologic frequency of esophageal cancer?	Adenocarcinoma has been increasing in frequency over the past four decades. In the 1960s, some 10% of esophageal cancers were adenocarcinomas. Currently nearly 50% of cases are adenocarcinoma.
What is the most common location of cancer of the esophagus?	The middle third (55%). The esophagus is divided into three portions: upper third, cervical (15%); middle third, upper and midthoracic (55%); and lower third, lower thoracic (35%).

GASTRIC CANCER

What are the two histologic presentations of gastric adenocarcinoma?	Intestinal and diffuse
Where do the intestinal manifestations arise from?	Intestinal manifestations arise from precancerous lesions, such as gastric atrophy or intestinal metaplasia.
What is the epidemiology of intestinal cancer?	Intestinal gastric cancer is found in epidemic areas (e.g., the Far East). There is a male predominance.
What are the symptoms of diffuse gastric adenocarcinoma?	Diffuse manifestations occur as symptoms of early satiety secondary to the diffuse involvement of the stomach wall.

What is the common name for this entity?

The name commonly given to this histologic subtype is linitis plastica, which refers to poor distensibility of the stomach as seen on an upper gastrointestinal series.

Where does gastric adenocarcinoma metastasize?

Local nodal metastases within the wall of the stomach extending to the duodenum and esophagus and direct extension to adjacent organs are the most common areas of involvement.

How commonly are gastric carcinomas found to be metastatic?

As many as 75% of lesions have spread in this fashion by the time of diagnosis.

What are the most common sites of distant metastasis?

The liver is the most common site of distant metastases. At autopsy, disease involves the liver in 50% of patients, the peritoneum in 25%, the omentum in 20%, and the lungs in 15%.

What is the prognosis for gastric adenocarcinoma?

Because most diagnoses are made late, the prognosis is poor: the 5-year survival rate is approximately 10%. Early gastric cancer confined to mucosa and submucosa with no metastases or lymph node involvement has a 90% 5-year survival rate.

Does adjuvant therapy improve survival in locally resected gastric cancer?

Intergroup 0116 is the largest of three randomized trials to show a survival benefit for patients who received postoperative chemoradiotherapy after complete surgical resection of their primary gastric carcinoma. Chemotherapy was 5-fluorouracil plus leucovorin. Current trials are under way to determine the optimal chemotherapy.

What is the treatment for advanced gastric cancer?

Palliation of symptoms. Gastric bypass and debulking procedures are sometimes useful. Combination chemotherapy can produce response in 30% of patients, but many of those responses are of short duration. Drugs used include 5-FU, leucovorin, doxorubicin (Adriamycin), methotrexate, cisplatin, and etoposide.

SMALL BOWEL NEOPLASM

What is a carcinoid tumor?	Tumor of neuroendocrine cells—90% are located in the gastrointestinal tract. Midgut carcinoid tumors are most common.
Where are carcinoid tumors located?	Appendix: 35% to 45%
	Ileum: 10% to 15%
	Right colon: 5%
	Other gastrointestinal locations include the rectum (10% to 15%), duodenum, stomach, gallbladder, pancreas, esophagus, biliary tract, and Meckel's diverticulum.
What is the treatment and prognosis for carcinoid tumors of the small bowel?	Surgical resection can cure small carcinoids, but cure is not possible with metastatic disease. Somatostatin analog controls the vasomotor symptoms and diarrhea.

COLORECTAL CANCER

What is the incidence and death rate of colorectal cancer?	There are approximately 148,610 new cases diagnosed in the United States each year and approximately 55,000 deaths due to colorectal cancer each year.
What are risk factors for developing colorectal cancer?	Age: 90% of cases are diagnosed after the age of 50 years.
	Genetic factors: familial adenomatous polyposis (FAP) and hereditary nonpolyposis colorectal cancer (HNPCC)
	Inflammatory bowel disease: ulcerative colitis or Crohn's disease
Is there anything that will reduce the risk of developing colorectal cancer?	Diets high in fruits and vegetables and low in animal fats
	Regular physical activity
	Nonsteroidal anti-inflammatory drugs (NSAIDs) and acetylsalicylic acid (ASA) have been associated with reduced risk.

How do the two staging systems of colorectal cancer compare?

Stage I (T1–2, N0, M0) = Duke's A

Stage IIA (T3, N0, M0) = Duke's B

Stage IIB (T4, N0, M0) = Duke's B

Stage IIIA (T1–2, N1, M0) = Duke's C

Stage IIIB (T3–4, N1, M0) = Duke's C

Stage IIIC (any T, N2, M0) = Duke's C

Stage IV (any T, any N, M1)

For the above staging system, what do T1, T2, T3, and T4 mean?

T1 = tumor invades submucosa.

T2 = tumor invades muscularis propria.

T3 = tumor invades through the muscularis propria into the subserosa or into nonperitoneal or perirectal tissues.

T4 = tumor directly invades other organs or structures and/or perforates visceral peritoneum.

For the staging system, what do N0, N1, and N2 mean?

N0 = no regional nodal metastases

N1 = metastasis in 1 to 3 regional lymph nodes

N2 = metastasis in 4 or more regional lymph nodes

What do M0 and M1 mean?

M0 = no distant metastasis

M1 = distant metastasis

How is colorectal cancer treated?

Surgical resection is the primary modality of therapy for stages I to III. For select cases of metastatic disease such as those with a solitary liver metastasis or lung metastasis, resection of the colorectal primary as well as the metastatic lesion can result in long-term survival.

What is the 5-year survival for colorectal carcinoma?

Stage I = 93%

Stage IIA = 85%

Stage IIB = 72%

Stage IIIA = 83%

Stage IIIB = 64%

Stage IIIC = 44%

Stage IV = 8%

In what stage of colorectal cancer has adjuvant chemotherapy been shown to prolong survival?

Stage III or Duke's C. Randomized trials evaluating adjuvant chemotherapy in patients with stage II or Duke's B have not consistently shown significant survival benefit in this group of patients; it is therefore not recommended.

Does treatment of metastatic colorectal cancer improve survival of these patients?

Median survival of patients with metastatic colorectal cancer who received best supportive care alone is 5 to 6 months. Median survival of patients with metastatic colorectal cancer who are treated with irinotecan or oxaloplatin in combination with 5-FU have a median survival around 20 to 24 months.

What are the chemotherapeutic options for patients with metastatic colorectal carcinoma?

5FU-based therapy has been the standard for decades. Several new drugs have recently been approved, including irinotecan, oxaliplatin, cetuximab [which is an antibody against epidermal growth factor receptor (EGFR)], bevacizumab [which is an antibody against vasculoendothelial growth factor (VEGF)], and panitumumab (which is also an EGFR inhibitor).

PANCREATIC CANCER

What is the most common histologic subtype of pancreatic carcinoma?

Ductal adenocarcinoma comprises >80% of pancreatic carcinoma.

Where in the pancreas are most ductal adenocarcinomas found?

70% arise in the head of the pancreas (possibly resulting in biliary obstruction).

Besides ductal adenocarcinoma, what other cell types are found?

Many other histologic subtypes are seen and have a better prognosis. These include carcinoid, lymphoma, sarcoma, nonfunctioning islet cell carcinomas, malignant and benign insulinomas, gastrinomas, and glucagonomas.

What tumor markers are used in pancreatic cancer?

Gastrin, carcinoembryonic antigen, AFP, beta-2 microglobulin, CA-125, and CA 19–9. None of these, however, is sensitive or specific enough to be used routinely.

What are the most common sites of metastatic disease in pancreatic cancer?

Porta hepatis, liver, peritoneum with malignant ascites, penetration into the splanchnic nerves, and local lymph nodes. Less commonly, lung and bone are affected.

Pancreatic carcinomas at what location and of what size are generally unresectable?

Tumors arising in the tail of the pancreas and those >4 cm are rarely resectable.

What percent of patients who undergo a resection are alive at 5 years?

<20%

Are there any proven adjuvant treatments that improve survival in resectable pancreatic cancer?

One prospective controlled study demonstrated an improvement in survival (21 months versus 11 months) with use of postoperative 5-FU and radiation therapy versus surgery alone.

What surgical approaches should be considered for locally unresectable disease?

Palliative and prophylactic biliary bypass surgery. Biliary stent placement either transhepatically or via ERCP is an alternative. Relief of gastric outlet obstruction and duodenal obstruction can be useful. Prophylactic gastric bypass procedures are useful in some scenarios. Splanchnic and celiac ganglion nerve blocks may relieve pain.

Are radiation and chemotherapy useful in the treatment of locally advanced pancreatic cancer?

Radiation therapy alone can improve pain and possibly prolong survival. Combined-modality therapy with 5-FU and radiation therapy in one study showed an improvement in survival from 5 to 10 months.

What is the most important treatment for patients with metastatic pancreatic cancer?

Palliation of symptoms

What standard treatments are there for metastatic pancreatic cancer?

5-FU is associated with a response rate of <20% and does not improve the survival rate. Gemcitabine was approved for metastatic pancreatic cancer because of its ability to improve quality of life. Combination chemotherapy such as 5-FU or gemcitabine plus cisplatin or oxaliplatin or irinotecan, for example, typically yield higher response rates; however, little or no difference in survival has been observed.

What other novel therapies are available for the treatment of metastatic pancreatic cancer?

Novel targeted therapies such as erlotinib (an oral epidermal growth factor inhibitor) or bevacizumab [an intravenous monoclonal antibody targeted against vascular endothelial growth factor (VEGF)] have been investigated in pancreatic cancer. A recent randomized phase III trial comparing gemcitabine $\pm$ erlotinib has recently been reported, showing improvement in survival for the patients treated with gemcitabine plus erlotinib. Another trial comparing gemcitabine $\pm$ bevacizumab was recently completed and no benefit was noted in the treatment group.

PANCREATIC ISLET CELL TUMORS

What are the types of pancreatic islet cell tumors?

Endocrine tumors of the pancreas are classified according to the type of clinical syndrome present: insulinoma, gastrinoma (Zollinger-Ellison syndrome), somatostatinoma, VIPoma (e.g., pancreatic cholera, Verner-Morrison syndrome), glucagonoma, PPoma, GRFoma, and nonfunctioning tumors.

How is the diagnosis of pancreatic islet cell tumor made?

Tumor localization

What is the sensitivity of the following tests in localizing islet cell tumors?

    Ultrasound · 10% to 20%

    Abdominal CT · 20% to 40%

    Selective angiography · 80% to 90%

    Intraoperative ultrasound · 90%

    OctreoScan · 40% to 100% (OctreoScan is indium-labeled pentetreotide used in a nuclear medicine study that is noninvasive; results depend on tumor type)

What is the malignant potential of pancreatic islet cell tumors?

Only 10% of insulinomas are malignant; at least 50% of all other histologic subtypes are considered malignant.

What is the treatment for pancreatic islet cell tumors?

All patients should be considered for possible surgical resection of the tumor. Medical treatment may be useful in unresectable or incompletely resectable tumors.

What is the specific medical treatment for the following:

    Insulinoma? · Diazoxide and frequent small meals

    Gastrinoma? · Omeprazole

    Glucagonoma? · Streptozocin chemotherapy

    Somatostatinoma? · Streptozocin has worked in a few cases.

    VIPoma, glucagonoma, GRFoma, insulinoma, Zollinger-Ellison syndrome? · Octreotide

What is the prognosis for pancreatic islet cell tumors?

Islet cell tumors have a far more favorable prognosis than ductal adenocarcinomas because they grow slowly and cause physical symptoms early. Survival is directly related to tumor extent: if no tumor is found at surgery, the 5- to 10-year survival rate is 90% to 100%; if there is complete tumor resection, the 5- to 10-year survival rate is 90% to 100%; if there is incomplete resection, the 5-year survival rate is 15% to 75%; in unresectable cases, the 5-year survival rate is 20% to 75%.

CHOLANGIOCARCINOMA

What is a Klatskin tumor?	Cholangiocarcinoma arising at the bifurcation of the right and left hepatic ducts
How is the diagnosis of cholangiocarcinoma made?	Ultrasound, abdominal CT, ERCP, and angiography may be useful in localizing the tumor and staging the disease.
Are serum AFP levels elevated in patients with cholangiocarcinoma?	No
What is the treatment for cholangiocarcinoma?	Surgery is the only definitive therapy. Resectable tumors of the distal bile duct are associated with a 60% 1-year survival rate. Arterial or portal vein involvement precludes resection. ERCP with stent placement and PTC with drainage may be useful palliative procedures to relieve biliary obstruction.
What chemotherapeutic options are there for patients with cholangiocarcinoma?	For patients with advanced cholangiocarcinoma and good performance status, improved survival has been observed with 5-FU or gemcitabine based regimens.

GENITOURINARY CANCER

RENAL CELL CARCINOMA

What are the paraneoplastic syndromes associated with renal cell carcinoma?	Some of the more common findings are pyrexia, cachexia, anemia, nonmetastatic liver dysfunction, amyloidosis, polycythemia, and hypercalcemia.

How is renal cell carcinoma staged?

Stage I: within kidney

Stage II: within Gerota's fascia

Stage IIIA: involvement of the renal vein or inferior vena cava

Stage IIIB: involvement of hilar lymph nodes

Stage IV: metastatic disease

What is the treatment of localized renal cell carcinoma?

Radical nephrectomy with lymphadenectomy. Two thirds of patients with stage I and stage II disease survive 5 years.

Can patients with metastatic renal cell carcinoma be cured?

Yes. Occasionally, patients with isolated pulmonary or brain metastasis can be cured with surgical resection of the metastatic foci.

BLADDER CANCER

What percentage of individuals with invasive tumors have distant metastatic disease at the time of diagnosis?

50%

What are some of the prognostic factors?

Major prognostic factors include the depth of invasion and degree of differentiation.

What are the treatment options for:

Carcinoma in situ or superficial tumors?

Transurethral resection. Intravesicular therapy with BCG is used for high-risk patients.

Muscle invasive tumors?

Radical cystectomy with bilateral pelvic lymph node dissection

Metastatic disease?

Typically treated with combination chemotherapy with regimens including methotrexate, cisplatin, doxorubicin, and vinblastine. Newer treatment agents include gemcitabine and the taxanes.

What are the 5-year survival rates for:

Superficial disease?	95%
Regional disease?	50%
Metastatic disease?	6%

PROSTATE CANCER

What is the most common histologic subtype of prostate cancer?

The proximal ducts of the prostate give rise to 98% of all prostate cancers, of which the most common histologic subtype is adenocarcinoma.

What other histologic subtypes of prostate cancer are there?

They include mucinous carcinoma, adenoid cystic carcinoma, carcinoid tumors, and undifferentiated cancers. The distal ducts give rise to 2% of cancers of the prostate, including the following histologic subgroups: transitional cell carcinoma, squamous cell carcinoma, papillary carcinoma, and ductal cancer.

How are prostate cancers graded?

The Gleason grade is used to provide additional prognostic information for prostate cancer.

How is the Gleason grade determined?

Tumors are graded from 1 to 5 based on the degree of glandular differentiation and structural architecture seen on the pathologic sample, 1 being small uniform cells and 5 being poorly differentiated cells. The final score is the sum of the two prominent cell types seen and ranges from 2 (best prognosis) to 10.

What test is effective in following up prostate cancer patients after treatment?

Serial measurement of PSA

TESTICULAR CANCER

Do all GCTs arise within the testicle?

No. As many as 5% of GCTs are termed extragonadal. Extragonadal GCTs arise as a result of malignant transformation of residual midline germinal elements, usually in the mediastinum and retroperitoneum but occasionally within the pineal gland and sacrococcygeal area.

What is the most common GCT?

Seminoma comprises 40% of GCTs. The other histologic subtypes are referred to as nonseminomatous germ-cell tumors (NSGCTs).

What percent of seminomas are confined to the testicle at presentation?

70%

What percent of NSGCTs are confined to the testicle at presentation?

30% to 40%

Which GCT typically results in elevation of beta-HCG?

Choriocarcinoma. Seminomas can have an elevated beta-HCG, but it is usually $<100 \mu$/L. Embryonal carcinoma can also have an elevated beta-HCG.

Which GCT typically has an elevated AFP?

Yolk sac and embryonal carcinoma. Pure choriocarcinoma and seminoma do not have an elevated AFP.

What other conditions can elevate beta-HCG?

Cancer of prostate, bladder, kidney, and ureter; also marijuana use and pregnancy

What other conditions can elevate the AFP?

Pregnancy, hepatocellular carcinoma, and gastric cancer

How are GCTs staged?

Stage I (A): tumor confined to the testicle

Stage IIA (B1): minimally bulky RPLNs

Stage IIB (B2): moderately bulky RPLNs

Stage IIC (B3): bulky RPLN

Stage III (C): supradiaphragmatic or visceral disease

How is stage I seminoma managed?

RTIO with 25- to 35-Gy radiation therapy to RPLNs. RTIO followed by close observation is a reasonable alternative, probably with an equivalent 5-year survival rate.

How is stage I NSGCT managed?	RTIO with RPLND. Surveillance in lieu of RPLND is an alternative but is not standard.
What is the management of stage II seminoma?	Radiation therapy
What is the management of stage II NSGCT?	Stages IIA and B: RPLND and chemotherapy Stage IIC: chemotherapy
What is the management of all stage III GCTs?	Chemotherapy
What chemotherapy is used?	Cisplatin, etoposide, and bleomycin
What is the 5-year survival rate of seminoma for the following:	
Stage I	>95%
Stage II	>95%
Stage III	80%
What is the 5-year survival rate of NSGCT for the following:	
Stage I	>95%
Stage II	90% to 95%
Stage III	70%
What is the treatment of EGGCT?	Chemotherapy

OVARIAN CANCER

Under what circumstances should a patient with an adnexal mass warrant consideration for surgical exploration?	The patient is premenarchal or postmenopausal. The mass is >8 cm. Complex cysts are shown on ultrasound.

There is an increase in size or persistence of the cyst through two to three menstrual cycles.

The masses are solid and irregular, fixed, or bilateral.

There is pain associated with the mass.

There is ascites.

Do all patients with ovarian cancer have elevated CA125 levels?

No. However, 80% of patients with advanced disease and 50% of patients with early-stage disease have elevated CA125 levels.

What are the most common sites of metastases for ovarian cancer?

Serosal surfaces of intra-abdominal tissues and RPLNs are the most common sites of metastases. Pelvic lymph nodes, liver, lung, bone, and brain metastases can occur.

What are the components of stage I ovarian cancer?

Stage I: tumor limited to the ovaries

Stage IA: one ovary, intact capsule, no ascites

Stage IB: both ovaries, intact capsule, no ascites

Stage IC: ruptured capsule, capsular involvement, positive peritoneal washings, or malignant ascites

What are the components of stage II ovarian cancer?

Stage II: ovarian tumor with pelvic involvement

Stage IIA: pelvic extension to the uterus or tubes

Stage IIB: pelvic extension to other pelvic organs (bladder, rectum, or vagina)

Stage IIC: pelvic extension and positive findings in stage IC

What are the components of Stage III ovarian cancer?

Stage III: tumor outside the pelvis or positive nodal involvement

Stage IIIA: microscopic seeding outside the pelvis

Stage IIIB: gross deposits ≤2 cm

Stage IIIC: gross deposits >2 cm or positive nodal involvement

What are the components of stage IV ovarian cancer?

Distant organ involvement including the liver or pleural space

What are the histologic subtypes of ovarian cancer?

Epithelial carcinomas comprise 85% of cases and all are approached in essentially the same way. GCTs and sex cord stromal tumors are the predominant nonepithelial tumors and are managed differently.

What is the surgical treatment for ovarian cancer?

Bilateral salpingo-oophorectomy, omentectomy with careful examination of all serosal surfaces, biopsy of suspicious and grossly involved areas, collection of ascites and peritoneal washings, and debulking of all gross disease. If the disease is limited to the ovary, an RPLND is performed for additional staging.

What paraneoplastic syndromes are seen in ovarian carcinoma?

Hypercalcemia, cerebellar degeneration (pancerebellar dysfunction associated with extensive Purkinje cell loss), sign of Leser-Trélat (sudden increase in the size and number of seborrheic keratosis), and Trousseau's sign (migratory thrombophlebitis)

What is the postoperative management of stage I and II patients?

For stage IA and IB good-risk patients (well- or moderately well-differentiated histologic grade), no further treatment is indicated. In poor-risk stage I and II, postoperative adjuvant chemotherapy with a cisplatin-based regimen is the standard.

What is the management of stage III and IV (advanced) ovarian cancer?

After an optimal surgical procedure, adjuvant chemotherapy is with cisplatin or carboplatin and paclitaxel or cyclophosphamide for six cycles. Intraperitoneal chemotherapy is a consideration in optimally debulked stage IIIA and IIIB patients.

**What are the survival rates
for the following:**

**Stage IA and IB with good
prognostic factors**

>90% cure rate with surgery alone

**Stage II patients or stage
I patients with poor
prognostic factors and
stage IC**

60% cure rate with surgery plus adjuvant
chemotherapy

Stage IIIA and IIIB

25% to 40% cure rate with surgery and
adjuvant chemotherapy

Stage IIIC and IV

<10% cure rate with surgery and adjuvant
chemotherapy

CARCINOMA OF UNKNOWN PRIMARY SITE

**What are the potential
histologic diagnoses?**

Adenocarcinoma, 70%; poorly
differentiated carcinoma, 15% to 20%;
poorly differentiated adenocarcinoma,
10%; squamous cell and neuroendocrine
are uncommon.

**In whom should a GCT
variant be suspected?**

In a young patient with predominantly
midline disease (mediastinal and
retroperitoneal lymphadenopathy).
However, in any patient with a good
performance status with the diagnosis of
PDA or PDC, it is not unreasonable to
obtain an AFP and beta-HCG and treat
with chemotherapy for an extragonadal
GCT.

**What is the management of
squamous cell carcinoma in
an isolated cervical lymph
node?**

This is usually the result of a head and
neck primary and can be cured with a
radical neck dissection, radiation therapy,
or both. A careful head and neck
examination should be undertaken.

**What is the management of
squamous cell carcinoma in
an inguinal lymph node?**

Careful evaluation of the anorectum,
vagina, cervix, and penis. These
malignancies are potentially curable with
surgery, chemoradiotherapy, or both.

What is the management of adenocarcinoma in an isolated axillary lymph node in a woman?

A mammogram should be performed, followed by a modified radical mastectomy with axillary node dissection. Adjuvant chemotherapy, radiotherapy, or both should be offered according to the final pathologic stage.

What is the management of peritoneal carcinomatosis and pathologic findings demonstrating adenocarcinoma in a woman?

Laparotomy with consideration of a debulking procedure as in patients with ovarian carcinoma. Postoperative chemotherapy is recommended if, after the debulking procedure, ovarian cancer is suspected.

Pulmonology

ABBREVIATIONS

A-a	Alveolar–arterial gradient
ABG	Arterial blood gas
ABPA	Allergic bronchopulmonary aspergillosis
AFB	Acid-fast bacillus
AHI	Apnea hypoxia index
AIDS	Acquired immunodeficiency syndrome
AIP	Acute interstitial pneumonitis
ANCA	Antinuclear cytoplasmic antibodies
ARDS	Adult respiratory distress syndrome
ASD	Atrial septal defect
BAL	Bronchoalveolar lavage
BiPAP	Bilevel positive airway pressure
BO	Bronchiolitis obliterans (also obliterative bronchiolitis)
BOOP	Bronchiolitis obliterans with organizing pneumonia
CAP	Community-acquired pneumonia
CF	Cystic fibrosis
CMV	Cytomegalovirus
CNS	Central nervous system

COP	Cryptogenic organizing pneumonia
COPD	Chronic obstructive pulmonary disease
CPAP	Continuous positive airway pressure
CSA	Central sleep apnea
C-T	Connective tissue
CT	Computed tomography
CTPA	Computed tomographic pulmonary angiogram
CXR	Chest x-ray
DLco	Diffusion capacity for carbon monoxide
DVT	Deep venous thrombosis
EDS	Excessive daytime sleepiness
FEV$_1$	Forced expiratory volume in 1 second
FIo$_2$	Fraction inspired oxygen
FVC	Forced vital capacity
HAP	Hospital-acquired pneumonia
HF or CHF	Heart failure or congestive heart failure
HIV	Human immunodeficiency virus
HRCT	High-resolution CT
HSP	Hypersensitivity pneumonitis
HTN	Hypertension
ICU	Intensive care unit
ILD	Interstitial lung disease
INH	Isoniazid
INR	International normalized ratio
IPF	Idiopathic pulmonary fibrosis
IPG	Impedance plethysmography
KS	Kaposi's sarcoma
LDH	Lactate dehydrogenase
LFT	Liver function test
MAC	*Mycobacterium avium* complex
NIPPV	Noninvasive positive-pressure ventilation
NSAID	Nonsteroidal anti-inflammatory drug
OP	Organizing pneumonia
OSA	Obstructive sleep apnea
PA	Pulmonary artery
PA gram	Pulmonary artery angiogram
PAH	Pulmonary arterial hypertension
PC	Pressure control
PCP	*Pneumocystis jiroveci* pneumonia
PE	Pulmonary thromboembolism
PEEP	Positive end-expiratory pressure
PEF	Peak expiratory flow
PFT	Pulmonary function test
PMN	Polymorphonuclear leukocytes
PPD	Purified protein derivative

PPH	Primary pulmonary hypertension
P-R	Pulmonary–renal
PS	Pressure support
PSG	Polysomnogram
PSI	Pneumonia severity index
PTT	Partial thromboplastin time
PZA	Pyrazinamide
RAST	Radioallergosorbent test
RDI	Respiratory disturbance index
RERA	Respiratory effort-related arousal
RV	Right ventricle (ventricular)
Sao$_2$	Oxygen saturation
SIMV	Synchronized intermittent mandatory ventilation
SIRS	Systemic inflammatory response syndrome
SLE	Systemic lupus erythematosus
TB	Tuberculosis
TLC	Total lung capacity
UARS	Upper airway resistance syndrome
VATS	Video-assisted thoracoscopic surgery
V̇/Q̇ scan	Ventilation/perfusion scan
WBC	White blood cell

HISTORY AND PHYSICAL EXAMINATION

What findings in someone with obstructive lung disease suggest that his or her FEV$_1$ is decreased to 30% or less?

Respiratory rate >30 breaths per minute and the use of accessory muscles of respiration; there may be evidence of CO_2 retention on ABG.

OBSTRUCTIVE LUNG DISEASE

CHRONIC OBSTRUCTIVE PULMONARY DISEASE

What causes the airflow obstruction in patients with COPD?

Decreased elastic recoil of the lung, increased airway resistance or dynamic airway collapse

Is clubbing a feature of COPD?

No, it is a feature of pulmonary fibrosis, among other things.

What is the first laboratory test to check when looking for a genetic cause of COPD?

Alpha-1 antitrypsin levels

What is the normal value for alpha-1 antitrypsin?

The threshold level is 80 mg/dL (11 μmol/L), which is 35% of predicted. Below this level, patients have increased risk of emphysema.

When should one order an alpha-1 antitrypsin level?

Emphysema in the absence of a known risk factor (in a minimal or nonsmoker, no occupational dust exposure); early-onset emphysema ($\leq$45 years old); emphysema favoring the lower lobes; symptomatic adult with emphysema; COPD or asthma with incompletely reversible airflow obstruction despite aggressive treatment; clinical findings or history of unexplained liver disease; bronchiectasis of unknown etiology; clinical findings or history of necrotizing panniculitis; antiproteinase 3–positive vasculitis [C-ANCA (anti-neutrophil cytoplasmic antibody)-positive vasculitis]; family history of emphysema, liver disease, bronchiectasis, or panniculitis

What are the indications for replacement therapy with alpha-1 proteinase inhibitor [human] (Prolastin)?

High-risk phenotype [PiZZ, PiZ(null), PiZ(null)] (normal is MM; SZ and MZ rarely have evidence of clinical pulmonary disease), obstructive lung disease (FEV_1 <80% predicted), serum alpha-1 antitrypsin levels <80 mg/dL (11 μmol/L), and smoking abstinence

Are mucolytics useful in patients with COPD?

No. Mucolytics such as acetylcysteine may be irritants and worsen cough and bronchospasm, especially if inhaled. Excessive intravenous hydration is not helpful either.

What are the mechanisms whereby supplemental oxygen causes hypercarbia in a patient with COPD?

In order of most to least important: $\dot{V}/\dot{Q}$ mismatch (increased dead-space ventilation), the Haldane effect, decreased hypoxic drive

What is the mechanism of action and effect of theophylline?

The exact mechanism of action remains controversial. Theophylline is a phosphodiesterase inhibitor and increases levels of intracellular cyclic adenosine monophosphate. Antagonism of adenosine receptors is another proposed mechanism. Theophylline may affect eosinophilic infiltration into bronchial mucosa as well as decrease T-lymphocyte numbers in the epithelium. Theophylline has numerous effects including bronchodilation, enhancement of mucociliary clearance, stimulation of the respiratory drive, increased cardiac function, pulmonary arteriole vasodilation, and augmentation of diaphragmatic contractility.

Which medications increase theophylline levels?

Macrolide antibiotics (erythromycin, clarithromycin), cimetidine, ticlopidine, and quinolones (e.g., ciprofloxacin)

Which medications decrease theophylline levels?

Phenobarbital, phenytoin, carbamazepine, and rifampin

What factors or medical conditions increase theophylline levels?

Hypoxia, cirrhosis, heart failure, systemic febrile viral illness, and advanced age

Why can overly aggressive nutritional therapy be detrimental in patients with severe COPD?

Intake of increased carbohydrate calories may lead to increased oxygen consumption and increased CO_2 production, leading to increased ventilatory requirements. Replacing carbohydrates with lipids will remedy this situation. However, not overfeeding the patient is probably more important than the relative percentage of carbohydrates and lipids in the diet.

What is the long-term prognosis for COPD patients hospitalized on mechanical ventilation who are discharged to home?

50% 1-year mortality rate

What is lung volume reduction surgery?

Lung volume reduction surgery removes emphysematous lung tissue.

What are the physiologic effects of lung volume reduction?

Improved pulmonary mechanics (increased lung recoil, decreased resistance, decreased hyperinflation, decreased air trapping), respiratory muscle strength (by making the diaphragms less "flat"), and gas exchange (decreased $PaCO_2$, increased PaO_2).

What improves the gas exchange in these patients?

Improved $\dot{V}/\dot{Q}$ mismatch and dead-space ventilation are the etiologies of the improved gas exchange.

Which patients are best candidates for lung volume reduction surgery?

Patients with predominantly upper lobe emphysema and low (<40% of predicted) maximum exercise capacity after pulmonary rehabilitation

ASTHMA[1]

Which allergens should be tested for?

Indoor allergens, including dust mite, animal dander, and cockroach antigens. Other important allergens include *Alternaria*, which is associated with an increased risk of fatal and near-fatal asthma attacks in the Midwest, and *Aspergillus* because of the syndrome of ABPA.

Pollen and other seasonal allergies are usually more obvious to the patient and therefore less of a problem.

What are the criteria for mild intermittent asthma?

Requires normal lung function, PEF variability <20%, using a beta-2 adrenergic agonist <2 times a week, and waking up <2 times a month

What are the criteria for mild persistent asthma?

PEF variability 20% to 30%, using a beta-2 adrenergic agonist >2 times a week but <1 per day, and waking up >2 times a month

What are the criteria for moderate persistent asthma?

PEF variability >30%, using a beta-2 adrenergic agonist daily, and waking up >1 times a week

---

[1] In collaboration with M. Reitmeyer, S. AlGazlan, and L. Wheatley.

What are the criteria for severe persistent asthma?

PEF variability >30%, continual daily symptoms and frequent nocturnal symptoms

In a patient uncontrolled on inhaled corticosteroids alone (400 μg or greater), what is the most appropriate next step?

Adding a long-acting beta-adrenergic agonist is superior to doubling the dose of inhaled corticosteroids or adding a leukotriene modifying agent.

What agents have been used as corticosteroid-sparing?

Methotrexate, gold, cyclosporine, anti–tumor necrosis factor-alpha agents, macrolides. Studies have failed to show a benefit of corticosteroid-sparing agents over steroids, but in selected patients, these agents may be useful to minimize corticosteroid side effects.

What are the contraindications to allergen testing?

Contraindications also include initiation during pregnancy and beta-adrenergic blocker therapy.

How is aspirin sensitivity testing performed?

Sensitivity is generally tested by challenging the patient with escalating concentrations of aspirin. Because such testing is dangerous, it should be done in a monitored unit. Similarly, aspirin desensitization is performed using graduating doses and is similarly dangerous.

Is aspirin desensitization effective?

Yes. Desensitization is effective in controlling asthma in some sensitized patients. There is little evidence to suggest that aspirin desensitization is effective for urticaria. Leukotriene-modifying agents may be useful in this population. However, aspirin and NSAIDs should still be avoided.

Is cromolyn useful in acute asthma?

No. Cromolyn is not a bronchodilator; rather, it works by inhibiting histamine release from mast cells and neurogenic mechanisms. It works as an NSAID and can take several weeks for improvement to occur. Although very safe, it is no longer frequently used even for stable asthma because it is a weak anti-inflammatory agent and must be taken three or four times a day.

What are the indications for hospital admission?

Incomplete response to emergency room therapy defined as persistence of mild to moderate symptoms and signs, hypoxemia, FEV_1 and PEF <50% to 70% (see findings in severe asthma)

What are the indications in acute asthma for initiating noninvasive (via nasal or oronasal mask) and invasive (via endotracheal tube) ventilatory support?

Asthmatics are very difficult to ventilate mechanically because of hyperinflation and airway resistance. Intubate for drowsiness or confusion, fatigue, progressive hypercapnia, refractory hypoxemia, or bradycardia. Paradoxical thoracoabdominal movement and absence of wheezing are also ominous.

What should a peak flow meter be used for?

To provide an objective measure of a patient's condition at home (a patient may have a decrement in airflow and be unaware of the change) and objective information about a patient's response to therapy in the emergency room

Do short-acting beta-adrenergic agonists increase the risk of death?

Although some studies suggest that high doses of short-acting beta-adrenergic agonists may be associated with increased mortality, their increased use was more likely a sign of uncontrolled asthma than a direct cause.

Do long-acting beta-adrenergic agonists increase the risk of death?

Long-acting beta-adrenergic agonists appear to be safe as long as they are utilized when needed for uncontrolled asthma and with an inhaled corticosteroid.

What are some areas of work associated with immunologically mediated occupational asthma?

Laboratory work; work in the pharmaceutical and food industries; sawmill, plastic, and metal work; farming; cosmetology (e.g., beauticians); longshoring; and clothing manufacturing. One should take a careful occupational and environmental history in all patients with asthma.

What symptoms should suggest a diagnosis of:

Work-aggravated asthma?

A history of asthma symptoms occurring in the workplace and improving when away from work (i.e., at night, on weekends, vacation).

Irritant-induced asthma?

For irritant-induced, either the exposure is massive and obvious or many workers are affected.

Immunologically mediated asthma?

For immunologically mediated, few workers are affected. Symptoms progressively worsen as the work week progresses.

What are the similarities and differences between HSP and immunologically mediated occupational asthma?

Both diseases are characterized by cough and shortness of breath, but HSP also causes systemic symptoms such as fever as well as pulmonary infiltrates and restrictive PFTs (decreased TLC, DLco). HSP is not IgE-mediated, whereas occupational asthma generally is.

What are the three types of HSP?

Acute, subacute, and chronic.

How does acute HSP present?

Acute HSP presents similarly to community-acquired pneumonia with the acute onset of both respiratory and systemic symptoms occurring 4 to 8 hours after exposure.

How does subacute HSP present?

Subacute HSP presents with a several-week to many-month history of respiratory and mild systemic symptoms.

How does chronic HSP present?

Chronic HSP presents more indolently over months to years, often without systemic symptoms.

What are the major criteria to diagnose HSP?

1. Exposure to a known offending agent (history, serum precipitating antibodies, or environmental analysis)
2. Compatible symptoms (i.e., recurrent episodes of symptoms occurring 4 to 8 hours after exposure)
3. Infiltrates on CXR

What are the minor criteria to diagnose HSP?

1. Crackles on physical examination
2. Decreased PaO_2, lung volumes, or DL_{CO}
3. Lung biopsy that demonstrates loosely formed granuloma and a lymphocytic alveolitis around airways
4. Positive challenge test
5. BAL may also be helpful, because there is an increase in $CD8^+$ T cells, as opposed to the increase in $CD4^+$ T cells seen in sarcoidosis.

What is required to diagnose HSP?

Requires all major and two minor criteria

BRONCHIECTASIS[2]

What is the first step in the diagnostic evaluation for ABPA?

Perform skin prick test to *Aspergillus;* if negative, perform intradermal injection. If both are negative, ABPA is ruled out. If positive, one must go on to the next step, because 20% to 30% of asthmatics may have a positive response.

What is the second step in the diagnostic evaluation for ABPA?

Measure total IgE and serum precipitating antibodies (IgG) to *Aspergillus* (serum precipitans).

---

[2]In collaboration with M. Reitmeyer, S. AlGazlan, and L. Wheatley.

What is the third step in the diagnostic evaluation for ABPA?

If total IgE >1000 ng/mL and serum precipitans is positive, check specific IgE to *Aspergillus* (e.g., by RAST) and HRCT; a positive specific IgE to *Aspergillus* or an HRCT demonstrating central or proximal bronchiectasis clinches the diagnosis of ABPA.

Other diagnostic criteria for ABPA include an eosinophil count ≥8%.

Which criteria above may be affected by remission or therapy?

All the criteria with the exception of positive RAST testing may be absent when patients are in remission. Also, peripheral eosinophilia and elevated total IgE may be absent in patients who are being treated with oral prednisone, although the total IgE level rarely returns entirely to normal.

INTERSTITIAL LUNG DISEASE

Which disorders are included in the idiopathic fibrosing interstitial pneumonia group?

Usual interstitial pneumonitis (UIP), desquamative interstitial pneumonitis (DIP), respiratory bronchiolitis—associated interstitial lung disease (RB-ILD), nonspecific interstitial pneumonitis (NSIP), AIP, and COP. COP is the new term for idiopathic BOOP. IPF is synonymous with usual interstitial pneumonitis from an unknown cause.

Which C-T diseases cause ILD?

SLE, rheumatoid arthritis, ankylosing spondylitis, progressive systemic sclerosis, Sjögren's syndrome, and polymyositis–dermatomyositis

Which P-R syndromes cause ILD?

Goodpasture's syndrome, Wegener's granulomatosis, microscopic polyangiitis, allergic angiitis, and granulomatosis (Churg-Strauss syndrome)

Which environmental substances cause ILD?

Inorganic dusts, fibers, and metals: asbestos, silica, coal, and beryllium

Organic dusts: cotton (byssinosis)

Toxic gases and fumes: nitrogen dioxide

Which ILDs are associated with granulomas?

Known causes: HSP, beryllium, silica, and medications (e.g., methotrexate)

Unknown causes: sarcoidosis, Langerhans cell granulomatosis (eosinophilic granuloma), granulomatous vasculitides (Wegener's, Churg-Strauss), and bronchocentric granulomatosis

Which inherited diseases cause ILD?

Tuberous sclerosis, Hermansky–Pudlak syndrome, neurofibromatosis, metabolic storage disorders (e.g., Gaucher's, Niemann–Pick), and hypocalciuric hypercalcemia

Which miscellaneous diseases cause ILD?

BO with or without organizing pneumonia (BOOP/COP), eosinophilic pneumonia, drugs, radiation, lymphangioleiomyomatosis, alveolar proteinosis, veno-occlusive disease, lymphangitic carcinomatosis, idiopathic pulmonary hemosiderosis, gastrointestinal or liver diseases (inflammatory bowel disease, primary biliary cirrhosis, chronic active hepatitis), graft-versus-host disease (bone marrow transplant), lymphocytic infiltrative diseases, and alveolar microlithiasis

What is Caplan's syndrome?

The association of rheumatoid arthritis and pulmonary nodules in patients with pneumoconiosis, particularly coal workers' pneumoconiosis

What pulmonary function abnormalities occur with BO and OP?

BO is obstructive, and OP is restrictive.

What are the ATS criteria to determine improvement?

>10% change in FVC or TLC; >15% change in DL_{CO}; >4% increase in O_2 sat; >4 mm Hg change in Pao_2 during exercise

What should you think of if your patient's illness worsens during treatment with prednisone and cytotoxic agents?

Infection or pneumonitis, including with unusual organisms such as *Pneumocystis jiroveci* (PCP). HF, pulmonary embolism, ARDS, and an acute exacerbation of ILD are other considerations.

CYSTIC FIBROSIS

What laboratory tests are performed for CF?	Chest radiograph PFTs Sweat chloride test Search for genetic mutations
What are the typical findings seen on the CXR in patients with CF?	Shows hyperinflation, bronchiectasis, and reticular nodular fibrosis; rarely shows atelectasis or pneumothorax
What are the typical findings seen on the PFTs in patients with CF?	Early, shows obstructive lung disease; late, shows restrictive lung disease
What are common organisms found in the sputum of patients with CF?	*Staphylococcus aureus, Haemophilus influenzae,* and *Pseudomonas aeruginosa*
What antibiotic class should be avoided and why?	Quinolones rapidly induce resistance.

PULMONARY THROMBOEMBOLISM AND DEEP VENOUS THROMBOSIS

What are the clinical indicators of a primary hypercoagulable state?	Family history of thrombosis, recurrent thrombosis without an obvious predisposing factor, thrombosis at an unusual anatomic site (e.g., artery), thrombosis at a young age, multiple miscarriages, and resistance to conventional antithrombotic therapy
How sensitive is Homans' sign?	No better than 50%
In what disease states are pulmonary infarctions more likely to occur?	More likely to occur with HF, COPD, and mitral stenosis
How reliable is the D-dimer?	Because of its good sensitivity (negative predictive value), a value <500 indicates a low probability of DVT or PE. Because of its poor specificity (positive predictive value), a positive value is not helpful and requires further evaluation.

What is the likelihood of PE if the V̇/Q̇ scan is one of the following:

    Low probability?   <10% to 20%

    Intermediate probability?   40% to 50%

    High probability?   90%

What is the sensitivity and negative predictive value for CTPA?

A recent study demonstrated a sensitivity of 83% and a negative predictive value of 95%; adding a CT venogram increased the sensitivity for diagnosing PE/DVT to 90% and the negative predictive value to 97%.

What is the imaging test to use if the D-dimer is elevated with or without a normal CXR?

CT angiogram if the pretest probability and D-dimer indicate further workup is needed, particularly if the CXR is abnormal and renal function is OK (creatinine ≤1.4)

What other test could be used to image the patient if the chest film was normal?

A V̇/Q̇ scan can also be performed at this step, particularly if the chest radiograph is normal and/or renal function significantly abnormal (creatinine >1.4). An MRPA may also be used in some centers.

When should a PA gram be considered?

Pulmonary angiogram if the pretest probability plus D-dimer plus the V̇/Q̇ or CT angiogram indicate further workup is needed despite negative IPG or Doppler ultrasound of the lower extremities

When the suspicion for PE is very high, one should continue evaluation until a positive result requiring treatment is obtained or a PA gram is performed.

When should thrombolysis be considered for DVT?

When iliac veins are involved

What are the treatment options for a hemodynamically significant PE?

Thrombolysis (indications are not based on prospective studies) when hemodynamically unstable patients are unresponsive to maximal medical management

Surgical embolectomy for hemodynamically unstable patients (PE) who are unresponsive to thrombolysis or with a contraindication to thrombolysis (as for thrombolysis, there are no prospective studies)

When should an IVC filter be considered?

For patients who have failed anticoagulation (rare) or in whom anticoagulation is contraindicated (i.e., patients with active gastrointestinal bleeding) or in patients with PE who are at high risk of dying should another PE occur (i.e., massive PE or chronic thromboembolic pulmonary hypertension)

PULMONARY HYPERTENSION

What are the 5 World Health Organization (WHO) categories for pulmonary HTN?

1. Idiopathic PPH
2. Associated with left heart disease (e.g., left ventricular failure, valvular heart disease, left atrial obstruction)
3. Associated with lung diseases and/or hypoxemia (e.g., ILD, COPD, sleep-disordered breathing, alveolar hypoventilation disorders, high altitude, neuromuscular diseases, thoracic cage abnormalities)
4. Due to chronic thrombotic or embolic disease
5. Miscellaneous (e.g., sarcoidosis, compression of pulmonary vasculature by adenopathy, tumor, fibrosing mediastinitis)

What other laboratory tests may be useful in detecting pulmonary HTN?

C-T disease serologic tests, LFTs, and HIV serologies

What other testing should be considered?

Sleep study for sleep-disordered breathing

$\dot{V}/\dot{Q}$ scanning to rule out chronic PE

In addition to history, what test can be helpful in determining the patients' functional class?

6-minute walk test

What is the definition of a significant response to vasodilators on cardiac catheterization?

Defined as a decrease in mean PA pressure by at least 10 mm Hg to a level ≤40 mm Hg and with a stable or increased cardiac output

What prostatcyclins can be considered for treatment?

Intravenous: epoprostinol, treprostinol

Subcutaneous: treprostinol

Inhaled: iloprost

What other oral medications can be considered for treatment?

Endothelin receptor antagonist (bosentan, sitaxetan in Europe); phosphodiesterase-5 inhibitor (sildenafil)

PULMONARY NEOPLASMS (SEE CHAPTER 9, "ONCOLOGY")

SLEEP-RELATED BREATHING DISORDERS

What is Cheyne-Stokes respiration?

A pattern of central apnea, characterized by periodic, regular waxing and waning of ventilation. During the waning phase, there is frank apnea. Major causes include HF, CNS lesions, renal failure, and high altitude.

What is the difference between obstructive and central apnea?

In obstructive apnea, there is no airflow with persistent respiratory effort.

In central apnea, there is no airflow with no associated respiratory effort (presumably secondary to the absence of the central drive to breathe).

Mixed apnea is a combination of the two.

What is a RERA?

A CNS arousal terminating obstructed events that do not meet the criteria for an apnea or hypopnea

What is the UARS?

A clinical syndrome of excessive sleepiness resulting from RERAs

What is the incidence of OSA?

Much more common than previously thought: 24% of men and 9% of women have sleep apnea; 4% of men and 2% of women have sleep apnea syndrome.

What is the AHI?

The AHI is the number of apneic plus hypopneic episodes per hour of sleep. It is a measure of the severity of sleep-disordered breathing.

What is the RDI?

The number of apneas plus hypopneas plus RERAs per hour of sleep.

What is the sleep apnea syndrome?

Sleep apnea (AHI >5) plus some physiologic consequence (e.g., EDS)

What are some of the consequences of hypoxia and hypercapnia?

Polycythemia, pulmonary HTN, cor pulmonale, chronic hypercapnia, morning and nighttime headache, HF, nocturnal arrhythmias, nocturnal angina, and systemic HTN

What is the therapy for patients who fail to respond to weight loss, CPAP, or BiPAP?

Tracheotomy is only rarely required and should be considered a last resort. Rapid-eye-movement (REM) sleep suppressant drugs (i.e., tricyclic antidepressants) should be used only in select cases. Respiratory stimulants (e.g., progesterone and acetazolamide) should also be used only in select cases.

What is the difference between CPAP and BiPAP?

With CPAP, the inspiratory and expiratory positive airway pressures are and must be the same; with BiPAP, the inspiratory positive airway pressure and the expiratory positive airway pressure can vary, allowing you to set the inspiratory higher then the expiratory positive airway pressure.

What is an additional use of BiPAP?

BiPAP also allows you to set a backup respiratory rate; consequently you can ventilate a patient with BiPAP.

When would you consider using BiPAP instead of CPAP?

When a patient with OSA has difficulty tolerating CPAP or when the patient has CSA or is hypoventilating

BRONCHITIS AND PNEUMONIAS[3]

BRONCHITIS

How is the diagnosis of acute bronchitis made?	Because cough is a symptom associated with a variety of pulmonary diseases, other causes must be ruled out before the diagnosis of acute bronchitis is made.

PNEUMONIA[4]

How is CAP defined?	CAP is defined as a pneumonia beginning outside the hospital or diagnosed within 48 hours after admission.
How is HAP defined?	HAP occurs more than 48 hours after admission to the hospital and excludes any infection that began before or was present at the time of admission.
What are risk factors for health care–associated pneumonia?	Hospitalization for ≥ 2 days in the preceding 90 days, residence in a nursing home or extended care facility, home infusion therapy (including antibiotics), chronic dialysis within 30 days, home wound care, family member with a multidrug-resistant pathogen
What is the clinical importance of health care–associated pneumonia?	These individuals are at risk for multidrug-resistant pathogens such as *Pseudomonas* and methicillin-resistant *Staphylococcal aureus*. Empiric therapy therefore must cover these organisms.
What clinical signs suggest chlamydial pneumonia?	Hoarseness and fever starting first, with respiratory tract symptoms not appearing for a few days
What symptoms and signs can suggest mycoplasmal pneumonia?	Ear pain, bullous myringitis, skin rashes, hemolytic anemia, and persistent, nonproductive cough

---

[3]In collaboration with N. Thielman, V. Shami, and C. Sable.
[4]In collaboration with N. Thielman, V. Shami, and C. Sable.

Is there a difference in prognosis for elderly patients with pneumonia?

Advanced age carries an increasing risk of fatal pneumonia with an increased risk of infection with more virulent pathogens, including *S. aureus* and gram-negative bacilli.

What noninfectious diseases can mimic CAP?

PE, HSP, ARDS, acute eosinophilic pneumonia, COP, drug-induced pneumonitis, systemic vasculitis, AIP, lung cancer, and atelectasis

For the following epidemiologic circumstances, list the typical pathogen(s):

    COPD?

H. influenzae and parainfluenza, *Moraxella catarrhalis,* and *S. pneumoniae*

    Health care–associated?

Gram-negative bacilli (many drug-resistant, including *Pseudomonas*), *S. aureus*, including methicillin resistant, pneumococcus, *C. pneumoniae*

    Rabbit exposure?

Tularemia

    Exposure to cats, cattle, sheep, and goats?

Coxiella burnetii (Q fever)

    Exposure to turkeys, chickens, and psittacine birds?

Chlamydia psittaci

    Caves?

Histoplasma

What are the risk factors for drug-resistant or nonsusceptible *S. pneumoniae*?

Extremes of age (>65 years, <5 years), beta-lactam antibiotic in the last 3 months, immunosuppressive illness (alcoholism, nephrotic syndrome, HIV, sickle cell disease, corticosteroids >10 mg/day), day-care attendance or family member of day-care attendee, and multiple medical comorbidities

What are the risk factors for *Legionella* pneumonia?

>10 mg/day of prednisone, renal failure, neutropenia, chemotherapy, malignancy, including hairy cell leukemia, transplants, and exposure to contaminated water sources such as cooling towers, air conditioning, or saunas. *Legionella* should also be considered in the late summer.

Who is likely to be infected with *Moraxella*?

Cigarette smokers, COPD patients, diabetics, patients with malignancies, alcoholics, and patients taking corticosteroids. Such infection is rare in normal adults.

What are the complications associated with severe pneumonia?

Approximately 10% of patients require admission to the ICU for respiratory (and often, multisystemic) failure with or without hemodynamic shock.

What are the pathogens associated with severe pneumonia?

The most common pathogens are *S. pneumoniae* and *Legionella pneumophila,* but it may also be caused by gram-negative bacilli or *M. pneumoniae.*

What are complications of anaerobic pneumonia?

If untreated, necrosis, cavitation, and empyema

What is the mortality rate of CAP?

5% to 25%

What do the following findings on CXR suggest:
    Lobar consolidation, cavitation, and effusion?

Bacterial pneumonia

    Diffuse bilateral involvement?

PCP, *Legionella* infection, mycoplasma, or virus

    Superior segment of the lower lobe or posterior segment of the upper lobe involvement?

Aspiration

What is CURB-65 and how can it assist in the management of patients with CAP?

Like the PSI, it is a clinical prediction rule that has been validated in nonimmunosuppressed adults and permits quantitative assessment of an individual patient's risk of dying during an episode of acute pneumonia.

What are the components of the CURB-65?

C = confusion; U = urea >20 mg/dL, B = blood pressure (systolic <90 or diastolic ≤60 mm Hg), age ≥65.

How do the CURB-65 point scores correlate with mortality and admission recommendation:

    0 to 1 points?

0.4% mortality: can treat as outpatient

    2 points?

7.6% mortality: hospitalize or closely supervised outpatient therapy

    3 points?

14.0% mortality: hospitalize, consider intensive care unit.

    4 to 5 points?

27.8% mortality: hospitalize, consider ICU.

What is the CRB-65?

CRB-65 correlates well with CURB-65 and avoids the need for laboratory studies.

How do the CRB-65 point scores correlate with mortality and admission recommendation -

    0 points?

0.9% mortality: can treat as outpatient.

    1 point?

5.2% mortality: consider hospitalization.

    2 points?

12.0% mortality: consider hospitalization.

    3 to 4 points?

31.2% mortality: high risk of death, hospitalize, consider ICU.

What are the determinants of severe CAP?

A patient has severe CAP if he or she has two of three minor criteria (PaO_2/FIO_2 <250, systolic blood pressure $\leq$90 mm Hg, multilobar involvement) or one of two major criteria (need for mechanical ventilation, septic shock)

What is a general rule for the treatment of CAP?

It is important to cover for both "typical" and "atypical" organisms. In addition, as a very general rule, the older a patient is, the more comorbid conditions he or she has, the sicker he or she is, the more likely he or she has a gram-negative bacillus, *Legionella,* or *S. aureus* as the cause of pneumonia.

For a patient with CAP and a PSI risk class of I, II, and some III, what would be reasonable antibiotic choices?

Include a macrolide (e.g., azithromycin, clarithromycin, erythromycin), tetracycline (doxycycline), or a respiratory fluoroquinolone (levofloxacin, gatifloxacin, moxifloxacin). Take into account risk factors for certain organisms. For instance, in outpatients with risk factors for Gram-negative bacilli, add a beta-lactam antibiotic to a macrolide or doxycycline, or treat the person with a respiratory fluoroquinolone alone. With risk factors for anaerobes, add amoxicillin-clavulanate, clindamycin, or metronidazole.

For hospitalized patients with CAP (risk class IV, V, some III), *without* severe CAP (outlined above), what would be reasonable antibiotic coverage?

Reasonable antibiotic choices for this group include a macrolide *or* doxycycline plus a third-generation cephalosporin (ceftriaxone, cefotaxime) *or* ampicillin/sulbactam or piperacillin-tazobactam *or* high-dose amoxicillin *or* a respiratory fluoroquinolone alone. These patients can usually be treated on a general medicine ward.

How should patients with *severe* CAP and no risk factors for *P. aeruginosa* be treated?

In general, they should be admitted to the ICU. A macrolide *or* a respiratory fluoroquinolone plus a third-generation cephalosporin (ceftriaxone, cefotaxime) *or* piperacillin-tazobactam or ampicillin/sulbactam is a reasonable regimen.

How should patients with *severe* CAP *and* risk factors for *P. aeruginosa* be treated?

In general they should be in the ICU. Recommended treatment includes a macrolide or respiratory fluoroquinolone *plus* an antipseudomonal beta lactam [cefepime, ceftazidime, carbapenem (imipenem, meropenem), piperacillin, piperacillin-tazobactam, or ticarcillin-clavulanate] *plus* an aminoglycoside; or antipseudomonal beta lactam plus fluoroquinolone.

What percentage of aspiration pneumonias become infected?

Approximately 40% of chemical aspirations become infected. Bacterial superinfection usually develops slowly over days and may evolve into necrotizing pneumonia, abscess, or empyema.

What are some of the other late consequences of aspiration?

Other consequences of aspiration include bronchospasm, bronchiectasis, pulmonary fibrosis, and ARDS.

NOSOCOMIAL (HOSPITAL-ACQUIRED) PNEUMONIA[5]

What are the features used to make the diagnosis of HAP?

CXR evidence of an infiltrate that is alveolar, has an air bronchogram sign, is new or progressive, plus two or more of the following: fever or hypothermia, purulent secretions, WBC >12,000 or <4000 or >10% band forms, or decreased PaO_2

Why is it more difficult to diagnose pneumonias in intubated patients?

Because of bacterial colonization of the upper airway and oropharynx, the development of tracheobronchitis in many intubated patients, the numerous causes of chest radiographic infiltrates, and the many causes of fever in hospitalized patients

What would be a typical regimen for:
    Patient with HAP and hospitalized for <5 days?

Unlikely to have *P. aeruginosa, Acinetobacter,* or methicillin-resistant

---

[5] In collaboration with N. Thielman, V. Shami, and C. Sable.

S. *aureus* causing the pneumonia. Therefore a second-generation cephalosporin (cefuroxime), nonpseudomonal third-generation cephalosporin, or beta lactam/beta-lactamase inhibitor would be recommended.

Same patient with a penicillin allergy?

Could use a fluoroquinolone or clindamycin plus aztreonam

Same patient with risk factors for *Pseudomonas*?

Treat as ≥5 days in hospital

Patient with HAP, hospitalized ≥5 days?

Need to double cover *P. aeruginosa* in this group; at least initially, it increases the likelihood that you are adequately covering the organism. Recommended regimens include an aminoglycoside or fluoroquinolone plus an antipseudomonal beta lactam or aztreonam plus vancomycin.

The prevalence as well as the antibiotic sensitivity in the individual hospital and in individual units must be taken into consideration as well.

Same patient with risk factors for anaerobes?

Add clindamycin, or treat with beta lactam/beta-lactamase inhibitor alone.

Same patient with risk factors for methicillin-resistant S. *aureus*?

Add vancomycin.

Same patient with risk factors for *Legionella*?

Add erythromycin with or without rifampin; consider a quinolone.

MYCOBACTERIUM TUBERCULOSIS[6]

What group is at higher risk of extrapulmonary TB?

It is more common in the HIV population.

---

[6] In collaboration with N. Thielman, V. Shami, and C. Stable.

What organ systems are involved with extrapulmonary TB?

Extrapulmonary TB occurs in approximately one in six cases and may involve the CNS, bone, genitourinary system, lymph nodes, or gastrointestinal tract.

How is the tuberculin skin test read?

Induration is read at 48 to 72 hours.

What does the tuberculin skin test identify?

Remember that the tuberculin skin test identifies people who have been infected with *M. tuberculosis* but does not distinguish between active and latent infections.

What groups are considered to have a positive PPD test if the induration is one of the following:

≥5 mm but <10 mm?

Persons in the high-risk group above

≥10 mm but <15 mm?

Persons in the intermediate group above

≥15 mm?

Individuals not at increased risk of becoming infected with or developing TB

What is MDR-TB?

Multidrug-resistant TB, defined as resistant to both INH and rifampin

Why is MDR-TB important?

Different drug regimens are needed for a longer time. Cure rates are much lower than for susceptible TB.

What is the association between HIV and TB?

Active TB is more likely to develop in HIV-positive patients once infected (50% first year versus 5% to 15% in general; 8% to 10% per year versus 0.3% per year). TB can develop at any time in patients with HIV.

What is different about the TB infections in HIV patients with lower CD4 counts?

Associated with atypical disease; such patients are less likely to have a positive PPD and more likely to have extrapulmonary TB.

How should HIV-positive patients be treated if they have:

    A positive PPD? — INH preventive therapy given for 9 months; alternative: rifampin for 4 months

    A negative PPD? — Preventive therapy if in recent contact with a patient with active TB, history of prior untreated or inadequately treated prior TB, unavoidable high-risk of TB exposure (e.g., residents of prisons or homeless shelters)

    Active disease? — Treatment of disease is with the same four-drug regimen given for 9 months.

PLEURAL EFFUSIONS

Why does egophony occur above the effusion? — Secondary to lung consolidation and/or atelectasis

Which way does the mediastinum shift with a pleural effusion? — Away from the side of effusion

Which way does the mediastinum shift with a pneumothorax? — Toward the side of effusion

How do you confirm the presence of a subpulmonic effusion? — Obtain a lateral decubitus film or do an ultrasound.

Which pleural effusions do not require thoracentesis? — Associated with HF; small, right-sided pleural effusion with ascites; small, asymptomatic effusions in the following circumstances: documented pneumococcal pneumonia, ARDS, the first few days after abdominal surgery

Which effusions in the setting of HF require a thoracentesis? — Presence of a fever, pleuritic chest pain, hemoptysis, pulmonary infiltrate or mass, unexplained elevated WBC count, or weight loss

How much pleural fluid may be removed at one time?

If pleural pressure is not monitored, up to 1500 mL of fluid may be removed for symptomatic relief.

What is the danger of removing too much pleural fluid?

Removal of more than 1500 mL may lead to postthoracentesis pulmonary edema.

Is there a way to remove more fluid without causing trouble?

With gravity drainage, one can remove as much of the pleural effusion as desired.

Give some examples of transudative effusions.

The most common cause of a transudative pleural effusion is HF. Other causes include nephrotic syndrome, cirrhosis, hypoalbuminemia, acute glomerulonephritis, urinothorax, peritoneal dialysis, superior vena cava obstruction, atelectasis, trapped lung, and constrictive pericarditis.

What are the three most common causes of exudative pleural effusions?

Infections, malignancy, and PE are the most common causes.

What are some of the other common causes of an exudative pleural effusion?

Other common examples are TB, trauma, collagen vascular disease, and abdominal disease.

What are some of the more unusual causes of an exudative pleural effusion?

Unusual causes include esophageal rupture, drug-induced, asbestos, postcardiac injury syndrome, chylothorax, uremia, radiation therapy, sarcoid, yellow nail syndrome, hypothyroidism, and Meig's syndrome.

What are examples of "classic" exudates that can present as transudates?

Malignancy, PE, sarcoidosis, hypothyroidism

What is a "classic" transudate that can present as an exudate?

Pleural fluid obtained after diuresing HF sometimes meets exudative criteria. It is important to note that any effusion tends to become exudative the longer it stays in the pleural space.

What should one measure to decide whether the effusion is a true exudate or an exudate from diuresis?

A serum to pleural fluid albumin gradient >1.2 g/dL indicates that diuresed HF is the cause of the exudate.

How much blood does it take to make an effusion look bloody?

A hematocrit of 1% to 2% is "bloody appearing" (and has no clinical importance), as little as 1 mL of blood can turn a 500-mL pleural effusion bloody.

What should be suspected with the following:
    Eosinophils (>10%)?

The most common cause is air, followed by blood in the pleural space. Examples include pneumothorax, hemothorax, PE or infarction, previous thoracentesis, pulmonary contusions, parasitic disease such as echinococcus, drug-induced such as nitrofurantoin, fungal disease such as histoplasmosis, postcardiac injury syndrome, asbestos, lymphoma (especially Hodgkin's disease) and carcinoma (uncommon).

    Brown fluid?

Amebic liver abscess and long-standing bloody effusion

    Black fluid?

Aspergillus

    Yellow-green fluid?

Rheumatoid pleurisy

    "Bloody" fluid?

A hematocrit should be performed on all "bloody" pleural effusions.

If the pleural/serum hematocrit is >2% but <50%: pulmonary embolism leading to pulmonary infarction, pleural carcinomatosis, trauma, benign asbestos pleural effusion, and postcardiac injury syndrome

What is a complicated parapneumonic effusion?

An effusion associated with a pneumonia that is nonpurulent

What are the characteristics of a complicated parapneumonic effusion?

One or more of the following characteristics:

pH <7.20

Glucose <60 mg/dL

Positive Gram's stain

Positive culture

Loculations

Are thrombolytics helpful in the treatment of these effusions?

Recent evidence has indicated that thrombolytics are not useful.

Which drugs can cause effusions?

Frequently: hydralazine, procainamide, isoniazid, phenytoin, and chlorpromazine

Infrequently: nitrofurantoin, bromocriptine, dantrolene, and procarbazine

What is the preferred method for a pleural biopsy?

The choice between a closed needle biopsy and a surgical pleural biopsy depends on clinical suspicion. If TB is likely, the less invasive closed needle biopsy is preferred. If malignancy is suspected despite negative cytology, VATS is more likely to yield a diagnosis.

When is bronchoscopy indicated?

If the patient has a parenchymal abnormality on chest film or CT scan or to rule out an obstruction if atelectasis is associated with the effusion

What chronic complications are associated with pleural effusions?

Pleural fibrosis, resulting from organization of the pleural effusion. Extensive fibrosis can pull the trachea to the affected side and cause trapped lung (late finding; see below).

What is the difference between "trapped" and "entrapped" lung?

A trapped lung results from remote pleural inflammation. An entrapped lung is secondary to active inflammation or malignancy.

What is the overall physiologic cause of both of these?

Both result from decreased visceral pleural compliance (increased stiffness).

What is the clue to suspect one of these has occurred?	A "trapped" or "entrapped" lung should be considered when a pleural effusion rapidly reaccumulates after thoracentesis.
What causes a trapped lung?	It results from remote pleural inflammation; this creates a negative intrapleural pressure.
Does a trapped lung cause transudate or exudate?	A transudative pleural effusion
What causes an entrapped lung?	An entrapped lung is secondary to active inflammation or malignancy.
Does an entrapped lung cause a transudate or exudate?	The resultant effusion is usually an exudate.
What is the treatment for trapped and entrapped lungs?	Treatment is of the underlying cause and possibly decortication.

IMMUNOSUPPRESSED PATIENTS

LUNG TRANSPLANTATION

What is the survival rate after lung transplantation?	75% at 1 year; 60% at 2 years
Why is the standard procedure for CF patients referred to as *bilateral sequential* as opposed to *double lung*?	A double lung involves a tracheal anastomosis and the bilateral sequential is two separate single-lung transplants.
Why is a bilateral sequential operation the preferred procedure?	A bronchial anastomosis heals better and there is less chance for phrenic injury.
What complications need to be watched for in the immediate posttransplant period?	Bleeding, air leak, and bronchial anastomotic dehiscence

How is acute rejection recognized?	Diffuse pulmonary infiltrates in the transplanted lungs, decreased PaO_2, rales, cough, dyspnea, and low-grade fever. After the first month or so, the chest radiograph may be normal.
When does acute rejection usually occur?	It is most common during the first 3 weeks after transplantation, with the peak incidence in the second week.
How is the diagnosis of acute rejection made?	The "gold standard" is the presence of perivascular infiltrate of lymphocytes on transbronchial biopsy.
What else causes BO?	Cytomegalovirus infection, ischemic reperfusion injury, and gastroesophageal reflux
What is the classification of BO?	BO is classified as stage 0 to 3 depending on the severity of decline in FEF_{25-75} and FEV_1 compared to baseline values after transplant.
What diseases recur in the transplanted lung?	Sarcoid, giant cell interstitial pneumonitis, and lymphangioleiomyomatosis

STEM CELL TRANSPLANTS

What is the most common pulmonary problem in stem cell transplantation?	Interstitial pneumonitis

OTHER IMMUNOSUPPRESSED PATIENTS

What are the major organisms responsible for pulmonary infections in each of the following:	
Primary neutrophil defects?	Gram-positive organisms, especially *S. aureus, Streptococcus viridans,* enterococci, and *Corynebacterium jeikeium;* Gram-negative organisms, especially Enterobacteriaceae and *P. aeruginosa;* anaerobes; and fungi, especially *Candida* and *Aspergillus*

Cell-mediated?	Intracellular organisms such as mycobacteria (*M. tuberculosis* and *Mycobacterium avium* complex) and *Nocardia;* fungi such as *Pneumocystis* and *Cryptococcus,* and endemic organisms like *Histoplasma;* viruses, especially DNA viruses such as CMV; and parasites and protozoa
Humoral?	Encapsulated bacteria, including *S. pneumoniae, H. influenzae, Neisseria* spp., and *E. coli*

ACQUIRED IMMUNODEFICIENCY SYNDROME

What is the likelihood of PCP with a low LDH and low ESR?	Patients with serum LDH levels of <220 U/L and an ESR <50 mm/hr are unlikely to have PCP and may be clinically followed.
How does KS present in the lung?	KS may present as infiltrates, interstitial disease, effusions, lymphadenopathy, or endobronchial involvement. Hemorrhage may occur. Gallium scans are negative, unlike those for infections and lymphoma.

CRITICAL CARE

What are the phases of shock?	1. Compensated hypotension (blood flow to brain, heart, liver, and kidney is maintained) 2. Decompensated hypotension (end-organ malperfusion) 3. Irreversible shock (microcirculatory failure and cell death)
What are the six causes of hypoxemia?	Hypoventilation Decreased inspired pressure of oxygen (PIo_2) (e.g., living at high altitude) $\dot{V}/\dot{Q}$ mismatch Shunt Decreased diffusion Decreased mixed venous oxygen saturation

How do you calculate an A-a gradient?

Simplified method:

$PaO_2 - PaO_2$

$PaO_2 = 7 \times FiO_2$

$PaO_2 = PO_2 - (PaCO_2 \times 1.25)$

Normal is <20.

What does a normal A-a gradient indicate?

That hypoventilation or decreased PIO_2 is the cause

What does complete improvement to 100% O_2 indicate?

Complete improvement indicates that the cause of the hypoxemia is $\dot{V}/\dot{Q}$ mismatch; incomplete improvement indicates that shunt is the mechanism.

What are the determinants of oxygen delivery?

O_2 delivery = cardiac output × arterial oxygen content (CaO_2)

$CaO_2 = (1.34 \times$ hemoglobin × oxygen saturation$) + (0.003 \times PaO_2)$

In a hypoxic patient, what is a good clue that shunting is occurring?

Because $\dot{V}/\dot{Q}$ mismatch responds well to increasing the concentration of oxygen, one typically requires no more than 2 to 4 L/min oxygen. If more oxygen is required, a component of shunt exists. Thus, if a patient with a COPD exacerbation is requiring more than 4 L/min oxygen, you should look for causes of shunt such as pneumonia, cardiac pulmonary edema, and atelectasis.

What are the four most common causes of ARDS?

Sepsis, multiple trauma with multiple transfusions, aspiration of gastric contents, and diffuse pneumonia

What are general indications for intubation?

Inability to protect airway (e.g., mental status changes)

Copious secretions

Hypoxemic respiratory failure (e.g., PaO_2 <50 mm Hg on 100% nonrebreathing face mask)

Ventilatory failure (e.g., $PaCO_2$ >45 mm Hg with a pH <7.2) caused by excessive work of breathing (e.g., asthma), neuromuscular weakness (e.g., myasthenia gravis), or a combination

Hypoperfusion or shock states

Treatment of increased intracranial pressure

Why is tube size important for weaning?

Resistance, which affects the patient's work of breathing, is directly related to tube length and inversely related to tube radius to the fourth power.

What is the peak airway pressure?

With volume-limited ventilator modes, the peak pressure is the maximum pressure generated at the completion of inspiration—e.g., after the entire tidal volume has been delivered by the ventilator

What is the significance of peak airway pressure?

Provides information about the resistance and compliance of the respiratory system. It is important to keep in mind that ventilatory pressures such as the peak airway pressure provide information about the entire respiratory system including the extrapulmonary structures and the ventilator circuit.

Besides lung-related issues, what can raise a peak airway pressure?

An obstructed endotracheal tube and a taut abdomen will cause elevated airway pressures.

What is the plateau or static pressure?

With volume-limited ventilator modes, the plateau or static pressure is measured by initiating an inspiratory hold or pause maneuver.

What is the significance of the plateau or static pressure?

The plateau or static pressure provides information about the compliance or stiffness of the respiratory system. The plateau pressure also provides an estimate of the average pressure to which most alveoli are exposed.

What would be the goal plateau pressure to maintain below?

Minimizing alveolar pressure by keeping the plateau pressure ≤ 25 to 30 cm H_2O pressure has been shown to decrease morbidity (e.g., pneumothorax) and mortality in patients with COPD and ARDS.

For pressure-limited modes of ventilation, what is a reasonable approximation of plateau pressure or mean alveolar pressure?

Set pressure + PEEP + auto-PEEP

What is the clinical significance of the peak inspiratory pressure minus the plateau pressure?

In patients on volume-limited ventilation, this measure provides information about the resistance of the respiratory system. One can calculate resistance by dividing this difference by inspiratory flow. As a very general rule, for an endotracheal tube size ≥ 7.0 cm and normal inspiratory flows (60 L/min), a normal peak inspiratory pressure minus plateau pressure difference is ≤ 5 to 10 cm H_2O. Higher values indicate increased respiratory system resistance.

How does one calculate the compliance of the respiratory system in a patient on a volume mode of ventilation?

Set tidal volume/(plateau pressure – PEEP – auto-PEEP)

How does one estimate the compliance of the respiratory system in a patient on a pressure mode of ventilation?

Although there is no "true" plateau pressure with pressure modes of ventilation, one can estimate the respiratory system compliance as exhaled tidal volume/set pressure.

What are chest radiographic signs of a pneumothorax in a mechanically ventilated patient?

Because most CXRs are anterior, one may not see "classic" findings such as a pleural line. Look for a deep sulcus sign, sharp heart border or diaphragm, absent lung markings, pleural reflection, and mediastinal shift.

What are the major determinants of PaCO$_2$?

PaCO$_2$ — $\dot{V}_{CO_2}/[\text{MV} (1 - \text{Vd/Vt})]$

Where $\dot{V}_{CO_2}$ is CO$_2$ production

MV is minute ventilation

Vd/Vt is the ratio of dead space to tidal volume

MV = tidal volume × respiratory rate

What adverse effects are associated with auto-PEEP?

Similar to those seen with positive-pressure ventilation. In addition, because the patient must overcome auto-PEEP before triggering the ventilator or air entering the lungs, auto-PEEP results in increased inspiratory work of breathing and, for those on a ventilator, patient-ventilator dyssynchrony.

What is the best mode for liberating a patient from the ventilator?

Possible methods include T-piece, CPAP, PS, and SIMV. Multiple studies have not demonstrated a clear advantage of any single technique. However, SIMV has been shown to be inferior.

What are appropriate situations for using noninvasive ventilation for acute respiratory failure?

Patients with COPD and HF achieve the best outcomes, although there are data supporting the use of noninvasive ventilation for all causes of respiratory failure.

What are inappropriate situations for using noninvasive ventilation for acute respiratory failure?

Patients with frank apnea or respiratory arrest, inability to protect the airway, voluminous secretions, facial trauma or other factors preventing a tight mask seal, upper airway obstruction, inability or refusal to cooperate, respiratory failure so severe that the patient cannot tolerate even a brief disconnect, and hemodynamic instability.

Chapter 11   Rheumatology

ABBREVIATIONS

ANA	Antinuclear antibody
ANCA	Antineutrophil cytoplasmic antibodies
APS	Antiphospholipid antibody syndrome
AS	Ankylosing spondylitis

AVN	Avascular necrosis
BUN	Blood urea nitrogen
CBC	Complete blood count
CH50	Total complement
CK	Creatine kinase
CNS	Central nervous system
CPP	Calcium pyrophosphate
CPPD	Calcium pyrophosphate dihydrate deposition disease
CTD	Connective tissue disease
dcSSc	Diffuse cutaneous systemic sclerosis
DGI	Disseminated gonococcal infection
DIL	Drug-induced lupus
DIP	Distal interphalangeal joint
DM	Dermatomyositis
DMARD	Disease-modifying antirheumatic drug
FMS	Fibromyalgia syndrome
ESR	Erythrocyte sedimentation rate
GC	Gonococcal
HIV	Human immunodeficiency virus
HTN	Hypertension
IBD	Inflammatory bowel disease
JRA	Juvenile rheumatoid arthritis
lcSSc	Limited cutaneous systemic sclerosis
LFT	Liver function test
MCP	Metacarpophalangeal
MCTD	Mixed connective tissue disease
MSU	Monosodium urate
NSAID	Nonsteroidal anti-inflammatory drug
OA	Osteoarthritis
PAN	Polyarteritis nodosa
PCP	Pneumocystic carinii
PIP	Proximal interphalangeal joint
PM	Polymyositis
PMN	Polymorphonuclear neutrophils
PMR	Polymyalgia rheumatica
PsA	Psoriatic arthritis
RA	Rheumatoid arthritis
RF	Rheumatoid factor
RNP	Ribonucleoprotein
ROM	Range of motion
SCLE	Subacute cutaneous lupus erythematosus
SjS	Sjögren's syndrome
SLE	Systemic lupus erythematosus
SSc	Systemic sclerosis
UA	Urinalysis
VAS	Vasculitis

HISTORY AND PHYSICAL EXAMINATION

What are the common diseases that present as monoarthritis?	OA Crystal-induced arthritis (gout, pseudogout, hydroxyapatite) Infection AVN Tumor Trauma Hemarthrosis Collagen vascular diseases
What are the common diseases that present as oligoarthritis (<4 joints)?	OA Collagen vascular diseases Infections Postinfectious arthritis Seronegative spondoarthropathy (e.g., PsA, AS) Hematologic disorders (leukemia, hemophilia, sickle cell disease)
What are the common diseases that present as polyarticular arthritis?	Viral infections (e.g., parvo, rubella, hepatitis B & C) RA SLE Sarcoidosis Other collagen vascular diseases Crystal-induced arthritis (polyarticular gout) Hypertrophic pulmonary osteoarthropathy
What are the common diseases that present with axial skeletal involvement?	AS PsA IBD-associated arthritis Reactive arthritis Degenerative arthritis

LABORATORY AND OTHER DIAGNOSTIC STUDIES

Why order a CBC?

A CBC can establish the presence of anemia (anemia of chronic disease, hemolytic anemia, drug side effect); leukopenia, lymphopenia, thrombocytopenia (all may be induced by autoimmunity or can be a drug side effect); thrombocytosis (can be a marker of inflammation)

Why order liver enzymes?

LFTs can be abnormal in autoimmune liver disease, liver disease associated with arthritis such as hemochromatosis or Wilson's disease. Preexisting liver disease can also impact the choice of drug therapy.

Why order a urinalysis?

A UA can demonstrate evidence of an inflammatory process involving the glomeruli (dysmorphic RBCs, RBC casts, protein in urine)

Why order a serum creatinine and BUN?

These studies can demonstrate evidence of renal involvement with an inflammatory process or evidence of medication toxicity. They can also estimate the current renal function, which can result in modification of therapy.

Why order genetic testing in autoimmune diseases?

Genetic testing can be suggestive of a condition like AS (HLA B27 gene).

What is the drawback of genetic testing?

Genetic testing is not diagnostic of any particular condition (a positive HLA B27 is found in up to 8% of the normal population) and a negative result does not necessarily rule out the possibility of a certain autoimmune disease.

AUTOANTIBODY AND DISEASE MATCH

What diseases are commonly seen with:
    ANA

Positive ANA can be found in SLE, lupus subsets, SjS, RA (target—nuclear proteins)

What percentage of healthy people have a positive ANA?	Up to 14% of healthy subjects may have low-titer ANA.
Anti-dsDNA	SLE (target—DNA) Double-stranded DNA antibodies are best examined by the Crithidia assay.
Anti-ENA (extractable nuclear antigens)	ENA is a test that examines the specificity of the ANA. Some of the commonly tested specificities are: anti-Smith, anti-SSA, anti-SSB, and anti-RNP.
Anti-Sm (Smith)	SLE (target—RNP proteins). This test should not be confused with SM (smooth muscle antibody), seen in autoimmune hepatitis.
Anti-RNP	SLE, MCTD (target—other RNP proteins)
Anti–SS-A (Ro)	SjS, SCLE, neonatal SLE, SLE (target—proteins associated with RNA)
Anti–SS-B (La)	SjS, SCLE, neonatal SLE, SLE (target—other RNA proteins)
Anticentromere	Raynaud's phenomenon, lcSSc, primary biliary cirrhosis (target—centromere proteins)
Anti–Scl-70	dcSSc (target—antitopoisomerase I)
Anti–Jo-1	Seen in PM > DM, especially with lung involvement (target—anti-histidyl-tRNA synthetase)
c-ANCA	Wegener's granulomatosis (target—proteinase 3)
p-ANCA	PAN and other vasculitides. However, this antibody can be found in a variety of nonvasculitic conditions (IBD, autoimmune hepatitis, RA, SLE, AS).

Anti-Mi2	DM and PM
Anti-Ku	SSc/PM overlap >SLE>SSc> PM and DM
Anti-PM-Scl	SSc/PM overlap > PM and DM
Anti-histone	SLE, DIL
Are there other serologic markers that are useful in patients with rheumatic complaints?	There are many other serologic tests that can be useful, such as TTG in celiac sprue.

IMAGING STUDIES IN RHEUMATOLOGY

What is the earliest sign on plain films of an inflammatory process?	Periarticular osteopenia
What radiographic sign on plain films are the hallmark of an inflammatory process?	Erosive joint changes
What are osteophytes?	Reactive bony changes seen in degenerative arthritis
What are syndesmophytes?	Osteophytes seen in the spondyloarthropathies
What else should be looked for on plain films?	Fractures
What if the plain films are negative in a patient with a suggestive clinical history?	In such cases an MRI (or ultrasound) may be useful in some clinical settings.
Why order a bone scan?	A bone scan measures abnormal metabolic processes involving the bone. This can occur in fractures, bone metastases, metabolic bone disease, and degenerative bone disease.

Why order an MRI?
It is a critical tool to demonstrate early erosive changes and pannus (synovitis). It is also useful to examine the spine, the neuroforamina, and the CNS. It is most useful to evaluate disc space infection, osteomyelitis, bone tumor, and insufficiency fractures. MRI and MRA are useful in evaluating patients with vasculitis.

Why order an angiogram?
This study is the "gold standard" in evaluating the presence of medium and large vessel vasculitis.

Why order an ultrasound?
This technique has gained a significant place in the evaluation of patients with inflammatory arthritis since it is less expensive than MRI, yet it can demonstrate synovitis and erosive changes early

TREATMENT OF RHEUMATIC DISEASES

What might a treatment plan for a patient with inflammatory rheumatic disease include?
1. Education
2. Physical therapy/occupational therapy
3. NSAIDs, which are used for their anti-inflammatory and analgesic effect
4. Corticosteroids, which are used when a strong anti-inflammatory effect is needed
5. DMARDs, when an immuno-suppressive drug is needed
6. Antibiotics such as doxycycline or minocycline and drugs that have immunomodulatory effect, such as sulfasalazine and hydroxychloroquine

What are biologic therapies?
These drugs are DMARDs. They include anti-TNF-α drugs, anti–B cell agents, and a drug that inhibits the costimulation of T cells.

What are the current anti–TNF-α drugs used in rheumatology?

1. Infliximab (Remicade) is a chimeric (hybrid) murine/human monoclonal antibody directed to TNF-α.
2. Etanercept (Enbrel) is a recombinant fusion protein consisting of the ligand-binding domains of the TNF-α receptor (the business end of the receptor) and the Fc portion of immunoglobulin (IgG1).
3. Adalimumab (Humira) is a humanized monoclonal antibody directed against TNF-α.

What is an anti–B cell drug?

Rituximab is a monoclonal antibody against CD20, a surface antigen found on B cells.

What is Abatacept?

Abatacept is a fusion protein that blocks the costimulation of T cells.

Do some rheumatologic illnesses pose a higher risk for malignancy?

Yes, there is an association between certain collagen vascular diseases and malignancy. In most cases an age-appropriate malignancy screening is adequate. However, in other cases (e.g., dermatomyositis and paraneoplastic syndromes), a more extensive evaluation for malignancy is needed at the time of diagnosis and periodically thereafter.

What should be screened for in patients who will require immunosuppressive therapy?

Evidence of infectious disease process. Vaccines need to be up to date (no live vaccine for patients who are immunosuppressed).

Should any prophylaxis be considered for patients on NSAIDs?

Gastroprotection for patients on high-dose corticosteroids and/or NSAIDs

For patients on long term immunosuppression, should any prophylaxis be considered?

PCP prophylaxis

In patients who have been on long-term steroids, what should be considered if they are to undergo surgery or medical stress?	Corticosteroid replacement

MAJOR TOXICITY OF RHEUMATIC DRUGS

What is a major toxicity of:

Hydroxychloroquine	Macular degeneration
Methotrexate	Myelosuppression, hepatic injury and cirrhosis, and pulmonary fibrosis
Azathioprine	Myelosuppression, hepatotoxicity, immunosuppression, and lymphoproliferative disorders
Leflunomide	Myelosuppression, hepatotoxicity, immunosuppression
Sulfasalazine	Myelosuppression and hepatic toxicity
Anti–TNF-α drugs	Immunosuppression, increased risk of malignancy
Cyclophosphamide	Immunosuppression, myeloproliferative disorders, malignancy, hemorrhagic cystitis, infertility
Rituximab	Immunosuppression

What is the time to onset of effectiveness for:

Intramuscular gold?	4 to 5 months
Methotrexate (MTX)?	1 to 2 months
Sulfasalazine (SSZ)?	Weeks to months
Hydroxychloroquine (Plaquenil)?	3 to 4 months
Cyclophosphamide (Cytoxan, CTX)?	Weeks

Azathioprine (Imuran, AZA)?	Weeks to months
Etanercept?	Weeks
Infliximab?	Weeks
Anakinra?	Weeks
Adalimumab?	Weeks
Rituximab?	Weeks
Abatacept?	Weeks

AVASCULAR NECROSIS

How does AVN present?	With pain
How is AVN diagnosed?	Radiographs (late) MRI (early) (classical surreptitious pattern)
What is the treatment of AVN?	Analgesics and orthopedic surgery consultation

BACK PAIN

What are physical examination features for disk disease at the following levels?	
L4–5	Decreased ability to walk on toes
L5–S1	Decreased ability to walk on heels
What are the major treatment options for back pain?	Education, physical therapy, optimizing weight, analgesics, pain clinic referral, orthopedic or neurosurgical consultation

OSTEOARTHRITIS

What is the incidence of OA?	OA occurs in 30% of adults and is the most common form of arthritis.

What is found on examination in OA?	Crepitus, bony enlargement, decreased ROM, pain with ROM, and mild inflammation. Distribution is bilateral and often asymmetrical, involving hands, feet, knees, and hips and usually sparing shoulders and elbows.

RHEUMATOID ARTHRITIS

What is the incidence of RA?	RA occurs in 1% to 2% of all adults. It is the most common autoimmune disease.
What risk factors are associated with RA?	Female gender and family history. Several genetic susceptibility markers have been identified, and some of these markers are associated with more aggressive disease (heterozygote for DRB1 0401 and DRB1 0404).
What does examination of the rheumatoid hand find early in the illness?	Synovitis (inflammation of the synovium) localized to the MCPs and PIPs (DIPs spared)
What does examination of the rheumatoid hand find late in the illness?	Ulnar drift caused by tendon laxity; subluxation of proximal phalanges under MCP heads; and nodules on bony prominences and extensor surfaces
What are some extra-articular manifestations of RA?	Interstitial fibrosis; pleural, pericardial and cardiac involvement; episcleritis/scleritis; Felty's syndrome (splenomegaly and leukopenia)
What are the laboratory test findings in RA?	RF is present in 80% of cases. Anti-CCP antibody is found in 60% of RA patients.
What other conditions are associated with RF?	Subacute bacterial endocarditis, viral and other infections (e.g., infectious mononucleosis, hepatitis C, tuberculosis, Lyme disease), increasing age, SLE, SjS, and sarcoidosis
What is anti-CCP?	An antibody directed against cyclic citrullinated peptide, more specific than RF for the diagnosis of RA

How is the diagnosis of RA made?	Documentation of inflammatory synovitis by the following: 1. Synovial fluid WBC count >2000/mm^3 2. Chronic synovitis on histologic study 3. Radiologic evidence of erosions 4. Symptoms present for longer than 6 weeks 5. Symmetric joint involvement
When are DMARDs started?	DMARD therapy should be initiated as soon as a definitive diagnosis is established. The goal is a clinical and laboratory remission.
In addition to DMARDs, what other therapies should be considered in RA?	The overall treatment plan should also include physical and occupational therapy, joint injections with steroids, and surgery for joint stabilization. For progressive disease, consider synovectomy (unresponsive to medical treatment) or joint replacement (advanced disease).
When are oral steroids used?	Oral steroids should be used for "bridge" treatment (i.e., while waiting for DMARDs to be effective).
When is treatment of RA urgent?	In cases of severe flares, vasculitis, relative steroid insufficiency, or joint or systemic infections
When is treatment of RA emergent?	When there is severe adrenal insufficiency (addisonian crisis) or atlantoaxial (C1-C2) instability

CONNECTIVE TISSUE DISEASE

SYSTEMIC LUPUS ERYTHEMATOSUS

What tests should be ordered for suspected SLE?	CBC, ESR, C-reactive protein, UA, electrolytes, BUN, creatinine, ANA (high sensitivity), anti-dsDNA (high specificity), anti-Smith, anti-RNP, anticardiolipin antibodies, CH50, and possibly C3 and C4

Once the diagnosis of SLE is established, what tests are used to follow up disease activity?

CBC, anti-dsDNA, CH50, UA, BUN, and creatinine. It is noteworthy that the usefulness of anti-dsDNA and CH50 as indicators of disease activity is limited.

What are urgent indications for treatment in SLE?

Increase in constitutional symptoms and other symptoms indicative of a flare

Infection

New signs of renal involvement—decreasing renal function, increasing BUN and creatinine from baseline, increasing proteinuria, and increasing urine RBCs, WBCs, and casts

Other laboratory evidence of a flare such as the development of hemolytic anemia or thrombocytopenia

What should also be considered in the following SLE emergencies?

Mental status change and/or headache?

CNS infection and vasculitis

Acute shortness of breath and/or chest pain?

Pericardial effusion, tamponade, or pulmonary embolus

Leg pain, shortness of breath, pulmonary embolus, and/or CNS changes?

Hypercoagulable state

Ischemic digits?

Raynaud's phenomenon, APS, vasculitis, and necrosis

Pregnant patient with flare?

Patients with preeclampsia also have proteinuria, CNS disease, and HTN, making it difficult to differentiate toxemia from an SLE flare; however, SLE has low complement levels, while the complement levels are usually normal in toxemia. Also, serum uric acid levels are usually elevated in preeclampsia and normal in an SLE flare.

LUPUS DISEASE SUBCATEGORIES

What is APS?	Antiphospholipid antibody syndrome. This is a hypercoagulable state that occurs in association with SLE, certain cancers, and infections, or it can occur as a primary disorder in itself.
What is required for the diagnosis of APS?	The diagnosis requires a history of a thrombotic event and a positive lab test (lupus anticoagulant, anticardiolipin, or B2-glycoprotein I antibody).
What is the treatment for APS?	Long-term anticoagulation with warfarin
What laboratory tests are ordered in the workup of APS?	Tests include anticardiolipin antibodies, prothrombin time, partial thromboplastin time, Venereal Disease Research Laboratory tests, and modified Russell's viper venom time, anti–beta-2 glycoprotein-I, or local test for "lupus anticoagulant."
What agents have been implicated in DIL?	Chlorpromazine, methyldopa, hydralazine, TNF-α inhibitors, procainamide, isoniazid, and interferon

SYSTEMIC SCLEROSIS

What is SSc?	A disorder of connective tissue characterized by overproduction of collagen (types I and III) and matrix proteins
What is the treatment for Raynaud's syndrome?	Calcium channel blockers, losartan, and sildenafil
What is the treatment for renal crisis?	Angiotensin-converting enzyme inhibitors, hydralazine
GERD?	H_2 blockers, omeprazole
Lung disease?	Cyclophosphamide
Pulmonary hypertension?	Sildenafil, bosentan, and/or epoprostenol

SJÖGREN'S SYNDROME

What are the laboratory findings in SjS?	ANA, anti–SS-A (anti-Ro), anti–SS-B (anti-La), RF, cryoglobulins, anemia, leukopenia, thrombocytopenia, increased ESR. SjS is known for high levels of multiple antibodies in nonspecific patterns.

VASCULITIS

POLYARTERITIS NODOSA

What are the laboratory findings in PAN?	Hepatitis B surface antigen or antibody is found in 15% of cases, urine RBCs, RBC casts, and proteinuria

WEGENER'S GRANULOMATOSIS

What are the laboratory findings in Wegener's granulomatosis?	UA—microhematuria, RBC casts, proteinuria, and increased BUN and creatinine c-ANCA—present in 80% of cases CXR—bilateral, nodular fixed infiltrates that usually cavitate

CHURG–STRAUSS SYNDROME

What are the three phases of Churg-Strauss disease?	1. Prodrome that can last for many years. Allergic manifestations include rhinitis, polyposis, and asthma. 2. Peripheral blood and tissue eosinophilia with infiltration of organs like the lungs and the GI tract 3. Systemic vasculitis (heralded by fever and weight loss) chest radiograph abnormalities, skin lesions, mononeuritis multiplex, congestive heart failure, abdominal symptoms, and renal disease
What are the laboratory findings in Churg-Strauss syndrome?	Peripheral blood eosinophilia in more than 10% of cases. Biopsy of lung or skin shows eosinophilic necrotizing granulomas and necrotizing small vessel disease.

OTHER VASCULITIDES

Name three to four distinctive features of each of the following vasculitides:

Giant cell arteritis

1. Headache, scalp tenderness, jaw claudication, constitutional symptoms, PMR, depression, dry cough, and ischemic optic neuritis
2. Occurrence in persons approximately 50 years of age and more commonly in women than in men
3. High ESR (>50)

Behçet's syndrome

1. Recurrent painful aphthous oral and genital ulcers
2. Uveitis and retinal vasculitis
3. Erythema nodosum and papulopustular skin lesions
4. Possible CNS involvement

Cryoglobulinemia

1. Immunoglobulins that precipitate at cold temperatures, and are usually RF.
2. Raynaud's phenomenon, purpura, and ischemic ulcers, which are a result of hyperviscosity and plugging of small vessels. Vasculitis is uncommon.
3. Mixed cryoglobulins are associated with CTDs, hepatitis A/B/C, parasites, many infections, and lymphoproliferative diseases.

Takayasu's arteritis

1. Chronic vasculitis of the aorta and its branches
2. Occurrence in young women and in persons of Asian descent
3. Asymmetrically decreased peripheral pulses

Henoch-Schönlein purpura

1. Occurrence usually in 5- to 15-year-old children with history of upper respiratory infection
2. Palpable purpura on buttocks and legs (IgA found on biopsy of the skin lesions)
3. Crampy umbilical pain and nephritis

Primary angitis of the CNS	1. Small and medium vessel vasculitis in the CNS 2. Laboratory workup usually negative 3. Diagnosis based on MRI, angiogram, and/or biopsy
Cholesterol emboli	1. Fever, livedo, digital ischemia, gangrene 2. Mononeuritis multiplex 3. Renal insufficiency

SERONEGATIVE SPONDYLOARTHROPATHIES

Name the five seronegative spondyloarthropathies.	1. Ankylosing spondylitis 2. Reactive arthritis 3. Reiter's syndrome 4. Psoriatic arthritis 5. Enteropathic arthritis

ANKYLOSING SPONDYLITIS

What are the imaging findings in ankylosing spondylitis?	The earliest changes may be erosions involving the sacroiliac joints and squaring of the vertebral bodies, especially at the thoracic-lumbar junction. Radiographs show symmetric ankylosis of sacroiliac joints and spine, absence of subluxation and cysts, and generalized osteopenia after ankylosis.
How is the diagnosis of ankylosing spondylitis made?	Clinical presentation and radiographic findings. In early cases, radiographs may be normal; MRI may be useful in establishing the diagnosis.
What are the medications used for ankylosing spondylitis?	Include NSAIDs (e.g., indomethacin), sulfasalazine (may be effective as a DMARD), and anti–TNF-α therapy
What are emergent considerations in ankylosing spondylitis?	The ankylosed spine is susceptible to fracture, usually transverse, at C5–C6 or C6–C7, with risk of spinal cord injury.

REACTIVE ARTHRITIS

What microbes are associated with reactive arthritis?	*Yersinia, Salmonella, Shigella,* and *Campylobacter* in the gastrointestinal tract; *Chlamydia* in the genitourinary tract
What are the laboratory findings in reactive arthritis?	There are no diagnostic tests, but the clinician should try to isolate pathogens and rule out septic arthritis and GC arthritis.

REITER'S SYNDROME

What is the classic triad of Reiter's syndrome?	Arthritis, urethritis (nongonococcal), and conjunctivitis

PSORIATIC ARTHRITIS

What are some of the clinical distinguishing features of PsA?	Involvement of the DIP, inflammation involving a ray distribution (DIP, PIP, MCP, of the same digit). Usually skin involvement precedes arthritis; however, approximately 15% of patients present first with joint inflammation.
What are the five disease patterns of PsA?	1. Oligoarticular (asymmetric), 50% 2. Spondyloarthropathy, 20% 3. Polyarticular (RA-like), 20% 4. DIP disease ("classic"), 8% 5. Mutilans (deforming), 2%
What is a distinguishing feature of radiographic findings?	Proliferative bone changes adjacent to the erosions

ENTEROPATHIC ARTHRITIS

How frequently does arthritis occur in Crohn's disease?	In 20% of cases
What is the distribution of the arthritis?	Distribution is pauciarticular, asymmetric, transient, and migratory.
Which joints are affected?	Affects large and small joints of lower extremities
What are the classic hand and foot changes?	"Sausage digits" (dactylitis) and heel enthesopathies

How does the arthritis correspond with the activity of the bowel disease?	They do not strictly coincide.
How frequently does arthritis occur in ulcerative colitis?	In <20% of cases
How do the arthritic features compare to those of Crohn's disease?	They are the same.
How does the timing of the bowel activity and the arthritis compare to that of Crohn's disease?	Has a more distinct temporal relationship between flares of arthritis and colitis

GOUT AND PSEUDOGOUT

GOUT

What are the four stages of gout?	1. Asymptomatic hyperuricemia 2. Acute gouty arthritis 3. Intercritical gout 4. Chronic tophaceous gout

ACUTE GOUTY ARTHRITIS

What are attack triggers for acute gouty arthritis?	Alcohol, surgical stress, trauma, acute medical illness, and drugs (diuretics, allopurinol, or probenecid without colchicine)
What is intercritical treatment of chronic gout?	Avoidance of alcohol, weight loss, and colchicine; probenecid (uricosuric); and allopurinol (xanthine oxidase inhibitor)

CHRONIC TOPHACEOUS GOUT

What are complications of chronic tophaceous gout?	Renal stones, proteinuria, HTN, and chronic renal insufficiency
What are some of the contraindications for uricosuric treatment?	Kidney stones Renal insufficiency Tophaceous gout

PSEUDOGOUT

What is the incidence of pseudogout?	Approximately half as common as gout
What are risk factors for pseudogout?	Aging, OA, amyloid, hypothyroidism, hyperparathyroidism, and hemochromatosis
What are the laboratory findings in pseudogout?	In synovial fluid, CPP crystals are short, cuboidal, and blue when parallel to axis.
What is the therapy for acute pseudogout?	NSAIDs, colchicines, or steroids

INFECTIOUS ARTHRITIS

List the infectious arthritis syndromes.	GC, nongonococcal, Lyme, and viral
What pathogens are associated with infectious arthritis?	*Neisseria gonorrhoeae* is most common in sexually active adults. *Staphylococcus aureus* is most common otherwise.
What are the microbiologic findings in nongonococcal bacterial arthritis?	*S. aureus* (60%), streptococci (15%), gram-negative rods (15%), *Pneumococcus* (5%), and polymicrobial (5%)
What is the differential diagnosis of increased WBCs and PMNs in synovial fluid?	RA and crystalline joint disease

GONOCOCCAL ARTHRITIS

What is the incidence of GC arthritis?	Of the 1 million cases of gonorrhea in the United States per year, 1% have bacteremia and arthritis.
What is the clue to the diagnosis of DGI?	Tenosynovitis and dermatitis are rare in nonneisserial bacterial arthritis.

NONGONOCOCCAL BACTERIAL ARTHRITIS

What are risk factors for nongonococcal bacterial arthritis?	Trauma, surgery, and arthrocentesis Chronic medical illness (e.g., RA, diabetes mellitus, SLE, and chronic liver disease)

Age extremes

Immunosuppression

Prosthetic joints

How often is the knee affected?
Distribution of 50% in knee

How often is it monoarticular?
80% monoarticular (polyarticular cases are usually associated with a risk factor)

Which microbes are usually associated with nongonococcal arthritis?
S. aureus, 60%; beta-hemolytic streptococci, 15%; gram-negative rods, 15%; *Pneumococcus,* 15%; and polymicrobial, 5%

LYME ARTHRITIS

What are the three stages of Lyme arthritis, and how are they characterized?

1. Early, localized—erythema migrans
2. Early, disseminated—migratory musculoskeletal pain, in joints, bursae, tendons, muscle and bone
3. Late—in 6 months, onset of brief attacks of oligoarthritis, usually involving large joints (knee). Episodes become longer, with erosion of cartilage and bone.

What laboratory tests are ordered for Lyme arthritis?
Enzyme-linked immunosorbent assay with Western blot to confirm. Both acute and convalescent titers should be evaluated.

VIRAL ARTHRITIS

Parvovirus B19

What are features of parvovirus B19 illness in adults?
Severe, self-limited flu-like illness with arthralgias and arthritis and a rheumatoid-like distribution

Hepatitis C Virus

List four rheumatic manifestations of hepatitis C.

1. Arthralgias
2. Arthritis, palpable purpura, and cryoglobulinemia
3. Fibromyalgia
4. Membranoproliferative glomerulonephritis

Hepatitis B Virus

List five arthritis features of hepatitis infection.

1. Clinical presentation is immune complex–mediated, occurring early in course.
2. Onset of arthritis is sudden and severe.
3. Distribution is symmetric, migratory, and additive.
4. Joints involved are hands and knees.
5. Urticaria is a feature.

Human Immunodeficiency Virus

List six rheumatic syndromes seen in HIV.

1. Sjögren-like syndrome
2. Lupus-like syndrome
3. Vasculitis
4. Fibromyalgia
5. Hypertrophic osteoarthropathy
6. AVN

ARTHRITIS SECONDARY TO SYSTEMIC DISEASES

DIABETES MELLITUS

What is the differential diagnosis of pain and weakness in the proximal thigh of a diabetic?

Acute mononeuritis (femoral nerve)

Meralgia paresthetica (lateral cutaneous nerve)

Diabetic amyotrophy (polyneuropathy)

Lumbar plexopathy

Herniated disk

Herpes zoster (before eruption)

OA in hip joint

AVN of femoral head

Trochanteric bursitis

THYROID DISEASE

Name five rheumatologic features of hyperthyroidism.

1. Osteoporosis
2. Onycholysis (separation of nail from bed)—differential diagnosis: Reiter's syndrome, psoriasis, PsA
3. Painless proximal muscle weakness with normal creatine phosphokinase— differential diagnosis: PM

4. Frozen shoulder
5. Thyroid acropachy (distal soft tissue swelling, clubbing, and periostitis of MCP joints)

Name four rheumatologic features of hypothyroidism.

1. Carpal tunnel syndrome
2. Polyarthritis
3. AVN of hip
4. Myalgias (may have elevated CK)

SARCOIDOSIS

What is the incidence of arthritis in sarcoidosis?

10%

AMYLOIDOSIS

How are types of amyloidosis classified?

By type of amyloid protein deposited (e.g., AA, AL, Ab2M, and Ab)

What is the mean age of onset of idiopathic and myeloma-associated (AL) amyloidosis?

Mean age at diagnosis, 60 years

What organs are commonly affected?

Heart and kidney

How common is arthropathy?

<5%

What is the shoulder-pad sign?

Amyloid infiltration of the shoulder, a nearly pathognomonic sign

What illnesses is reactive amyloid (AA) seen with?

Seen with RA, JRA, and ankylosing spondylitis

What rheumatologic illnesses is AA rarely seen with?

Extremely rare in SLE and PM

What inflammatory bowel disease is AA seen with?

Seen in Crohn's disease; rare in ulcerative colitis

What general category of patients develop beta$_2$-microglobulin amyloid?

Seen in long-term dialysis patients

What peripheral neuropathy is seen?	Carpal tunnel syndrome
What bony manifestations are seen?	Arthropathy, cystic bone lesions, and pathologic fractures
Where are the amyloid deposits of aging-associated amyloid seen?	Localized microdeposits in joints
What other arthritis syndromes may occur with aging associated amyloid?	OA and CPPD

ARTHRITIS ASSOCIATED WITH MALIGNANCIES

Name five ways in which musculoskeletal syndromes may be related to malignancies.	1. Metastatic disease to bone 2. Primary malignant disease (rare) 3. Paraneoplastic syndromes [e.g., PM, scleroderma, lupus-like syndrome, and Sweet's syndrome (fever; abrupt onset of painful plaques on arms, neck and head; and neutrophilia)] 4. Increased incidence of malignancy in preexisting CTDs (e.g., SjS) 5. Malignancy as a complication of treatment (e.g., with cyclophosphamide, methotrexate, biologics or radiotherapy) or rheumatic disease

ARTHRITIS SECONDARY TO SICKLE CELL DISEASE

What are the most common sites of arthritis in sickle cell disease?	Knees and ankles
What are the most serious complications of arthritis in sickle cell disease?	AVN (hip, 10%); osteomyelitis (*Salmonella*)

ARTHRITIS SECONDARY TO HEMOPHILIA

What is the incidence of hemarthrosis (bleeding into a joint) in hemophilia?	85%. It is the most common major hemorrhagic event in the disease.

What are features of an acute hemarthrosis?

Swollen, warm, exquisitely painful

Held in flexion from muscle spasm

Progressive loss of form and function

What are features of a chronic hemarthrosis?

Bony enlargement with atrophic muscle affecting knees, then elbows, ankles, and shoulders

Flexion contracture

Asymmetric, sporadic distribution

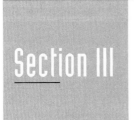

Section III   Related Specialties

Dermatology

ABBREVIATIONS

ANA	Antinuclear antibody
EN	Erythema nodosum
H&P	History and physical examination
HHV	Human herpesvirus
HIV	Human immunodeficiency virus
HPV	Human papillomavirus
HSV	Herpes simplex virus
KOH	Potassium hydroxide
MF	Mycosis fungoides
MM	Multiple myeloma
MMR	Measles, mumps, rubella
NL	Necrobiosis lipoidica
NSAID	Nonsteroidal anti-inflammatory drug
PUVA	Psoralen plus ultraviolet light of A wavelength
RMSF	Rocky Mountain spotted fever
RPR	Rapid plasma reagin
SCC	Squamous cell carcinoma

SLE	Systemic lupus erythematosus
SPF	Sun protection factor
SSSS	Staphylococcal scalded skin syndrome
STD	Sexually transmitted disease
TEN	Toxic epidermal necrolysis
TPN	Total parenteral nutrition
UV	Ultraviolet
VZV	Varicella zoster virus
VZVIg	Varicella zoster immunoglobulin

INTRODUCTION

What are the general rules of dermatology?	If it is wet—dry it. If it's dry—wet it. When in doubt—cut it out. If they are not on steroids—add them.

TOPICAL THERAPY

What is a shake lotion?	A powder in water
What is a shake lotion used for?	To cool and dry the skin (e.g., calamine lotion)
What is a milky lotion?	A liquid mix of oil in water
What is a milky lotion used for?	To cool and dry the skin or lubricate it (more oil or lubrication)
What is a cream?	A mix of oil in water
What is a cream used for?	Acts as an intermediate agent between a lotion and an ointment. The higher the oil content, the more lubricating the cream.
What is an ointment?	A mix of water in oil
What is an ointment used for?	To lubricate and occlude the skin
What is a gel?	Oil in water and alcohol
What is a gel used for?	Often used on hairy areas or when drying is desired (e.g., fungus between toes)

PRIMARY SKIN LESIONS

What is a macule?
A flat, discolored, nonpalpable skin lesion <1 cm in diameter

What is a patch?
A flat, discolored, nonpalpable skin lesion >1 cm in diameter

What is a papule?
An elevated, circumscribed, palpable lesion <0.5 cm in diameter

What is a nodule?
An elevated, circumscribed, palpable lesion >0.5 cm in diameter

What is a plaque?
A flat-topped elevated lesion >0.5 cm in diameter with elevation

What is a pustule?
A circumscribed elevated lesion or papule containing pus

What is a vesicle?
A small blister <0.5 cm in diameter

What is a bulla?
A large blister >0.5 cm in diameter

What is a wheal (hive)?
An edematous elevated skin lesion, usually migratory, lasting 24 to 48 hours

What is a cyst?
A cavity with an epidermal lining containing fluid or cheesy material

What is a telangiectasia?
A dilated superficial blood vessel, usually blanchable

SECONDARY SKIN LESIONS

What is a crust?
A dried skin exudate

What is a scale?
A superficial group of dead epidermal cells

What is an erosion?
The focal loss of superficial epidermis

What is an ulceration?
Loss of epidermis and some dermis

What is a fissure?
A deep split through the epidermis into the dermis

What is atrophy?	Skin thinning
What is a scar?	Fibrous tissue laid down in response to skin injury
What is an excoriation?	A skin abrasion caused by scratching
What is lichenification?	Thickening of the skin in response to rubbing, with increased skin markings
What are petechiae?	Small, nonblanchable lesions caused by extravasated blood
What is purpura?	Larger areas of extravasated blood

CONFIGURATION AND MORPHOLOGIC TERMS

How are the following lesions shaped?	
Nummular	Coin-shaped
Serpiginous	Snake-like
Herpetiform	Grouped vesicles resembling HSV (but may also result from noninfectious etiology)
Annular	Ring-shaped
Targetoid	Concentric rings
Dermatomal	Follows the distribution of a cutaneous sensory nerve
Verrucous	Warty
Discoid	Oval or round
Morbilliform	Maculopapular, resembling the exanthem of measles

HISTORY AND PHYSICAL EXAMINATION

What 15 key questions should be asked in a dermatologic history?	What are the age and gender of the patient? When did the problem start?

Where on the body did the lesion start, and where is it now?

How did the condition appear at first, and how has it changed?

What are the symptoms?

Is anyone else at home affected?

Have there been any occupational or hobby exposures?

Has this or something like it happened before?

Does the patient have any chronic medical problems?

Has the patient had any particular life stresses?

What medication is the patient taking?

Does the patient have allergies?

Are there any diseases that run in the family?

What treatments have been tried?

Did any treatment help?

What six rashes should be considered when the rash involves the palms and soles?
RMSF, secondary syphilis, Stevens-Johnson syndrome, erythema multiforme, toxic shock syndrome, and SSSS

COMMON DERMATOLOGIC DIAGNOSTIC TOOLS

What does a Tzanck prep help diagnose?
Usually HSV and VZV infection

How is a Tzanck test done?
The base of an intact vesicle is scraped with a scalpel blade onto a slide. It is air-dried, fixed in methanol, stained with Giemsa or Wright's stain, and then examined under a microscope.

When are results of a Tzanck test positive?
When multinucleated giant cells are seen

What does a KOH prep help diagnose?
Dermatophyte and yeast infections

When should a KOH test be done?	When a lesion has pustules, vesicles, or scales (if it scales, scrape it)
How is a KOH test done?	Skin scales on the edge of a lesion or on the roof of a vesicle or pustule are scraped onto a slide with a no. 15 scalpel blade or another slide, 1 to 2 drops of KOH are applied, the sample is covered with a coverslip and gently heated over an alcohol lamp. The sample is allowed to sit for a few minutes and is then examined under a microscope.
When are the results of a KOH test positive?	When hyphae, pseudohyphae, or yeasts are seen
How is a scabies scraping done?	A papule or burrow is scraped with a no. 15 blade moistened with a drop of oil. The scrapings are transferred to a slide, covered, and examined. A positive result shows mites, eggs, or feces.
How is a Wood's lamp used?	As the lamp is held over a skin lesion, typical colors are seen. Certain infections fluoresce, and hypopigmented lesions are accentuated.

TOPICAL CORTICOSTEROIDS

How are topical steroids rated?	From class VII (weakest) to class I (strongest)
What determines the strength of a topical corticosteroid?	Chemical structure, vehicle, and concentration
What are some commonly used weak, medium, potent, and superpotent topical steroids?	
Weak	Hydrocortisone
Medium	Triamcinolone acetonide

Potent	Fluocinonide
Superpotent	Clobetasol propionate
How strong a steroid can be used on the face?	Typically, weak steroids in class VII; sometimes, medium- or high-potency steroids for 2 weeks or less
What are the side effects of topical steroids?	Striae, atrophy, acne, rosacea, perioral dermatitis, pigmentation abnormalities, glaucoma, and systemic absorption
What factors may promote systemic absorption of topical steroids?	Prolonged treatment, use of potent topical steroids, large treated areas, and inflamed skin (disrupts barrier function)

INFECTIOUS DISEASES

VIRAL INFECTION

What is an exanthem?	Acute generalized cutaneous eruption, often symmetric, associated most commonly with viral infection or drug reaction, occasionally with bacterial infection
What are some common exanthems?	Rubella, roseola infantum, adenovirus, echovirus, measles, scarlet fever, coxsackievirus A and B, and mononucleosis
What is an enanthem?	Lesions on the oral mucosa (e.g., Koplik's spots in patients with measles)

Chickenpox and Herpes Zoster

What is chickenpox?	Highly contagious, primary infection of VZV (herpes family)
What is the route of transmission for chickenpox?	Respiratory route
What is the incubation period?	10 to 21 days

What are the symptoms of chickenpox?

Fever, malaise, and pruritic vesicular rash. The rate of morbidity increases in adults and immunocompromised patients.

What is the appearance of chickenpox?

"Dewdrop on a rose petal." Crops of vesicles with surrounding erythema that are often excoriated and crusted. An important feature is presence of lesions in all stages of evolution.

What is the distribution of chickenpox?

Starts on the head, then "rains down" the body

How is the diagnosis of chickenpox made?

Usually clinically. Tzanck smear or culture can verify the diagnosis.

What is the duration of chickenpox?

New lesions erupt for approximately 5 days, and then crusting begins.

What is Reye's syndrome?

A sometimes fatal combination of encephalopathy and hepatitis, most often in children with VZV who have received aspirin

How is chickenpox prevented?

A live attenuated varicella vaccine is available in the United States. Vaccination is recommended for children aged 12 to 18 months and anyone over 13 years old with a VZV-negative titer.

What is herpes zoster (shingles)?

Acute, usually painful reactivation of the VZV from a dorsal root ganglion in a unilateral dermatomal pattern

Where is the source for herpes zoster (shingles)?

Sensory nerve ganglia harbor latent infection.

What is the appearance of herpes zoster?

Grouped vesicles along a dermatome progressing to crusted papules

What are the most common locations for herpes zoster on the body and on the face?

Thoracic dermatomes and the ophthalmic branch of the fifth cranial nerve (V1)

What is Hutchinson's sign and why is it of concern?

Vesicles on the nasal tip indicate involvement of the nasociliary nerve and can herald eye involvement.

What is the most common complication of herpes zoster?

Postherpetic neuralgia, in which pain may last for weeks, months, or years after resolution of the rash

What demographic group is most affected by postherpetic neuralgia?

The incidence of postherpetic neuralgia increases with advancing age.

What is the treatment for herpes zoster?

Oral acyclovir, famciclovir, or valacyclovir or intravenous acyclovir for severe cases. Sometimes steroids may be used to decrease inflammation.

Is there a preventive therapy?

A vaccine for shingles is available for patients aged 60 and over.

Warts

What are warts?

Also known as verrucae vulgaris, warts are caused by infection of the epithelium by HPV, which causes epithelial hyperplasia. Warts are common in children and immunosuppressed persons.

What is the appearance of warts?

Appearance varies with location. Often, warts appear as firm keratotic papules with typical black dots (thrombosed capillaries) and an irregular surface.

What are complications of warts?

Some types of HPV (e.g., 6, 11, 16, 18, 31, 33), especially genital, predispose the patient to malignancy. If warts are perianal, vulvar, or perimeatal, an internal examination is necessary because there may be mucosal involvement.

What are the treatment options for warts?

Treatments include cryotherapy, topical acids, imiquimod, podophyllin, cantharidin, and laser.

Molluscum Contagiosum

What is molluscum contagiosum?

Small papules usually with central umbilication caused by a poxvirus infection. These are very common.

What are the risk factors for molluscum contagiosum?

Attendance at day-care centers, sexual activity, and HIV infection

What are the symptoms of molluscum contagiosum?

Usually none, but the lesions may itch and become eczematized.

What is the distribution of molluscum contagiosum?

Anywhere on the body, but the genital area raises suspicion of sexual transmission.

What is the duration of molluscum contagiosum?

Months to years. They usually regress spontaneously.

How is the diagnosis of molluscum contagiosum made?

Usually clinically. Lesions may also be curetted and placed on a slide for identification of "molluscum bodies."

What is the treatment for molluscum contagiosum?

Curettage and freezing with liquid nitrogen are the most common treatments. Imiquimod and cantharidin may be used in children (less painful).

What diagnosis should be considered in a patient with many mollusca in unusual locations?

HIV infection, especially when lesions are on the face. Many mollusca may also be seen in patients with atopic dermatitis.

Measles (Rubeola)

What is measles?

Paramyxovirus infection that is rarely seen as a result of administration of the MMR vaccine

What is the incubation period for measles?

8 to 13 days

What are the symptoms of measles?

The three C's: cough, coryza, and conjunctivitis, plus high fever and rash

What is the appearance of measles?	Petechiae on the soft palate, then white Koplik's spots on the mucosa adjacent to the second molars, followed 1 to 2 days later by erythematous macules and papules
What is the distribution of measles?	The rash starts postauricularly, then moves down to the trunk as the upper rash fades in 24 to 48 hours.
What is rubella, and how does it differ from rubeola?	Because of the vaccine, German measles (rubella) has become a rare viral infection. It is milder than rubeola but significant because it can cause serious congenital defects if infection occurs during pregnancy.
When should rubella be suspected?	In a patient with an exanthem plus posterior cervical lymphadenopathy

Roseola Infantum

What is roseola infantum?	A common infection in children aged 6 months to 2 years, which is caused by HHV-6 or occasionally HHV-7
What is the rash in roseola called?	Exanthem subitum
How is the diagnosis of roseola made?	Clinical diagnosis is made by "the rash that follows the fever." Fever lasts 3 to 5 days; then, 1 to 2 days after defervescence, an exanthematous rash appears. Infants generally appear well.

Erythema Infectiosum

What is erythema infectiosum?	An exanthem common during the winter in children 5 to 15 years old. It is caused by parvovirus B19 infection and is also called fifth disease.
What are the symptoms of erythema infectiosum?	Children are often asymptomatic but may have fever, sore throat, and malaise, followed 1 to 4 days later by a rash. Adults have more severe constitutional symptoms and transient arthralgias.

What is the appearance of erythema infectiosum?

Diagnosis is made by the classic "slapped cheek" appearance, which evolves into reticulate erythema on the trunk, proximal arms, and legs.

What is the treatment for erythema infectiosum?

None is necessary; however, infected pregnant women need to be followed for the possibility of fetal complications.

BACTERIAL INFECTION

Folliculitis

What infectious agents are associated with folliculitis?

Primarily *Staphylococcus aureus*, also gram-negative organisms and *Pityrosporum*

What are the risk factors for folliculitis?

Shaving, hot-tub use (gram-negative organisms), prior steroid use, and antibiotics (*Pityrosporum*)

What is the appearance of folliculitis?

Pruritic or painful scattered erythematous papules and pustules around hair follicles

What is the distribution of folliculitis?

Any hair-bearing area (e.g., scalp, extremities, beard area)

How is the diagnosis of folliculitis made?

Clinically or by culture

What is the treatment for folliculitis?

S. aureus—antistaphylococcal antibiotics

Gram-negative—usually clears spontaneously with cessation of hot-tub use or correction of the tub pH

Pityrosporum—topical antifungal preparations

Cellulitis

What infectious agents are associated with cellulitis in:
  Patients who are immunocompetent?

Group A beta-hemolytic streptococci, followed by *S. aureus*

  Immunocompromised patients?

Gram-negative rods, including *Pseudomonas*

Periorbital location in children?	*Haemophilus influenzae*
After dog or cat bite?	*Pasteurella multocida*
After saltwater trauma?	*Vibrio vulnificus*
What are the risk factors for cellulitis?	Diabetes mellitus, intravenous drug use, immunocompromised state, trauma, venous stasis, and lymphedema
What are the symptoms of cellulitis?	Fever, chills, mild pain, lymphadenopathy, nausea, vomiting, and confusion, especially in the elderly
What is the appearance of cellulitis?	An erythematous, warm, indurated plaque
What is the distribution of cellulitis?	Extremities are most commonly involved.
What is St. Anthony's fire?	Erysipelas—a rapidly spreading superficial cellulitis most often on the face with well-defined margins
What is the most common cause of St. Anthony's fire?	Group A streptococci
What clues help determine the need for surgical consultation in cases of cellulitis?	Crepitus (a sign of gas from bacterial metabolism), extreme pain, rapid extension, dusky cyanosis, and superficial gangrene may be signs of necrotizing fasciitis.
What is necrotizing fasciitis in the genitalia called?	Fournier's gangrene
What diagnostic tests are ordered for cellulitis?	Blood cultures, Doppler ultrasound if a severe infection or clot is suspected. The yield from aspiration culture of the leading edge is low.
How is the diagnosis of cellulitis made?	Usually clinically

What is the treatment for cellulitis?

In the uncomplicated patient, staphylococcal or streptococcal coverage is needed; broader coverage is needed in patients with medical problems such as diabetes to cover gram-negative rods.

Abscesses

What is the most common bacterial cause of skin abscesses?

Staphylococcus aureus

What type of skin infection is commonly misdiagnosed as a spider bite?

Methicillin-resistant *S. aureus* (MRSA) infection

What is the most common presentation of MRSA infection of the skin?

An abscess or furuncle

What is the treatment for community-acquired MRSA abscess of the skin?

Drainage of the abscess and coverage with either trimethoprim/sulfamethoxazole or minocycline

Erythrasma

What is erythrasma?

A common chronic superficial bacterial infection of the intertriginous areas caused by *Corynebacterium minutissimum*

What is the appearance of erythrasma?

Sharply demarcated pink to brown macules coalesced into confluent patches with a fine scale

How is the diagnosis of erythrasma made?

Wood's lamp shows coral-red fluorescence.

Impetigo

What is impetigo?

A contagious superficial bacterial skin infection common in children in the summer

What infectious agents are associated with impetigo?

Staphylococci, group A beta-hemolytic streptococci

What are the risk factors for impetigo?	Poor hygiene and trauma
What is the appearance of impetigo?	A honey-colored crusting of erosions. The presence of bullae implies infection with *S. aureus.*
What is the distribution of impetigo?	Face is most common but any site is possible.
How is the diagnosis of impetigo made?	Usually clinically. Occasionally cultures are obtained.
What is the treatment for impetigo?	Usually oral antibiotics for coverage of staphylococci and streptococci. Topical mupirocin may be given if the lesions are localized.
What is the duration of impetigo?	Lesions should clear in approximately 1 week with treatment.
What complication can follow impetigo?	Poststreptococcal glomerulonephritis, which is caused by certain strains of *Streptococcus pyogenes*
What is scarlet fever?	Toxin produced by *S. pyogenes,* usually in the setting of streptococcal pharyngitis
What characteristics help in the diagnosis of scarlet fever?	Sandpaper texture of the exanthem, "strawberry tongue," linear petechiae in skinfolds (called Pastia's lines), and desquamation, which usually follows the rash

FUNGAL INFECTION

Candidiasis—Mucocutaneous and Intertriginous

What are the risk factors for candidiasis?	Diabetes, immunosuppression, oral contraceptive use, obesity, pregnancy, and antibiotics
What are the symptoms of candidiasis?	Pruritus and occasionally pain. Or the patient may be asymptomatic.
What is the distribution of candidiasis?	Any mucosal surface and intertriginous skin (e.g., groin and under breasts)

What is the appearance of candidiasis in the:

    Oral cavity?   White patches on mucosal surfaces and tongue that can be scraped off

    Vagina?   White cheesy discharge with vaginal inflammation

    Intertriginous areas?   Erythematous plaques, papules, and pustules; well-demarcated raw surface with satellite lesions

What does involvement of the scrotum imply in cases of superficial fungal infection?   *Candida* affects the scrotum; tinea cruris does not.

How is the diagnosis of candidiasis made?   Clinically, by KOH prep, and sometimes by culture

What is the treatment for candidiasis?   A wide variety of oral and topical antifungal regimens. Griseofulvin is not effective against yeast, and nystatin is not effective against dermatophytes.

Tinea (Dermatophytosis)

What is tinea?   A common superficial fungal infection of keratin-containing skin structures

What three genera of fungi commonly cause tinea?   *Microsporum, Epidermophyton*, and *Trichophyton*

What are the risk factors for tinea?   Diabetes mellitus and immunosuppression

What is the appearance of tinea?   Scaly erythematous plaque with an active border and central clearing

What are the laboratory findings in tinea?   KOH prep of scraping reveals hyphal elements. In resistant or questionable cases, fungus may be cultured. Some types of microsporum fluoresce bright green under a Wood's lamp.

What is the cause of dystrophic nails?

Many are caused by dermatophytes; other causes include inflammatory diseases (e.g., psoriasis) or trauma. Therefore, before initiating systemic treatment for fungus of the nail, positive KOH or culture must be demonstrated.

What is the treatment for tinea?

Topical or oral antifungals, depending on location and severity

What is "two foot, one hand" syndrome?

Common pattern of tinea involvement usually caused by *Trichophyton rubrum*. Both soles and one palm are scaly and erythematous.

What is a kerion?

A boggy, inflamed mass, usually on the scalp, representing an immunologic reaction to tinea infection. Treatment is with oral antifungals and often prednisone.

What is an "id reaction"?

A hypersensitivity reaction to a dermatophyte or cutaneous bacterial infection that is most often manifest as vesicles or pustules on the palms and soles

Tinea Versicolor

What is tinea versicolor?

A common superficial yeast infection caused by *Malassezia furfur*. The rash is asymptomatic or occasionally pruritic with pigment alterations.

What is the appearance of tinea versicolor?

Scattered sharp round–oval macules with a fine scale made more obvious by scraping. On sun-protected skin, lesions are hyperpigmented; on sun-exposed skin, lesions are hypopigmented.

What is the distribution of tinea versicolor?

Usually the upper trunk and back

How is the diagnosis of tinea versicolor made?

KOH scraping demonstrates "spaghetti and meatballs" hyphae.

What is the treatment for tinea versicolor?	A 2.5% selenium sulfide shampoo to the affected area is cost-effective, although most antifungal agents are adequate. Reinfection is common. Normal pigmentation may take months to return.

SEXUALLY TRANSMITTED DISEASES

What is the differential diagnosis of genital ulcers?	Think: "Always Show Caution Getting Lunch From The Hospital":
	Aphthous ulcers
	Syphilis
	Chancroid
	Granuloma inguinale
	Lymphogranuloma venereum
	Fixed drug eruption
	Trauma (zipper or factitial)
	Herpes

Syphilis

What are the classic skin signs of primary syphilis?	Painless chancre—ulcer with an indurated border
What are the classic skin signs of secondary syphilis?	Condylomata lata—soft, fleshy papules in the genital region
	"Moth-eaten" alopecia
	Copper penny macules or papules with erythema on the palms, soles, and trunk
What are the classic skin signs of tertiary syphilis?	Noduloulcerative syphilides—plaques and nodules with scalloped edges, with or without ulcers and scale
	Gummatous syphilis—punched-out ulcers on an erythematous base on the scalp, face, and lower extremities
	Both skin findings are extremely rare
What is the treatment for syphilis?	Intramuscular penicillin G for primary syphilis. RPR tests should be repeated periodically to confirm a decreasing titer, which indicates successful treatment.

Gonorrhea

What are the symptoms of gonorrhea?

In men, urethral discharge; in women, discharge, pain, fever, or no symptoms

What is the appearance of gonorrhea?

In men, periurethral edema and discharge; in women, vaginal discharge, endometritis, and salpingitis

How is the diagnosis of gonorrhea made?

On clinical grounds plus demonstration of gram-negative intracellular diplococci on Gram's stain

Herpes Simplex

What are the risk factors for herpes simplex?

Fever blisters are likely acquired in childhood from relatives. Genital infection is transmitted sexually.

What are the symptoms of herpes simplex?

Initial symptoms include fever, malaise, pain, or no symptoms. In recurrent cases, symptoms include pruritic or painful vesicular lesions (systemic symptoms are uncommon in recurrent cases).

What is the appearance of herpes simplex?

Clusters of vesicles or erosions on an erythematous base. In immunocompromised patients, atypical presentation and location may occur.

What is the distribution of herpes simplex?

Mucous membranes, lips, and nose, but any location is possible

How is the diagnosis of herpes simplex made?

Clinically or by Tzanck smear or culture

What is the treatment for herpes simplex?

Acyclovir, valacyclovir, and famciclovir may shorten the duration, but they may be ineffective if not started in the first 24 hours. Generalized infection or infection in an immunocompromised host may require higher dosing or intravenous therapy.

What is the most common cause of recurring erythema multiforme?

A hypersensitivity reaction after herpes infection

What is herpetic infection of the finger called?

Herpetic whitlow, classically seen in dental hygienists who do not wear protective gloves

What is eczema herpeticum?

Widespread florid herpes infection, usually in patients with eczema (atopic dermatitis)

What is the significance of viral shedding?

Herpes can be detected in (and probably transmitted by) infected individuals even when they are asymptomatic.

Condylomata Acuminata

What is condylomata acuminata?

HPV infection of the genital epithelium

What is the incidence of condylomata acuminata?

It is the most common sexually transmitted disease.

What is the appearance of condylomata acuminata?

Soft, flesh-colored, verrucous papule or plaque that may be pedunculated or cauliflower-shaped

How is the diagnosis of condylomata acuminata made?

Clinically, by application of acetic acid on suspicious lesions or by biopsy

What is the treatment for condylomata acuminata?

Freezing with liquid nitrogen or application of topical podofilox, imiquimod, or podophyllin. Large lesions may require surgical or laser removal. They often recur because the wart virus is in surrounding normal skin.

What else is essential after making the diagnosis of condyloma acuminata?

Sexual partners require examination; many do not realize that they are infected. Women require gynecologic examination, and perirectal involvement requires rectal examination. Association with cancer risk should be discussed with the patient.

What types of HPV does the papillomavirus vaccine target?

6, 11, 16, and 18

Human Immunodeficiency Virus

What are some skin conditions associated with HIV infection?	Condylomata acuminata, seborrheic dermatitis, psoriasis, pruritus, molluscum contagiosum, verrucae, cryptococcosis (mimicking molluscum), and Kaposi's sarcoma
Is there a rash associated with primary HIV infection?	Yes, a morbilliform exanthem in one third of patients
What is Kaposi's sarcoma?	A tumor derived from proliferative endothelial cells. Recent polymerase chain reaction studies have found HHV-8 particles in all types of Kaposi's sarcoma.
What are the three subvariants of Kaposi's sarcoma seen in patients who are HIV-negative?	1. Classic—occurs in elderly Mediterranean men 2. Immunosuppressed—especially occurs with cyclosporine use 3. African
What is the appearance of Kaposi's sarcoma?	Vascular-appearing macules or nodules that may require biopsy for confirmation
What is the distribution of Kaposi's sarcoma?	Any location, especially the face in HIV-positive patients and lower extremity in classic variants
What is the treatment for Kaposi's sarcoma?	Because all the treatments have side effects and do not provide a cure, treatment varies per patient. Treatments range from observation (if disease is localized) and antiretroviral therapy to radiation, surgical excision, laser, bexarotene, cryotherapy, intralesional or systemic vincristine, paclitaxel or docetaxel (if disease is extensive or debilitating).
What skin lesions may be confused with Kaposi's sarcoma in AIDS patients?	Skin lesions of bacillary angiomatosis
What is bacillary angiomatosis?	Skin lesions resulting from the proliferation of small blood vessels

What are the two most common causes of bacillary angiomatosis?	*Bartonella henselae* and *Bartonella quintana*
What is the treatment for bacillary angiomatosis?	Doxycycline
What is oral hairy leukoplakia?	White, asymptomatic, verrucous thickening of the inferolateral surface of the tongue caused by Epstein-Barr virus. It is virtually pathognomonic for HIV infection.
How can oral hairy leukoplakia be differentiated from thrush?	Thrush can be scraped off; hairy leukoplakia cannot.

INFESTATIONS

Scabies

What is scabies?	Common infestation of the skin with a burrowing mite, *Sarcoptes scabiei*, transmitted by skin contact
What is seen on physical examination in scabies?	Linear burrows, papules, and excoriations
What are the symptoms of scabies?	Extreme pruritus, especially at night
What is the distribution of scabies?	The wrists and ankles and the webs of fingers and toes are the most classic locations, but scabies also occurs in the pubic area (scrotum in men), lower abdomen, trunk, and legs.
What diagnostic tests are performed for scabies?	Scabies scraping
What is the treatment of scabies?	A variety of scabicides are available. Permethrin is first-line, lindane and crotamiton are less used due to concerns about toxicity. A single dose of oral ivermectin also appears to be effective.

What is Norwegian scabies?

Whereas typical infestation involves approximately 20 mites, in Norwegian scabies, thousands of mites infest the patient. It is seen in mentally impaired persons, immunosuppressed patients, and patients with decreased sensation.

Pediculosis (Lice)

What is pediculosis?

Lice infestations of the scalp, body, or pubic area

How are lice transmitted?

Scalp lice can be epidemic in school children, or they may occur in adults after close contact. Body lice are usually seen in patients with poor hygiene and reside in clothing seams or sheets. Pubic lice are typically sexually transmitted.

What are symptoms of pediculosis?

Pruritus

What is the appearance of pediculosis on the:
    Scalp?

A few lice and many nits are seen firmly attached to hairs. Nits are glued to hair shafts close to the scalp. If they appear more than 1 cm from the scalp, they are probably hatched eggs.

    Body?

Itchy papules may be seen anywhere on the body. The lice are rarely seen because they are nocturnal.

What is the distribution of pubic lice?

Pubic lice are seen clinging to individual pubic hairs. They may also be found on axillary hair, chest hair, and eyelashes.

How is the diagnosis of pediculosis made?

On clinical grounds, with visualization of a louse

What is the treatment for lice on the:
    Scalp?

Permethrin cream is first line and is applied for 10 minutes, then nits are combed out after loosening with vinegar. Treatment is repeated in 7 days. Close contacts should be examined and fomites cleaned. Malathion, pyrethrins, lindane, and oral ivermectin are alternatives.

Body?

Clothing and bedding are washed in scalding water or discarded.

Pubic area?

As for scalp lice. The eyelashes should be checked for nits, and treated with petroleum jelly if present. As these represent an STD, the patient should be checked and treated for other STDs.

Cutaneous Larva Migrans

What is cutaneous larva migrans?

Lesion caused by migration of a nematode larva (commonly *Ancylostoma braziliense*) under the skin

What is the epidemiology of cutaneous larva migrans?

Common in southeastern U.S. coastal areas

What are the risk factors for cutaneous larva migrans?

Walking barefoot or sitting on infested sand or soil

What are the symptoms of cutaneous larva migrans?

Extreme pruritus

What is the appearance of cutaneous larva migrans?

A thin serpiginous, erythematous trail that advances

What is the distribution of cutaneous larva migrans?

Feet and buttocks

What is the duration of infection in cutaneous larva migrans?

Larvae die in 4 to 6 weeks because humans are not the natural host.

How is the diagnosis of cutaneous larva migrans made?

Clinically

What is the treatment for cutaneous larva migrans?

Thiabendazole applied topically under an occlusive wrap or administered orally

ECZEMATOUS DERMATITIS

CONTACT DERMATITIS

What is contact dermatitis?

Pruritic acute or chronic inflammation of the skin caused by contact with either a primary irritant or an allergen

What is the difference between an allergen and an irritant?

Allergens cause type IV hypersensitivity reactions and require prior antigen exposure for reaction to develop. Irritants probably represent 80% of contact dermatitis and do not require prior sensitization. Allergic reaction occurs 1 to 3 days after exposure, whereas irritant responses tend to occur soon after exposure.

What are common causes of allergic contact dermatitis?

Poison ivy, nickel, rubber, fragrances, and preservatives

What is the appearance of contact dermatitis?

Erythematous, scaly skin. Allergic contact dermatitis may be more indurated and less vesicular. Poison ivy causes linear streaks; sometimes oxidized black sap is seen on the skin.

What is the distribution of contact dermatitis?

Location may give clues to the cause; for example, nickel (earrings)— earlobes, perfume—neck, toothpaste— perioral.

What diagnostic tests are done for contact dermatitis?

Patch testing. A prepackaged kit, the T.R.U.E. Test, contains the 24 most common allergens.

What is the treatment for contact dermatitis?

In acute cases, topical corticosteroids two to three times per day and cool compresses. The precipitant should be identified and avoided. If the case is severe, a prednisone taper may be indicated. The reaction of poison ivy generally lasts 3 weeks from exposure.

Atopic Dermatitis

What is atopic dermatitis?

A chronic, pruritic eczematous skin disease associated with asthma, hay fever, and allergic rhinitis

What is the natural history of atopic dermatitis?

Commonly starts in infancy and usually (but not always) improves with time

What is the major risk factor for atopic dermatitis?

Family history of asthma, hay fever, or eczema

What are the symptoms of atopic dermatitis?

Pruritus, which may be severe enough to disrupt normal life and may worsen in winter or with stress. Exposure to allergens (e.g., dust mites, food antigens, and pollens) may exacerbate the condition.

What is the appearance of atopic dermatitis?

Erythematous scaly plaques and papules with excoriations and lichenification of affected skin

What is the typical distribution of atopic dermatitis?

In infants, extensor surfaces and face; in children, flexural areas (popliteal and antecubital fossae); in adults, hands

What tests are helpful in atopic dermatitis?

Scratch test to specific antigens, serum IgE level, and bacterial cultures of infected excoriations

How is the diagnosis of atopic dermatitis made?

Clinically

What is the typical treatment for atopic dermatitis?

"Soak and grease": avoidance of soap, wool, and fragrance

Tepid baths with bath oil and followed immediately by effective lubricants (e.g., petroleum jelly)

Topical corticosteroids to relieve inflammation

Allergen avoidance in the home

Antibiotics for secondary infection

**What complications may be
seen in patients with atopic
dermatitis?**

Generalized HSV infection and S. *aureus*
superinfection

Stasis Dermatitis

What is stasis dermatitis?

Edema resulting from venous
insufficiency with eczematous skin
changes of the lower legs

**What are symptoms of stasis
dermatitis?**

Pain, pruritus, or no symptoms

**What is the appearance of
stasis dermatitis?**

Edema, mild scale, weeping,
hyperpigmentation (hemosiderin
deposits), and lichenification. Lesions may
progress to ulceration, particularly at the
medial malleolus.

**What is the treatment for
stasis dermatitis?**

Leg elevation, oral antibiotics for
superinfection, pressure stockings of 30 to
40 mm Hg (not on active ulcers), and
Unna's boot (zinc gelatin) to decrease
edema and help healing of ulcers
(Silvadene cream or DuoDERM may be
applied to ulcers under Unna boot)

Lichen Simplex Chronicus

**What is lichen simplex
chronicus?**

Chronic inflammation and thickening of
the skin from constant scratching

**What is the incidence of
lichen simplex chronicus?**

It is a common condition, especially in
those with atopic dermatitis.

**What is the cause of lichen
simplex chronicus?**

An itch-scratch-itch cycle is set up and the
patient cannot stop scratching. Stress
exacerbates the condition.

**What is the appearance of
lichen simplex chronicus?**

Solitary or multiple well-demarcated
plaques of itchy, thickened, often
hyperpigmented dry skin

**What is the distribution of
lichen simplex chronicus?**

Hairline, wrists, neck, anal area, and
extensor forearms and shins

How is the diagnosis of lichen simplex chronicus made?	Clinically
What is the treatment for lichen simplex chronicus?	The patient should attempt to keep from scratching, so as to break the cycle. Topical corticosteroids are helpful. Topical doxepin and oral antihistamines may also be useful.

Nummular Eczema

What are the symptoms of nummular eczema?	Localized pruritus
What is the appearance of nummular eczema?	Coin-shaped pink plaques, dull red in color with dry scale; may ooze and form a crust
What is the distribution of nummular eczema?	Any skin surface, especially lower legs and arms
How is the diagnosis of nummular eczema made?	On clinical grounds after fungus has been ruled out by a KOH preparation
What is the treatment for nummular eczema?	Lubrication of the skin with or without topical hydrocortisone to relieve inflammation and antibiotics for secondary infection. Despite treatment, the condition is likely to recur.

PAPULOSQUAMOUS DISEASES

PSORIASIS

What is psoriasis?	A skin disease of multifactorial causes, in which epithelial proliferation is increased
What is the incidence of psoriasis?	Common, occurring in 2% of Caucasians in the United States
What are the risk factors for psoriasis?	Psoriasis is a disease of Western populations and may be hereditary. Severe psoriasis can occur in HIV-infected patients.

What are the symptoms of psoriasis?

Possible pruritus, arthritis in 10% of cases, and dystrophic nails

What is the appearance of psoriasis?

Discrete erythematous plaques with silvery white scale. When scale is removed, typical spots of bleeding occur underneath. Pitting of nails and the appearance of "oil spots" underneath may be seen, and there may be generalized exfoliative erythroderma.

What is the name of the sign when a scale of psoriasis is removed and bleeding occurs?

Auspitz sign

What is the distribution of psoriasis?

Elbows, knees, scalp, umbilicus, and buttocks are most common.

What is Köbner's phenomenon?

Psoriatic lesions that may be induced by trauma (a nonspecific sign, as it may occur in lichen planus)

How is the diagnosis of psoriasis made?

Clinically

What are the treatments for mild to moderate psoriasis?

Topical—tar, anthralin, steroids, calcipotriol, salicylic acid, PUVA, and UVA and UVB light

What are the treatments for moderate to severe psoriasis?

Oral—methotrexate, etretinate, and cyclosporine

Subcutaneous and intravenous injections; biologic therapies include alefacept, efalizumab, etanercept, infliximab

How do the biologic therapies work?

Either by reducing the number or activation of T cells or inhibiting tumor necrosis factor alpha made by activated T cells

What is guttate psoriasis?

Explosive eruption of small psoriatic papules and plaques, often after streptococcal pharyngitis

PITYRIASIS ROSEA

What is pityriasis rosea?	A common erythematous, scaling eruption of unknown cause, usually occurring in young adults. It is generally asymptomatic.
What is the appearance of pityriasis rosea?	Starts with an erythematous scaly "herald patch" several centimeters in diameter, then erupts with pink, oval, scaly macules on the trunk in a "Christmas tree" pattern
How is the diagnosis of pityriasis rosea made?	Clinically
What is the treatment for pityriasis rosea?	None. The condition generally resolves spontaneously in 3 to 12 weeks.
What infection can mimic pityriasis rosea?	Secondary syphilis (which lacks a herald patch) should always be considered in the differential diagnosis. If there is doubt, an RPR should be ordered.

SEBORRHEIC DERMATITIS

What is seborrheic dermatitis?	A chronic inflamed scaling condition of unknown cause. *Pityrosporum ovale* infection has been implicated as a contributing factor.
What is the incidence of seborrheic dermatitis?	Very common, beginning at puberty (common dandruff); also common in the newborn (cradle cap and diaper dermatitis)
What is the appearance of seborrheic dermatitis?	Erythematous, sometimes pruritic rash with greasy scales
What is the distribution of seborrheic dermatitis?	Scalp, eyebrows, nasolabial folds, ear canals, chest, and groin
How is the diagnosis of seborrheic dermatitis made?	Clinically

What is the treatment for seborrheic dermatitis?

Ketoconazole, selenium sulfide, or other dandruff shampoo three times per week can be applied to scalp, eyebrows, and skin. Topical steroids are used to control inflammation. The goal is control, not cure.

What diagnosis should be considered in adults with sudden, florid seborrheic dermatitis?

HIV infection. In the elderly, it may be associated with Parkinson's disease or other central nervous system disorders.

INFLAMMATORY DISEASE

ACNE

What is acne?

Inflammation of the sebaceous glands of multifactorial cause, including *Propionibacterium acnes* infection and hormones, commonly the first sign of puberty

What are the risk factors for acne?

Family history

What is the appearance of acne?

Open (whitehead) and closed (blackhead) comedones, erythematous papules, and pustules

Cystic acne—deep nodules and pus-filled cysts. Even though all lesions can cause scarring, it is more common in cystic acne.

What is the distribution of acne?

Face, chest, back, and neck

How is the diagnosis of acne made?

Clinically

What is the treatment for mild cases of acne?

Topical tretinoin (Retin-A), adapalene, benzoyl peroxide, erythromycin, clindamycin, azelaic acid, sulfur, and salicylic acid

What is the treatment for moderate cases of acne?	Topical agents as for mild cases plus oral antibiotics (tetracycline, erythromycin, doxycycline, or minocycline). Trimethoprim/sulfamethoxazole is effective for resistant acne but is associated with a higher incidence of severe allergic reactions (e.g., Stevens-Johnson syndrome).
What is the treatment for severe or cystic cases of acne?	Isotretinoin

ROSACEA

What is rosacea?	Chronic inflammation of the central face, commonly involving flushing erythema and intermittent acneiform eruptions. There is a wide spectrum of severity from flushing and telangiectasias to disfiguring papules and pustules.
Whom does rosacea affect?	Especially fair-complexioned persons of Celtic origin
What is the appearance of rosacea?	Erythema with papules, pustules, and telangiectasia but no comedones
What is rhinophyma?	Rhinophyma is seen almost exclusively in older men. The nose has a bulbous "W.C. Fields" appearance, which is caused by chronic hyperplasia of the sebaceous glands secondary to rosacea.
What are the aggravating factors for rosacea?	Conditions that induce flushing—consumption of alcohol (red wine more than beer, beer more than liquor), hot beverages, and spicy foods
What is the treatment for rosacea?	Avoidance of aggravating factors, tetracycline, doxycycline, and minocycline. Topical metronidazole, sulfur plus sulfacetamide lotion, and many alternative therapies that are similar to

acne treatments. Surgical or laser therapy can be used to treat rhinophyma. Vascular lesion lasers can be used to treat telangiectasias.

GRANULOMA ANNULARE

What is granuloma annulare?	Chronic granulomatous inflammation of the dermis
Whom does granuloma annulare most commonly affect?	Children
What are the symptoms of granuloma annulare?	None
What is the appearance of granuloma annulare?	Annular dermal papules spreading outward, varying from flesh-colored to pink or violaceous, with no scale present
What is the distribution of granuloma annulare?	Most commonly, lesions occur on the hands, feet, wrists, and ankles, but they may occur in a generalized form.
How is the diagnosis of granuloma annulare made?	On clinical grounds and by biopsy
What is the treatment for granuloma annulare?	Lesions tend to be recalcitrant, although many treatments have been tried.

LICHEN PLANUS

What is lichen planus?	A common, usually pruritic inflammation of the skin and mucous membranes, with a characteristic clinical and histopathologic appearance
What is the pathogenesis of lichen planus?	It is usually idiopathic but may be associated with hepatitis C. Lichen planus, especially when extensive, has been associated with many drugs (e.g., thiazides).

What is the appearance of lichen planus?	Think the **5 P's**: **P**urple **P**olygonal **P**ruritic **P**apules **P**laques
What is the appearance of healing lesions?	Lesions heal with hyperpigmentation. In the mouth, lacy reticular white lesions are seen. Chronic, painful mucosal ulcerations occur in both the mouth and vagina. There may be nail loss or pterygium formation.
What is the distribution of lichen planus?	Symmetric, most common in flexor areas, wrist, oral cavity, and genitalia
What are Wickham's striae?	White, lacy lines on the surface of lichen planus lesions, best visible with a hand lens after applying oil to the surface of the lesion
How is the diagnosis of lichen planus made?	There is a distinctive clinical picture; occasionally biopsy is done. Lesions demonstrate Köbner's phenomenon at sites of trauma.
What is the treatment for lichen planus?	Topical steroids are used frequently and may help pruritus, but the condition is poorly responsive to treatment. Most cases resolve spontaneously in <1 year; 50% of oral lesions recur.

DERMATOLOGIC MANIFESTATIONS OF SYSTEMIC DISEASE

SKIN METASTASES

Which cancers commonly metastasize to skin?	Breast (no. 1 in women), lung (no. 1 in men), colon, and lymphoma

To what areas of the skin do the following cancers metastasize?

    Breast

Local skin (*peau d'orange, en curasse* [superficial spreading cancer nodules across the trunk]) and scalp

    Lung

Trunk along intercostals and scalp

What is Sister Mary Joseph's nodule?

A round, dark, periumbilical nodule representing a cutaneous metastasis, usually of gastric cancer

What is erythema gyratum repens?

A "wood grain" pattern of annular, migrating erythematous bands on the trunk associated with internal malignancy

What is necrolytic migratory erythema?

Erythema, pustules, and erosions typically of the groin that mark a glucagon-producing pancreatic tumor. Necrolytic migratory erythema can mimic candidal infection.

CUTANEOUS T-CELL LYMPHOMAS

What is cutaneous T-cell lymphoma?

Cutaneous lymphomas are predominantly T-cell lymphomas. Mycosis fungoides (MF) is probably the most common and well described; it is a malignancy of the $CD4^+$ helper T cells.

What is the incidence of cutaneous T-cell lymphoma?

Uncommon but not rare. Occurs in middle-aged people, in men more than women, and in blacks more than whites.

What are the risk factors for cutaneous T-cell lymphoma?

Human T-lymphocyte virus has been detected in some patients.

What is the initial appearance of mycosis fungoides?

Variable, often starting as nonspecific large, erythematous, superficial patches with fine scale. It can be serpiginous or annular.

What can the lesions of mycosis fungoides mimic?

The lesions may mimic eczema or tinea infection.

What is the late appearance of mycosis fungoides?

Later MF evolves into plaques and reddish purple nodules with lymphadenopathy. There may also be hyperkeratosis of the palms and soles and alopecia.

What is the distribution of mycosis fungoides?

Often starts on buttocks, thighs, and abdomen and later becomes generalized

What is the course of mycosis fungoides?

Variable progression

What is Sézary's syndrome?

A variation of MF including erythroderma, lymphadenopathy, and more than 10% atypical lymphocytes in the buffy coat

What is large plaque parapsoriasis?

An eczematous condition involving erythematous patches >5 cm with fine scale

What is the potential late complication of large plaque parapsoriasis?

Progression to MF occurs in 10% of cases.

How is the diagnosis of cutaneous T-cell lymphoma made?

On clinical grounds and by biopsy. The diagnosis of MF may require multiple samples over time; biopsy is required for cell typing.

What is the treatment for indolent cases of mycosis fungoides?

Topical nitrogen mustard, topical steroids, topical retinoids and UVB therapy

What is the treatment for aggressive cases of mycosis fungoides?

Aggressive or widespread disease—PUVA, electron beam, extracorporeal photophoresis, and chemotherapy

ACANTHOSIS NIGRICANS

What is acanthosis nigricans?

A common hyperpigmented, velvety thickening of intertriginous skin, especially at the back of neck and in the axillae

What conditions are associated with acanthosis nigricans?	Diabetes mellitus, Cushing's disease, oral contraceptive use, Addison's disease, obesity, hypothyroidism, niacin therapy, and malignancies (90% are abdominal)
What is the most common cancer associated with acanthosis nigricans?	Gastric adenocarcinoma
How is the diagnosis of acanthosis nigricans made?	Clinically
What is the treatment for acanthosis nigricans?	Although no treatment is necessary, ammonium lactate may be used; obese patients should be encouraged to lose weight.

NECROBIOSIS LIPOIDICA

What is necrobiosis lipoidica?	Granulomatous disease of unknown cause
Whom does necrobiosis lipoidica affect?	Usually occurs in young adults and in women more than men
What are the risk factors for necrobiosis lipoidica?	Diabetes mellitus and trauma. (Whereas <1% of diabetics have necrobiosis lipoidica, most patients with necrobiosis lipoidica have diabetes.)
What are the symptoms of necrobiosis lipoidica?	Usually none, but lesions are painful if ulcerated.
What is the appearance of necrobiosis lipoidica?	Starts as an erythematous macule, then enlarges into a yellow-brown plaque with a waxy atrophic center, telangiectasia, and an elevated shiny border.
What is the distribution of necrobiosis lipoidica?	Most are pretibial.
How is the diagnosis of necrobiosis lipoidica made?	Usually clinically, with biopsy undertaken if there is doubt
What is the treatment for necrobiosis lipoidica?	Minimal success has been achieved with any treatment, including glucose control.

SKIN MANIFESTATIONS OF DIABETES MELLITUS

What skin conditions are associated with diabetes mellitus?	Think CENTURY: **C**ellulitis **E**ruptive xanthomas **N**ecrobiosis lipoidica diabeticorum **T**ense bullae on lower legs (diabetic bullae) **U**lcers **R**ubeosis—chronic flushed appearance of face caused by decreased vasoconstrictor tone and pooling of blood **Y**ellow skin—increased levels of beta-carotene

PRURITUS

What is the differential diagnosis of generalized pruritus?	Think DOC HELP X THE DAMN ITCHES: **D**rugs (opiates) **O**nchocerciasis **C**rabs **H**ookworms **E**xpecting (pregnancy) **L**ymphoma (Hodgkin's disease, MF) **P**araproteinemia **X**erosis **T**hrombocytosis **H**epatic disease **E**lusive infections **D**iabetes mellitus **A**llergies (food) **M**ultiple myeloma **N**euroses **I**ron deficiency **T**hyroid (hyper or hypo) **C**hronic renal failure **H**yperparathyroidism **E**rythrocytosis **S**cabies

RHEUMATIC FEVER

What is the classic rash of rheumatic fever?	Erythema marginatum
What is the appearance of erythema marginatum?	Transient, asymptomatic, faint, migratory serpiginous rash

BACTERIAL ENDOCARDITIS

What are Osler's nodes?	Painful purple-red subcutaneous nodules on finger and toe pads
What are Janeway lesions?	Nonpainful petechial and nodular lesions on the palms or soles
Are Janeway lesions more common in acute or subacute bacterial endocarditis?	Acute
What is the most common cause of splinter hemorrhage of the nails?	Trauma. However, bacterial endocarditis is also in the differential diagnosis, especially when multiple nails are involved and the splinters are near the nail bed.

SARCOIDOSIS

How commonly is the skin involved in patients who have sarcoidosis?	25% of patients have skin involvement. It is possible to have cutaneous sarcoid without systemic involvement.
What are the skin signs of sarcoidosis?	Sarcoidosis is considered a "great imitator," with a wide spectrum of appearances. All lesions are "apple jelly" color when blanched with a glass slide:
	Erythema nodosum—most common
	Lupus pernio
	Scarring alopecia, pruritus, ichthyosis, papules, hypopigmented macules, and ulceration
What is lupus pernio?	Cutaneous sarcoidosis manifested as small pink, tan, or violaceous papules on the nose and acral areas that are often associated with upper respiratory disease and granulomas in the bones

Are any of the skin signs pathognomonic of sarcoidosis?	No. Even when sarcoid is clinically suspected, biopsy is almost always done for confirmation.
What does the skin biopsy of sarcoidosis show?	Biopsy shows classic noncaseating granulomas.
What is Löfgren syndrome?	A combination of sarcoid, eosinophilia, erythema nodosum, bilateral hilar adenopathy, and fever. Prognosis is good.

ERYTHEMA NODOSUM

What is erythema nodosum?	The most common panniculitis, it is an acute inflammation of the subcutaneous fat.
In what group is erythema nodosum seen?	More common in young women
What are the common causes of erythema nodosum?	Streptococcal infection, sarcoidosis, oral contraceptive use, ulcerative colitis, and idiopathic
What are the symptoms of erythema nodosum?	Pain, fever, and malaise
What is the appearance of erythema nodosum?	Diffuse, warm, erythematous nodules that are indurated to touch, producing a very characteristic clinical examination
What is the distribution of erythema nodosum?	Pretibial more than arms, and usually symmetric
What is the duration of erythema nodosum?	Days to weeks
What diagnostic tests are ordered for erythema nodosum?	Culture for *Streptococcus* and chest film for sarcoid
How is the diagnosis of erythema nodosum made?	Clinically, with confirmation by biopsy if necessary

What is the treatment for erythema nodosum?

NSAIDs, rarely systemic steroids, potassium iodide, treatment of the underlying disease, and bed rest. The condition often recurs.

NUTRITIONAL DEFICIENCIES

What is the vitamin C deficiency syndrome?

Scurvy

What are the skin signs of scurvy?

Think **RIPE-C**:

Red, bleeding gums

Impaired wound healing

Perifollicular petechiae

Ecchymoses on arms and legs

Corkscrew hairs

What is the zinc deficiency syndrome?

Acrodermatitis enteropathica, which is characterized by acral and perioral eczematous lesions

What are the common causes of zinc deficiency/ acrodermatitis enteropathica?

Generally occurs in infants as an inability to absorb zinc (can be fatal) or can be acquired through malnutrition

What is the disease of niacin deficiency?

Pellagra. Certain drugs such as INH (a niacin analog) can induce a similar state, as can carcinoid (because of tryptophan consumption).

What are the symptoms of pellagra?

The **3 D's**:

Diarrhea

Dementia

Dermatitis

What are the skin signs of pellagra?

Erythematous, hyperpigmented scaling eruption in a photodistribution

What is the rash around the neck called?

Casal's necklace

Can pellagra be a serious problem?

Yes. Patients can die if not treated.

A bright-red atrophic tongue indicates what deficiencies?	Folic acid and B12 (among others)
What causes vitamin B6 deficiency?	Alcoholism and INH use
What are the skin signs of vitamin B6 deficiency?	Seborrheic dermatitis of the face, angular cheilitis, and glossitis
Which essential fatty acid deficiency can result from prolonged use of total parenteral nutrition?	Linoleic acid, causing dry, scaly, easily bleeding lesions
How can this be treated?	By rubbing the skin with sunflower oil
What is koilonychia?	Spoon-shaped nails
What deficiency is koilonychia associated with?	Iron deficiency, which may be seen in Plummer-Vinson syndrome
What are the cutaneous signs of kwashiorkor (protein malnutrition)?	"Flag sign"—alternating bands of light and dark hair "Enamel paint" dermatosis—hard, scaly erythema
What causes a yellow discoloration to the skin in anorexia?	Excessive carrot eating. This is also often seen in otherwise healthy babies who are fed large amounts of cooked carrots and sweet potatoes.
How is this skin discoloration distinguished from jaundice?	There is no involvement of the sclera.

PORPHYRIA CUTANEA TARDA

What is porphyria cutanea tarda?	The most common of the porphyrias, it is a disease of accumulation of porphyrin metabolites in the skin.
What are the risk factors for porphyria cutanea tarda?	Alcoholism and other liver disease, iron overload, HIV infection, drugs (e.g., furosemide, tetracycline, estrogens, and chloroquine), and genetic predisposition

What is unique about porphyria cutanea tarda?	It is the only porphyria that can be either acquired or genetic.
What is the deficiency in the genetic form of porphyria cutanea tarda?	Heterozygous uroporphyrinogen decarboxylase deficiency
What viral illness is the acquired form of porphyria cutanea tarda associated with?	Strong association with hepatitis C
What is the appearance of porphyria cutanea tarda?	Scarring blisters on the dorsal hands with milia formation, hypertrichosis of the temples, and variable signs (sclerodermal-like plaques, alopecia, and pigmentary changes)
What is the distribution of porphyria cutanea tarda?	Photodistribution—blisters usually first appear on the dorsa of the hands.
What do diagnostic tests demonstrate in porphyria cutanea tarda?	Urine darkens on exposure to air. Samples fluoresce orange-red under Wood's lamp. Quantitative porphyrin analysis shows uroporphyrins to coporphyrins in a 3:1 ratio.
What is the treatment for porphyria cutanea tarda?	Avoidance of hepatotoxins (stop alcohol consumption)
	Phlebotomy (1 unit per week) until a hemoglobin of 10 is reached; expect improvement in 3 to 6 months
	Low-dose hydroxychloroquine

LYME DISEASE (SEE ALSO CHAPTER 7, "INFECTIOUS DISEASE")

What is the classic rash of Lyme disease?	Erythema chronicum migrans (or erythema migrans)
What is the appearance and clinical course of Lyme disease?	Expanding annular rash >5 cm with central clearing at the site of a tick bite. The rash of erythema chronicum migrans takes several days to enlarge; if there is an immediate rash after tick bite, this may be a hypersensitivity reaction to the bite.

What bacterial species is the cause of Lyme disease?	*Borrelia burgdorferi*
What type of tick bite transmits this bacterium to humans?	*Ixodes scapularis*—eastern United States *Ixodes pacificus*—western United States
How is the diagnosis of Lyme disease made?	It is usually made clinically. A minority of patients notice the tick bite.
What is the treatment for Lyme disease?	Doxycycline, 100 mg twice a day for 21 days

THYROID DISEASE

What are the skin manifestations of hyperthyroidism?	The **10 P's:** **P**retibial myxedema **P**almar erythema **P**eriorbital swelling **P**ersistent facial flush **P**oor hair growth **P**ink papules, plaques, and nodules **P**igmentation increased **P**roptosis (exophthalmos) **P**alms are sweaty **P**lummer's nails
What are Plummer's nails?	Onycholysis (nails separating from nail bed) and a scooplike upward curve on nails
What are the skin manifestations of hypothyroidism?	Think **COLD MAN:** **C**oarse hair and skin **O**range palms **L**arge tongue **D**ry skin **M**yxedema **A**lopecia of the lateral one third of the eyebrow **N**ails brittle

CUSHING'S DISEASE

What are the skin manifestations of Cushing's disease?	Think **STEROID BLAST:** **S**triae **T**elangiectasia **E**cchymoses **R**ound facies **O**besity, central **I**ncreased hair growth **D**ermatophyte infections **B**uffalo hump **L**arge clitoris **A**cne **S**kin atrophy **T**inea versicolor

NEUROFIBROMATOSIS TYPE I (VON RECKLINGHAUSEN'S DISEASE)

What are four skin signs of neurofibromatosis type I?	Café au lait spots—hyperpigmented macules on the trunk and legs Neurofibromas—soft, fleshy nodules (up to thousands) Axillary freckling—Crowe's sign Lisch nodules—hamartomas of the iris (the most common manifestation of neurofibromatosis type I)
What is the buttonhole sign?	Invagination of neurofibromas when pressed
Are café au lait spots pathognomonic for neurofibromatosis?	No. Diagnostic criteria require more than six lesions of >1.5 cm; 10% of normal individuals have one to three café au lait spots.
What anatomic location of neurofibroma is almost always pathognomonic for neurofibromatosis type I?	Female areola and nipple

What are the characteristics of neurofibromatosis type II?

Bilateral acoustic neuromas, schwannomas, and neurofibromas but no café au lait spots or axillary freckling

What diagnosis should be considered with extensive café au lait macules with a "coast of Maine," or irregular, edge?

Albright's syndrome, which is manifest by bone lesions and precocious puberty in girls. The large macules respect the midline and rarely involve the face.

TUBEROUS SCLEROSIS

What is tuberous sclerosis?

A genodermatosis inherited in an autosomal dominant pattern with mental retardation, seizures, and specific skin changes

What are skin manifestations of tuberous sclerosis?

Ash leaf spots—often the first sign, hypopigmented macules shaped like a thumbprint on thighs and legs

Adenoma sebaceum

Facial angiofibromas

Shagreen patches

Periungual fibromas on the nails

MISCELLANEOUS SYSTEMIC DISEASE

What is the differential diagnosis of diffuse hyperpigmentation?

Think **HYPERPIGMENTS:**

Hemochromatosis

m**Y**xoma

Porphyria

Expecting (pregnancy)

a**R**senic

Pheochromocytoma

Iatrogenic—drugs, PUVA therapy

Gut—malabsorption, Peutz-Jeghers

Melanoma

Excess thyroid hormone

Neurofibromatosis

Tumors—secreting adrenocorticotropic hormone and melanocyte-stimulating hormone

Scleroderma

What are Cullen's and Grey–Turner's signs?

Periumbilical and flank pooling of blood resulting from hemorrhagic pancreatitis (or ruptured tubal pregnancy)

NAIL SIGNS AND SYSTEMIC DISEASE

What are nail signs of cirrhosis?

Terry's nails—opaque white proximal nail plate with normal-colored distal nails

Muehrcke's nails—transverse white bands across nails seen in hypoalbuminemia

What are Beau's lines?

Transverse nail ridges secondary to arrested nail growth during severe illness

What are half-and-half nails?

Lindsey's nails—proximal half of nail bed is white and distal half is brown, as seen in chronic renal failure

What are Mees' lines?

White, transverse nail plate lines secondary to arsenic poisoning or renal failure

BULLOUS DISEASE

What is the differential diagnosis of bullae?

Bullous erythema multiforme, TEN, dermatitis herpetiformis, porphyria, renal disease, diabetes, carbon monoxide toxicity, barbiturate use, pemphigus vulgaris, bullous pemphigoid, and epidermolysis bullosa

PEMPHIGUS VULGARIS

What is pemphigus vulgaris?

The most dramatic and serious of the family of pemphigus diseases, pemphigus vulgaris is a chronic, life-threatening autoimmune bullous disease of mucous membranes and skin, with defective cellular adhesion of epidermal cells.

What is the incidence of pemphigus vulgaris?	Uncommon, occurs at any age
What are the risk factors for pemphigus vulgaris?	Jewish or Mediterranean ethnicity
What is the appearance of pemphigus vulgaris?	Flaccid blisters that break easily and become weeping erosions
Where does pemphigus vulgaris start?	On mucous membranes in more than 50% of cases—a distinctive feature that helps in the diagnosis
What is the distribution of pemphigus vulgaris?	It may remain localized to mucous membranes or spread to scalp, face, chest, axilla, and groin.
What is Asboe–Hansen's sign?	The ability to extend a pemphigus vulgaris blister by pressing on the lateral edge
What is Nikolsky's sign?	Creation of a new pemphigus vulgaris blister by pressing on uninvolved skin
How is the diagnosis of pemphigus vulgaris made?	Skin biopsy
What is seen on the biopsy?	Histologic examination reveals a suprabasilar blister; immunofluorescence shows intracellular IgG.
What is the treatment for pemphigus vulgaris?	Systemic steroids, azathioprine, and cyclophosphamide
What is the prognosis for pemphigus vulgaris?	Fatal if untreated and 10% mortality rate with treatment. Exacerbations and remissions occur.

BULLOUS PEMPHIGOID

What is bullous pemphigoid?	Seen in older patients, bullous pemphigoid is a chronic autoimmune blistering disease that is usually not life-threatening.

What is the incidence of bullous pemphigoid?	Much more common than pemphigus vulgaris
What is the appearance of bullous pemphigoid?	Large tense bullae on erythematous or normal skin. A minority of patients have mucous membrane involvement.
What is the distribution of bullous pemphigoid?	Common on lower extremities and flexural areas but can be generalized
How is the diagnosis of bullous pemphigoid made?	Clinical suspicion is confirmed by biopsy.
What is seen on the biopsy?	Histologic examination reveals a subepidermal blister. Immunofluorescence shows deposition of IgG and C3 in the epidermis along the basement membrane.
What is the treatment for bullous pemphigoid?	Tetracycline in mild cases; systemic steroids, azathioprine, and methotrexate in more severe cases
What is the prognosis for bullous pemphigoid?	It is a self-limited disease that characteristically remits after years.

OTHER BULLOUS DISEASES

What is dermatitis herpetiformis?	An intensely pruritic, vesicular eruption over extensor surfaces
What is associated with dermatitis herpetiformis?	A gluten-sensitive enteropathy. Lesions disappear when a strictly gluten-free diet is followed.
What is the treatment of choice for dermatitis herpetiformis?	Dapsone
What is SSSS?	Staphylococcal scalded skin syndrome infection. It is caused by *S. aureus*, which releases an epidermolytic toxin that can act at distant sites, causing a generalized desquamative disease in young children, whose kidneys cannot clear the toxin.

How can SSSS be differentiated from TEN?

At times it is difficult to distinguish between the two by clinical examination, but biopsy reveals a higher cleavage plane in SSSS than in TEN.

From where should the culture be obtained in SSSS?

Mucous membranes

BENIGN SKIN TUMORS

KELOID

What is a keloid?

Overgrowth of scar tissue extending beyond the original site of injury, more common in dark-skinned people

What is the appearance of a keloid?

Skin-colored, shiny, protuberant firm nodule

What is the distribution of keloids?

Earlobe and areas of high skin tension (chest, shoulders, and knees)

How is the diagnosis of keloids made?

Clinically. Biopsy should be avoided unless necessary because it may cause further overgrowth.

What is the treatment for keloids?

Intralesional steroids or surgery plus intralesional steroids. Pressure dressings using silicone may help.

DERMATOFIBROMA

What is a dermatofibroma?

A firm dermal papule or nodule. It is skin-colored or hyperpigmented, often occurring on the legs. It exhibits "dimpling" when surrounding skin is pinched and may form at sites of insect bites or trauma.

What is the treatment for dermatofibromas?

Treatment is not required unless it is desired for cosmetic reasons.

SEBORRHEIC KERATOSIS

What is a seborrheic keratosis?	Benign epidermal proliferation with a greasy "stuck on" appearance, which may contain keratin horns. Keratoses can be tan, gray, or black and occur most commonly in elderly white patients.
What is the treatment for seborrheic keratoses?	None necessary; however, cryotherapy is effective if desired for cosmetic purposes.
What is the sign of Leser–Trélat?	Explosive growth of seborrheic keratoses associated with gastrointestinal malignancy

SKIN TAG (ACROCHORDON)

What is a skin tag?	A benign pedunculated skin growth associated with obesity and aging. Intertriginous sites and eyelids are the most common sites.
What is the treatment for a skin tag?	Removal by snipping or freezing, only for cosmesis

SUN DAMAGE AND CANCERS

How do sunscreens work?	They block UVB (short-wavelength) and sometimes UVA (long-wavelength) light by either a chemical or physical process.
Which range of UV light causes sunburn?	UVB is the most important cause outdoors, but UVA is used in tanning salons; both contribute to aging and skin cancer.
What does SPF 15 indicate?	Protection from sunburn 15 times longer with the sunscreen than without

ACTINIC KERATOSIS

What is an actinic keratosis?	Precancer of epidermis caused by chronic sun exposure (actinic = sun)
What is the appearance of actinic keratoses?	1-mm to 1-cm rough, scaling pink patches and papules with indistinct margins

How is the diagnosis of actinic keratosis made?	Clinically. The lesion is often more easily felt by palpation than it is seen. If there is induration, biopsy rules out SCC.
What is the treatment for actinic keratosis?	Reduction of sun exposure, freezing with liquid nitrogen, or curetting. If there are many lesions, topical 5-fluorouracil can be used.
What is the prognosis for actinic keratosis?	It is suspected that 1 in 1000 lesions progresses to SCC per year, but SCC develops eventually in 20% of patients with actinic keratoses.

BASAL CELL CARCINOMA

What is basal cell carcinoma?	Malignant neoplasm of epidermal basal cells
What is the incidence of basal cell carcinoma?	It is the most common form of cancer in the world.
What are risk factors for basal cell carcinoma?	Sun exposure and fair skin
What are symptoms of basal cell carcinoma?	Bleeding, itching, or no symptoms
What is the appearance of nodular basal cell carcinoma?	Most common of the group, with a pearly translucent papule with surface telangiectasias
What is the appearance of pigmented basal cell carcinoma?	Shiny blue-black nodule
What is the appearance of a superficial basal cell carcinoma?	Red, scaly, eczematoid patch with or without crust or ulcer
What is the appearance of a morpheaform basal cell carcinoma?	A sclerotic plaque

What is the distribution of basal cell carcinoma?

Nose, then nasolabial fold, ear, face, back, and chest, but may occur anywhere

How is the diagnosis of basal cell carcinoma made?

Clinical concern necessitates biopsy or excision.

What is the treatment for basal cell carcinoma?

Excision with margin if small.

Mohs' micrographic surgery if larger or in a difficult area.

Radiation if surgery is not practical.

Curettage or imiquimod may be effective for superficial basal cell carcinoma.

What is the prognosis for basal cell carcinomas?

Good, as they spread by direct extension and rarely metastasize

What is nevoid basal cell carcinoma syndrome?

An autosomal dominant genodermatosis with a susceptibility to forming many basal cell carcinomas throughout life

SQUAMOUS CELL CARCINOMA

What is SCC?

Malignant neoplasm of epidermis

What is the incidence of SCC?

20% of all cutaneous malignancies

What are the risk factors for SCC?

Sun exposure, family history, and immunosuppression after transplantation

What is the appearance of SCC?

Erythematous, scaling, indurated plaque or hard nodule with smooth, keratotic, or ulcerated surface

What is the distribution of SCC?

Sun-exposed skin and in burns and scars

What is the term for SCC arising in a wound or burn scar?

Marjolin's ulcer

What is the term for SCC in situ of the glans penis?

Erythroplasia of Queyrat

What is the term for SCC in situ of the skin?	Bowen's disease, which may also occur in non–sun-exposed skin
How is the diagnosis of SCC made?	Clinical suspicion necessitates biopsy.
What is the treatment for SCC?	Excision
What is the prognosis for SCC?	Metastasis is location-dependent. Most common in high-risk areas such as the lip and ear.

MELANOMA[1]

What is melanoma?	Malignant neoplasm of melanocytes
What is the incidence of melanoma?	In 1930, the lifetime risk of an American developing invasive melanoma was 1 in 1500. The risk in the year 2000 was 1 in 74.
What are the risk factors for melanoma?	Caucasian race, red and blonde hair, fair skin, exposure to light (especially UVB), tendency to develop sunburn, frequent sunburn as a child or adolescent, dysplastic nevus syndrome, xeroderma pigmentosum, family history, and immunosuppression
What other factors should raise suspicion of melanoma?	A new pigmented lesion (or skin-colored in the case of amelanotic melanoma); a change in color, size, shape, or surface (ulcer, scaling, crusting, or bleeding) of an existing mole; and itching, burning, or pain of an existing mole
What characteristics of a mole suggest melanoma?	Think **ABCDE:** **A**symmetry **B**order (irregular, indistinct)

---

[1] In collaboration with S. Meisfeldt and D. Woytowitz

Color (variegated or dark black)

Diameter (>0.6 cm)

Elevated from skin surface

What are the four clinical and histologic subtypes of melanoma?

1. Superficial spreading (70%)
2. Nodular (15% to 30%)
3. Lentigo maligna (4% to 10%)
4. Acral lentiginous (2% to 8%)

What is a Hutchinson's freckle?

Lentigo maligna—a large flat brown macule on an older patient.

What is the incidence of malignant melanoma with lentigo maligna?

In 10 years, MM develops in one third of these patients.

What is Hutchinson's sign?

Periungual pigmentation associated with subungual (under the nail plate) MM

What is the distribution of melanoma?

Anywhere on the body. Legs are the most common site in women; the back is the most common site in men.

What is the approach to biopsy a suspicious cutaneous lesion?

Excisional biopsy. An incisional biopsy can be used if the lesion is of a size or in a location that would result in disfigurement if an excisional biopsy was performed.

How deep should the biopsy extend in suspected MM?

Biopsy should extend to subcutaneous tissue to allow depth measurement, because tumor thickness is the most important prognostic factor.

What margins are used in reexcision of melanoma?

For melanoma in situ, 0.5 cm. For <2-mm-thick lesions, 1 cm; for 2-mm-thick lesions, 2 cm.

What are poor prognostic factors in melanoma?

Tumor thickness and depth of vertical invasion (Breslow's thickness and Clark's level); location on scalp, feet, soles, head, neck, and trunk; male gender; nodular and acral lentiginous histologic subtypes; ulceration; increased mitotic rate; larger tumor volume; microscopic satellites of tumor; older age; and DNA aneuploidy

What are the common sites of metastases for melanoma?

Subcutaneous tissue, skin, lymph nodes, bone, liver, spleen, and central nervous system

What is the workup of a patient with melanoma?

Routine lab tests and imaging studies are not necessary for melanomas <4 mm thick in asymptomatic patients. Sentinel node biopsy may be indicated for melanoma with a tumor thickness between 1 and 4 mm.

Is there any adjuvant treatment for melanoma?

Yes. Interferon-alpha-2b has been approved for the adjuvant treatment of melanoma stages IIB and III. Studies show increased disease-free survival but no increase in overall survival. Treatment is associated with significant toxicity.

What is the treatment for metastatic melanoma?

The disease is incurable at this time; therefore palliation of symptoms is the goal. Surgical resection of symptomatic metastases, if possible, is the best option. Melanoma is relatively radioresistant and chemoresistant; however, local radiotherapy can offer some benefit. Melanoma vaccines are being studied.

IMMUNE AND AUTOIMMUNE DISEASE (SEE ALSO CHAPTER 11, "RHEUMATOLOGY")

SJÖGREN'S SYNDROME

What is the appearance of Sjögren's syndrome?

Keratoconjunctivitis sicca (denuded epithelium of the conjunctiva)

What are the symptoms of Sjögren's syndrome?

Dry mouth and eyes, difficulty speaking, and dyspareunia

How is the diagnosis of Sjögren's syndrome made?

On clinical grounds plus biopsy of salivary gland

What is the treatment for Sjögren's syndrome?

Immunosuppressants and artificial lubricants

SYSTEMIC LUPUS ERYTHEMATOSUS

What is the appearance of SLE?	Skin involvement in 75% of patients, with lesions being photosensitive; brightly erythematous, macular malar butterfly rash; erythematous papules; bullae; Raynaud's phenomenon; palpable purpura (vasculitis); and periungual telangiectases
What is the appearance of discoid lupus?	Scarring plaques usually localized above the neck, with dilated follicles and horny plugs
What is the appearance of subacute lupus?	Polycyclic, annular, or psoriasiform lesions on sun-exposed surfaces and upper trunk
What is the distribution of SLE?	Face is most common, but symmetric lesions are seen on arms, legs, fingers, chest, and back.

SCLERODERMA

What are the features of the following subtypes of scleroderma:	
Progressive systemic sclerosis?	Occurs in elderly women. More than 95% of patients have Raynaud's phenomenon. There is internal involvement, especially of the heart, lung, and kidney. Sclerosis of the skin is a major diagnostic feature.
CREST?	**C**alcinosis cutis
	Raynaud's phenomenon
	Esophageal dysfunction
	Sclerodactyly
	Telangiectasias
Morphea (localized scleroderma)?	Violaceous macules advance to hard, smooth, ivory-colored lesions most common on trunk, with possible motion-limiting joint involvement.
Linear?	Lines of sclerosis on extremities or scalp (*en coup de sabre*), with possible bone atrophy beneath

PYODERMA GANGRENOSUM

What is pyoderma gangrenosum?	A chronic ulcerative condition of the skin
What are the risk factors for pyoderma gangrenosum?	Inflammatory bowel disease, hepatitis, Behçet's disease, rheumatoid arthritis, SLE, and monoclonal gammopathy. One half of cases are idiopathic.
What is the appearance of pyoderma gangrenosum?	Pustule progressing to a painful necrotic ulcer with purple overhanging border
What is the distribution of pyoderma gangrenosum?	Legs, buttocks, and abdomen most common
How is the diagnosis of pyoderma gangrenosum made?	Clinically suspected but biopsy needed to rule out other diseases
What is the treatment for pyoderma gangrenosum?	Steroids, dapsone, minocycline, and cyclosporine

VITILIGO

What is vitiligo?	An autoimmune disorder resulting in destruction of melanocytes and depigmentation
What is the appearance of vitiligo?	Depigmented patches that are more disfiguring in dark-skinned patients
What diseases are associated with vitiligo?	Graves' disease and Addison's disease
What is the distribution of vitiligo?	Starts distally on fingers, face, or genitalia and may spread anywhere
How is the diagnosis of vitiligo made?	Clinically—the lesions are more obvious under a Wood's lamp
What is the treatment for vitiligo?	In light-skinned patients, no treatment may be necessary other than skin protection; in dark-skinned patients, topical steroids may be given for local disease. PUVA therapy may be effective in restoring skin pigment; in severe cases, chemical depigmentation of the remaining skin may be necessary.

ALOPECIA AREATA

What is alopecia areata?	Autoimmune process characterized by localized loss of hair
What is the incidence of alopecia areata?	Most common in young people
What is the appearance of alopecia areata?	Round area of hair loss without skin lesions and with no scarring. There may be diagnostic "exclamation point" hairs, which are thinner at the base than at the end. Alopecia areata can progress to complete body hair loss in alopecia universalis. There may also be nail pitting.
How is the diagnosis of alopecia areata made?	Usually clinically
What is the treatment for alopecia areata?	There is no cure, but intralesional steroid injections may stimulate hair growth at least temporarily. It takes approximately 1 month to see results, and new hairs may initially be white. Sometimes oral steroids are used.
What is the prognosis for alopecia areata?	In 75% of patients, hair regrows after treatment. In many patients, regrowth is spontaneous. Younger age, more extensive loss, atopic diathesis, and ophiasis (hat-band loss) are poor prognostic indicators.

DERMATOMYOSITIS

What is dermatomyositis?	A systemic autoimmune disease with inflammation of skin and muscles
What is the age of onset for dermatomyositis?	Occurs from infancy to old age
What association is made with dermatomyositis?	In patients >60 years, there is a strong association with internal malignancy.
What are the symptoms of dermatomyositis?	Fever, weight loss, arthralgias, and proximal muscle weakness

What is the appearance of dermatomyositis?

May have butterfly malar rash, photosensitivity, periorbital heliotrope rash; periorbital edema; periungual telangiectasias; Gottron's papules (flat-topped violaceous papules); calcinosis cutis (more common in juvenile diabetes mellitus); and Raynaud's phenomenon (one third of patients)

How is the diagnosis of dermatomyositis made?

On clinical grounds, plus laboratory findings of elevated creatine kinase and ANA. Skin biopsy may be helpful, but histologic findings are indistinguishable from cutaneous lupus.

What is the treatment for dermatomyositis?

Steroids plus immunosuppressants

DERMATOLOGIC URGENCIES AND EMERGENCIES

What are some of the dermatologic urgencies and emergencies?

Bullous pemphigoid, pemphigus vulgaris (see "Bullous Disease," above), SSSS, toxic shock syndrome, cutaneous vasculitis, RMSF, and meningococcemia

ERYTHEMA MULTIFORME

What are the causes of erythema multiforme?

HSV-1 infection is by far the most common cause; other factors include hepatitis A or B infection, pregnancy, drugs, streptococcal infection, other infections, poison ivy, or idiopathic.

What is the appearance of erythema multiforme?

Erythematous "target lesions," papules, and plaques

What is the distribution of erythema multiforme?

Often localized to extremities, especially elbows, knees, the dorsum of the hands, palms, and soles.

What is the treatment for erythema multiforme?

Stop any potentially offending drug. Prophylactic acyclovir should be considered in recurrent HSV-induced erythema multiforme.

| **What is the prognosis for erythema multiforme?** | Episodes usually resolve in 2 to 3 weeks. The major concern is progression to Stevens-Johnson syndrome. |

STEVENS–JOHNSON SYNDROME

| **What is Stevens–Johnson syndrome?** | Extensive cutaneous and mucosal involvement, often with atypical target lesions, vesicles, and erosions. Stevens–Johnson is predominantly a drug reaction and may be fatal. |
| **Which medications are the most common culprits in Stevens–Johnson syndrome?** | Phenobarbital, phenytoin, beta lactams, sulfonamides, and NSAIDs |

TOXIC EPIDERMAL NECROLYSIS

What is TEN?	Severe, extensive, full-epidermal-thickness necrosis associated with a high mortality rate
What is the appearance of TEN?	Bullae, exfoliation, mucosal involvement, and nail loss are common.
What is the cause of TEN?	Generally a drug reaction
What is the treatment for TEN?	Stop all medications, correct electrolyte imbalances, administer pain control, and give antibiotics as needed. Supportive and aggressive skin care in a burn unit is recommended. Use of systemic corticosteroids is controversial.

EXFOLIATIVE ERYTHRODERMA

| **What is exfoliative erythroderma?** | A severe, generalized red inflammation and exfoliation of the skin |
| **What are the common causes of exfoliative erythroderma?** | Think **D-SCALPP:** **D**rug eruptions **S**eborrhea **C**ontact dermatitis **A**topic dermatitis **L**ymphoma **P**ityriasis rubra pilaris **P**soriasis |

What are the symptoms of exfoliative erythroderma?	Pruritus, chills, fevers, or no symptoms
What is the treatment for exfoliative erythroderma?	Admit patient to hospital, stop all medications, give topical or oral steroids, "soak and grease," and monitor fluids and electrolytes. Skin biopsy may help confirm the diagnosis.
What severe consequence may follow erythroderma?	High-output cardiac failure from increased blood flow through skin

MENINGOCOCCEMIA

What are the skin signs of meningococcemia?	Petechiae and purpura on the lower extremities and trunk. Larger lesions with stellate, sharp, angulated borders with central necrosis are caused by septic emboli.

ROCKY MOUNTAIN SPOTTED FEVER

What is the rash of RMSF?	Petechiae and ecchymoses begin on the wrists and ankles and spread to the palms and soles. They later generalize and become purpuric.

DRUG ERUPTIONS

What are the three most common drug eruptions?	1. Morbilliform exanthem 2. Urticaria 3. Fixed drug eruption
How common are drug eruptions?	Occur in 3% of hospitalized patients

FIXED DRUG ERUPTION

What is a fixed drug eruption?	Localized inflammation of the skin resulting from ingested drug
What is the appearance of fixed drug eruption?	Well-circumscribed red to purple macule on the skin or mucous membranes
What is the distribution of fixed drug eruption?	Same location each time the drug is taken

How is the diagnosis of fixed drug eruption made? Clinically

What is the treatment for fixed drug eruption? Stop the offending drug

PALPABLE PURPURA

What is palpable purpura? Vasculitic inflammation (vasculitis)

What is the differential diagnosis for palpable purpura?

Connective tissue disease

Henoch-Schönlein purpura

Internal malignancy (lymphoma and leukemia)

Polyarteritis nodosa

Wegener's granulomatosis

Infection

Cryoglobulinemia

Churg-Strauss disease

Drugs

Idiopathic

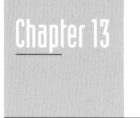

Chapter 13

Environmental Medicine: Diseases Resulting From Environmental and Chemical Causes

ABBREVIATIONS

ACLS	Advanced cardiac life support
ADME	Absorption, distribution, metabolism, or elimination
ALT	Alanine aminotransferase
ARDS	Adult respiratory distress syndrome
AST	Aspartate aminotransferase
AV	Atrioventricular
BUN	Blood urea nitrogen
CNS	Central nervous system
D5W	Dextrose 5% in water
DT	Delirium tremors
ECG	Electrocardiogram
EtOH	Ethyl Alcohol
INH	Isoniazid
LFT	Liver function test
LSD	Lysergic acid diethylamide
MCV	Mean corpuscular volume
PCI	Percutaneous intervention
PCP	Phencyclidine
PT	Prothrombin time
SR	Sustained release
TCA	Tricyclic antidepressant
THC	Tetrahydrocannabinol

POISONING

GENERAL INFORMATION

What is the incidence of toxic exposures reported in the United States?

According to the 2004 annual report of the American Association of Poison Control Centers, approximately 2.5 million toxic exposures were reported in humans and 141,000 toxic exposures in animals.

What percentage of these exposures were in young children?

Approximately 50% of these were reported in children below 6 years of age with 40% being children below age 3.

How often were the exposures severe?

Roughly 10,000 of the exposures were severe, and death occurred in more than 1200 cases.

What is the most common route of exposure?

In 2004, ingestion accounted for approximately 75% of exposures.

Of the common poisonings that occur, approximately what percentage are caused by:

    Medications? 50%

    Cosmetics, pesticides, petroleum products, and turpentine? 20%

    Cleaning and polishing agents? 15%

    Other substances? 15%

What can be done to reduce the incidence of toxic exposure?

Education, proper marking of containers, and removal of poisonous substances from areas with small children

What are some of the sources of information available to investigate diagnosis and treatment of toxic exposures?

Local poison control center; hospital drug information centers, pharmacists, and the following computer and text references:
Poisindex
www.micromedex.com

Shannon MW, Stephen Barrm, Michael Burns. *Haddad and Winchester's Clinical Management of Poisoning and Drug Overdose,* 4th ed. Philadelphia: Saunders, 2007.

Olson KR. *Poisoning and Drug Overdose,* 4th ed. McGraw-Hill, 2004.

Flomenbaum NE, Goldfrank LF, Hoffman RS, et al. *Toxicologic Emergencies,* 8th ed. McGraw-Hill, 2006.

BASIC PRINCIPLES

What is the first rule to remember in toxic exposure?

First, stabilize the patient using the **ABCs: A**irway, **B**reathing, and **C**irculation. Provide continual monitoring and support of vital signs throughout treatment.

After stabilizing the patient, what should be done next?

Information about the exposure should be obtained and supportive care given. A physical examination should be performed and clinical assessment made. Laboratory screening and analysis should be considered, as should gastric decontamination. Improving elimination from the body and checking for antidotes should also be considered.

What are important features of the history of exposure?

Time, type, and amount of exposure as well as past medical history. Allergies, previous admissions, and access to medication and chemicals are important to know. Ingestions of multiple substances are common in suicide attempts and gestures, and alcohol is commonly used to wash down pills.

In cases of suicide attempt or gesture, what additional steps are needed once the patient is medically stable?

Psychiatric consultation should be obtained. Patients thought to be at risk to themselves or others should be detained against their will if necessary (requires legal intervention).

What physical examination features suggest exposure to the following poisons:

Cyanide

Cyanide odor

Carbon monoxide

Cherry-red flush of the skin and mucous membranes

Lead

Lead line and paralysis of extensor muscles

What are the characteristic physical examination findings in the following common toxic syndromes:

Anticholinergics (e.g., atropine, belladonna alkaloid, TCAs, antipsychotics, antiparkinsonian medications, and antihistamines)?

"Red as a beet, hot as a hare, dry as a bone, blind as a bat, mad as a hatter, crazy as a loon" (i.e., dry, flushed skin and mucous membranes, fever, dilated pupils, and delirium)

Cholinergics (e.g., organophosphates)?

Think **SLUDGE:**

Salivation

Lacrimation

Urination

Defecation

Gastrointestinal upset

Emesis

Opiates (e.g., morphine, codeine, heroin, and methadone)?

Triad of miosis, depressed mental status, and depressed respiration

Barbiturates (e.g., phenobarbital and pentobarbital)?

Depressed mental status and respiration, bradycardia, hypothermia, hypotension, pulmonary edema, and areflexia

Stimulants (e.g., amphetamines, cocaine, and aminophylline)?

Excitation and agitation, tachycardia and arrhythmias, hypertension, mydriasis, and seizures

Substance withdrawal?	Agitation, confusion, mydriasis, tachycardia, hypertension, abdominal pain, nausea and vomiting, and seizures
What are the four times when qualitative tests are useful in patients with toxic exposure?	1. When no patient history is attainable 2. When clinical signs and symptoms differ from patient history 3. When multiple toxins are suspected 4. When medicolegal documentation is needed. Such documents can be used in court only if the legal chain of custody is observed.
What are the three times when quantitative tests are useful in patients with toxic exposure?	1. When the drugs have documented associations between adverse effects and therapeutic concentration 2. When there is rapid analysis time 3. When levels of drug present may direct medical management
Do pharmacokinetic alterations change laboratory variables or clinical signs?	Yes. Drug pharmacokinetics may be unpredictable in toxic exposures. In general, all variables—ADME—may be prolonged over those of the normal dose. Volumes of distribution are altered, and metabolism may invoke pathways that are not commonly used for normal doses of substances.
Why consider gastric decontamination in patients with toxic exposure?	To inhibit further adsorption from ingested toxins that may be present in the gastrointestinal tract. This prevents or decreases continued toxicity.
What determines the efficacy of gastric decontamination?	(1) The substance ingested, (2) length of time for exposure, (3) patient age, and (4) underlying medical problems
What are the different types of gastric decontamination?	Gastric lavage, activated charcoal, cathartics, and whole bowel irrigation
How is gastric lavage performed?	Typically, with the airway protected, a large-bore tube is used to remove the stomach contents. Serial aliquots of warm lavage solution (saline or tap water) are

used. The procedure is repeated until the fluid removed is clear.

In whom should gastric lavage be used?

Patients who are obtunded or intubated, those with life-threatening ingestions or patients with very recent ingestions, or patients who have ingested a substance that decreases gastric motility (e.g., anticholinergic agents)

What are contraindications to gastric lavage?

Gastric contents are larger than the lavage tube or hose, are alkalotic, or are sharp; or when the airway cannot be protected

What are complications of gastric lavage?

Accidental tracheal intubation, perforation of the esophagus or gastric area, and adverse cardiorespiratory effects

What are indications for the use of activated charcoal?

In most toxic exposures, use as a single agent or after gastric emptying

What are the contraindications to the use of activated charcoal?

Should be used with caution in patients at risk for aspiration and those with decreased gastrointestinal motility

What are the complications with the use of activated charcoal?

Activated charcoal may complicate endoscopy.

What are the limitations to the use of activated charcoal?

In cases of caustic ingestion, activated charcoal has questionable efficacy. Activated charcoal is incapable of adsorbing cyanide, ferrous sulfate, lithium, boric acid, dichlorodiphenyl-trichloroethane, and carbamate insecticides.

How should activated charcoal be dosed in adults?

60 to 100 g

Approximately what ratio of activated charcoal to toxin is needed to absorb the entire ingested toxin?

An approximate 10-to-1 ratio. This ratio may be unattainable in some ingestions.

What else is administered with the activated charcoal and why?

Administer with 70% sorbitol to reduce gastrointestinal transit time and prevent charcoal from remaining in gut (to decrease time for gut absorption of toxin).

Can multiple doses of activated charcoal be used?

Yes. The premise is to disrupt enterohepatic circulation such that available free toxin may be absorbed from the bloodstream back into the gastrointestinal tract for adsorption by charcoal.

What doses are used for multiple dosing of activated charcoal?

1.0 to 1.5 g/kg, then 0.5 to 1.0 g/kg every 2 to 6 hours. Sorbitol is given with the initial dose but not with every dose.

What are indications for multiple dosing of activated charcoal?

Large ingestions, ingestion of extended-release products, and especially overdose of theophylline and digoxin

What are additional cautions and limitations of using activated charcoal?

Use may increase the risk of perforation, cause diarrhea (and consequently electrolyte disturbances), or cause constipation.

What is the rationale for whole bowel irrigation?

To shorten gastrointestinal transit time and to reduce the absorption of toxic substrate

In what patients should whole bowel irrigation be used?

Patients in whom toxic substances are not adsorbed by activated charcoal, patients who have ingested a large amount of extended-release drug products, and patients who have packed body orifices with drug

What are contraindications of whole bowel irrigation?

Gastrointestinal ileus, obstruction, bleeding, and perforation

What is the dosing for whole bowel irrigation?

Oral or nasogastric polyethylene glycol electrolyte solution (e.g., GoLYTELY or Colyte) is given until rectal fluid is clear. Use up to 0.5 L/hr for children and 2 L/hr for adults.

What is the rationale for cathartic use of whole bowel irrigation?

To shorten gastrointestinal transit time in order to reduce absorption of toxic substances

What types of cathartics are used in whole bowel irrigation?	Most common—saline and osmotic agents (i.e., sorbitol) Other agents—sodium sulfate, magnesium sulfate, magnesium citrate
What are indications for cathartics?	The primary indication is for use of sorbitol with activated charcoal. Otherwise, they are seldom used because of adverse effects and questionable efficacy.
What are complications of cathartics?	Fluid and electrolyte alterations—sodium products may produce hypernatremia and should be avoided in heart failure; magnesium products may cause magnesium toxicity in patients with renal failure and dehydration.
What methods may be used to promote renal elimination of toxins?	Extracorporeal removal by hemodialysis or hemoperfusion, alterations in urinary pH and forced diuresis
When are extracorporeal methods used for renal elimination of toxins?	When toxins can be removed by hemodialysis or hemoperfusion, when clinical status declines after appropriate initial management, and in cases of life-threatening hyperkalemia with or without renal dysfunction
What types of drugs are removed by hemodialysis?	Drugs with low molecular weight Low plasma protein–binding drugs Drugs with volume of distribution <1.0 L/kg Un-ionized, uncharged substances
How does hemoperfusion work?	Toxic substances are extracted from blood as it washes over a column of activated charcoal or carbon.
What are complications of hemoperfusion?	Those related to placement of the large-bore line (depending on location; bleeding, hemo/pneumothorax,

infection, etc.), hypotension, thrombocytopenia, hypocalcemia, and embolus (air or charcoal)

What is the premise of forced diuresis?

To increase removal of toxin by reducing the time for renal reabsorption. Forced diuresis can be done with any crystalline fluid with or without altering urinary pH.

Why use alterations in urinary pH with forced diuresis?

To increase urine output. Toxin is trapped as an ion in the urine, therefore inhibiting reabsorption (i.e., weak acids are inhibited by alkalotic urine, and weak bases are inhibited by acidotic urine).

What agents are used to promote forced diuresis?

Sodium bicarbonate and ammonium chloride

What are complications of forced diuresis?

Fluid overload, electrolyte imbalance, altered urinary pH, and serum acid–base disturbances

COMMON PHARMACOLOGIC TOXINS

Acetaminophen

What are the clinical stages of acetaminophen toxicity— when does each stage occur, and what are its symptoms?

Stage 1

Ingestion to 24 hours after ingestion. Symptoms include nausea, vomiting, gastrointestinal irritation, lethargy, diaphoresis, and malaise.

Stage 2

24 to 48 hours after ingestion (a deceptive asymptomatic phase). There may be slight elevation of hepatic enzymes and right-upper-quadrant pain.

Stage 3

72 to 96 hours after ingestion. Symptoms include severe nausea, vomiting, jaundice, CNS changes ranging from lethargy to coma, elevated AST and ALT (may be >10,000 IU/L), coagulation dysfunction, and renal failure.

Stage 4

4 to 14 days after ingestion. Symptoms and laboratory values resolve or hepatic dysfunction progresses.

What type of gastric decontamination is used in acetaminophen toxicity?

Gastric lavage may be useful if administered within 4 hours of exposure; sometimes activated charcoal may help.

What are the considerations for the use of activated charcoal in acetaminophen toxicity?

Activated charcoal effectively adsorbs acetaminophen. It may also reduce the systemic absorption of the antidote acetylcysteine, but it can cause nausea and vomiting, making it difficult to give the acetylcysteine. If administration of acetylcysteine is delayed by at least 1 hour for some reason, then activated charcoal is an appropriate option for decontamination.

What is the mechanism for acetylcysteine antidotal therapy in acetaminophen overdose?

Acetylcysteine is administered to replace the sulfhydryl substance that detoxifies the N-acetylimidoquinone metabolite. Also, acetylcysteine may prevent liver damage by replenishing the glutathione stores, thereby stopping the accumulation of the toxic intermediary.

What are indications for acetylcysteine antidotal therapy in acetaminophen toxicity?

1. Serum levels of acetaminophen in the possibly toxic range
2. Ingestion exceeding 140 mg/kg
3. Unclear time of ingestion but a predicted half-life exceeding 4 hours

It is best to substantiate the predicated half-life and the amount of ingestion with serum acetaminophen levels. Delaying initiation of antidote for > 10 hours escalates the risk of toxicity. Acetylcysteine therapy may be ineffective if begun more than 24 hours after ingestion.

What is the antidotal dose of acetylcysteine in acetaminophen toxicity?

140 mg/kg orally, then 70 mg/kg every 4 hours for 17 doses. The solution is manufactured as 10% and 20%. The 20%

solution is mixed with soda or orange juice to a 5% solution before administering for oral use. The dose may be increased by 30% if activated charcoal is used.

What are additional monitoring concerns in acetaminophen toxicity?

LFTs should be monitored every 24 hours for approximately 3 to 4 days. Serum bilirubin should be measured in stages 1 and 2. AST and ALT levels typically peak 3 to 4 days after ingestion; levels >1000 IU/L may signify liver cell damage. Electrolytes and fluid status should be monitored for supportive care. BUN and creatinine should be measured because kidney damage may also occur.

What are adverse effects of acetylcysteine?

Nausea and vomiting (acetylcysteine has a rotten-egg odor)

What is alcohol–acetaminophen syndrome?

People with underlying liver disease, whether clinical or subclinical and usually caused by alcohol use, are at high risk for acetaminophen-induced hepatic necrosis. Less than 1 g of acetaminophen may be toxic. This is an often underrecognized cause of acute hepatic failure.

What is the prognosis for acetaminophen toxicity in alcohol–acetaminophen syndrome?

Serum transaminase levels may reach >10,000 and do not correlate with prognosis. Because the patient may be acutely encephalopathic and significant hepatic necrosis portends a poor prognosis, transplant consideration should be initiated early in the course of hospitalization.

Beta Blockers

What are the symptoms and signs of beta-blocker overdose?

Bradycardia, hypotension, and shock. Neurologic findings include delirium, coma, and seizure. Other effects include bronchospasm and hypoglycemia.

How is beta-blocker toxicity treated?

Gastric decontamination. Fluids and atropine for hypotension and bradycardia. If those are ineffective then calcium, insulin plus glucose, vasopressor agents, and inotropes. Glucagon may also be effective.

How does glucagon work in beta-blocker toxicity?

It activates the formation of cAMP independent of the beta-receptor mechanism, causing normal intracellular calcium exchange to occur.

What is the glucagon dose for beta-blocker toxicity?

One (or two boluses if needed) of 5 mg over 1 minute each (15-minute interval between doses), followed by an infusion of 1 to 5 mg/hr.

What is a common side effect of glucagon used in this way?

Vomiting

Cyclic Antidepressant Toxicity

What drugs are cyclic antidepressants?

Traditional TCAs (e.g., amitriptyline, imipramine, doxepin, nortriptyline, desipramine), monocyclics (e.g., bupropion), tetracyclics (e.g., maprotiline), and amoxapine (a dibenzoxazepine)

What are the mechanisms behind cyclic antidepressant–induced toxicity?

Inhibition of norepinephrine and serotonin reuptake, alpha-adrenergic blockade, cardiac membrane stabilization (an anesthetic-like property), and anticholinergic effects. Toxicity is then exhibited through CNS, cardiac, and anticholinergic manifestations.

What are CNS effects of cyclic antidepressant toxicity?

Anticholinergic effects and central adrenergic effects, possibly beginning with agitation and progressing to delirium, hallucinations, lethargy, and coma. Hyperreflexia, myoclonus, and seizures may occur. When seizures develop, they are typically brief, occurring within the initial 6 to 8 hours.

What are cardiovascular manifestations of cyclic antidepressant toxicity?

Hypotension may result from peripheral alpha-adrenergic blockade and from catechol depletion. Cardiac arrhythmias result from the membrane-stabilizing and anesthetic property.

What are the most frequent signs of cardiac toxicity with cyclic antidepressants?

Sinus tachycardia, QRS prolongation, AV blocks (including complete heart block), prolongation of the QT interval, and bundle branch blocks

What are the non-CNS anticholinergic effects of cyclic antidepressant toxicity?

Gastrointestinal symptoms (decreased bowel sounds, reduced motility, and prolonged gastric emptying, making absorption of overdose erratic and unpredictable), urinary retention, respiratory depression, mydriasis, blurred vision, tachycardia, dry skin, and flushing

Does the amount of cyclic antidepressant ingested predict severity of toxicity?

No. The dose ingested is a poor indicator of patient outcome.

What is the treatment for cyclic antidepressant toxicity?

Supportive care (a major component), gastric decontamination, and treatment of cardiac, CNS, and respiratory manifestations

What types of gastric decontamination are used in cyclic antidepressant toxicity?

Gastric lavage, single-dose activated charcoal, multiple-dose activated charcoal, and lavage followed by charcoal

Is extracorporeal removal of toxins helpful in treatment of cyclic antidepressant toxicity?

No. Cyclic antidepressants are highly protein-bound and have large volumes of distribution, making extracorporeal removal ineffective.

Is cardiac toxicity an important part of cyclic antidepressant toxicity?

Cardiac toxicity is responsible for most of the deaths.

What is the treatment for cardiac toxicity with cyclic antidepressants?

Treatment is with intravenous sodium bicarbonate, 1 to 2 mEq/kg bolus, then continuous infusion (isotonic—150 mEq sodium bicarbonate/L D5W) titrated to systemic pH 7.45 to 7.5.

How does sodium bicarbonate work in cyclic antidepressant treatment?

Sodium loading to reverse the inhibition of slow sodium channels in cardiac tissue. Alkalinization may help decrease binding of cyclics to cardiac tissue.

What are indications to treat cardiac toxicity with sodium bicarbonate in cyclic antidepressant toxicity?

Acidosis, resistant hypotension, abnormal cardiac conduction, ventricular arrhythmias, significant QT prolongation, and cardiac arrest. Some sources recommend use with QRS duration ≥0.10 second, whereas others recommend use with QRS ≥0.16 second.

How should cardiac arrhythmias be treated in cyclic antidepressant toxicity?

Hypoxia, hypotension, and acidosis should be treated; then sodium bicarbonate therapy should begin.

Lidocaine may be used for ventricular arrhythmias.

Beta-adrenergic blockers have been used successfully to treat supraventricular and ventricular tachycardias, but adverse effects of hypotension, bradycardia, and cardiac arrest may occur.

Isoproterenol or pacemakers may be needed for bradyarrhythmias and heart block.

What cardiac antiarrhythmic medications should be avoided?

Class IA (quinidine, procainamide, diisopyramide) and IC (flecainide, propafenone, moricizine) should not be used because they act similarly to the cyclic antidepressants. Atropine also cannot be used to treat cyclic antidepressant bradycardia.

Why is atropine ineffective?

Because these antidepressants inhibit muscarinic receptors

How is refractory hypotension treated in cyclic antidepressant toxicity?

Fluids and sodium bicarbonate if required, then norepinephrine, phenylephrine, and dopamine may be used as pressor agents.

What is the treatment for CNS toxicity in cyclic antidepressant toxicity?

Supportive care. Agitation and seizures respond to benzodiazepines. Second-line seizure treatment is phenobarbital.

Iron—Acute Intoxication

What dose of iron is considered toxic?

$\geq$20 mg/kg of elemental iron. Doses of 20 to 60 mg/kg typically produce mild to moderate toxicity; doses exceeding 60 mg/kg produce severe toxicity.

How does iron cause gastrointestinal toxicity?

Locally, iron may cause injury to the gastrointestinal mucosa ranging from irritation to ulceration, bleeding, loss of oxygenation, and perforation. Hepatic necrosis may occur as the portal circulation receives the initial toxic iron concentration from the blood.

What are the systemic toxicities of iron?

Multiple systemic effects may occur, including venodilation (decreased systemic and central venous pressures), enhanced capillary membrane permeability (third spacing and hypotension), interference with serum proteases (may increase PT), cellular destruction, and metabolic acidosis.

What are symptoms and signs of iron toxicity for the following stages, and how long do the stages last?

Stage I

Nausea, vomiting, diarrhea, and abdominal pain. Fluid losses with or without bleeding may result in decreased perfusion, hypotension, and acidosis. Symptoms occur rapidly after ingestion and may be relieved after 6 to 12 hours.

Stage II

Lethargy, metabolic acidosis, and possibly hypotension occurring in the period between relief of gastrointestinal symptoms and development of severe systemic effects. Onset is 6 to 12 hours after ingestion; duration is 12 to 24 hours.

Stage III

Multiple-organ dysfunction, including cerebral damage, coma, cardiac depression, renal dysfunction, liver failure, and ischemic bowel. Liver failure may result in coagulopathy or decreased blood glucose.

Stage IV	Gastrointestinal scarring resulting in gastric outlet and small bowel obstruction
What is most important to remember when making the diagnosis of iron toxicity?	Diagnosis is based on clinical presentation regardless of time since ingestion or laboratory test results.
What are the normal iron levels and what levels cause toxicity?	Normal serum iron is 50 to 150 μg/dL; levels >300 to 350 μg/dL typically result in toxicity; levels >500 μg/dL may cause severe toxicity.
When do peak serum iron levels occur?	Peak serum iron levels occur approximately 2 to 6 hours after ingestion.
Is the serum concentration of iron the etiology of the toxicity?	No. The intracellular concentration of iron creates the toxicity.
Do the iron levels predict symptoms?	Association between level and symptoms varies among patients.
Is measuring TIBC helpful in cases of iron toxicity?	Total iron-binding capacity is not a helpful measurement because it may be inappropriately high when serum iron levels are high.
How are blood glucose and white blood cell counts helpful in monitoring iron toxicity?	Blood glucose levels and white blood cell counts may become elevated with serum iron >300 μg/dL and may give additional information about severity of toxicity.
What is the treatment for iron toxicity?	1. Stabilization of the patient. 2. Gastric decontamination: gastric lavage may be used, but activated charcoal is ineffective. 3. Chelation therapy with deferoxamine. 4. Supportive care: fluid and electrolyte replacement, management of acid–base abnormalities, and coagulopathy.
How does deferoxamine work?	It acts as a chelating agent by converting ferric ions in the blood to ferrioxamine, which is renally eliminated.

What are indications for deferoxamine therapy?

1. Serum iron >300 to 350 $\mu g/dL$ in symptomatic patients or >400 $\mu g/dL$ in asymptomatic patients
2. Ingestion of >180 to 300 mg of elemental iron
3. Moderate level clinical symptoms and signs (i.e., more than one bout of emesis or more than one soft stool)

What is the most effective dose and route of delivery of deferoxamine for iron toxicity?

Therapy is most effective if given as 15 mg/kg/hr via continuous IV infusion for adults or approximately 4 mg/kg/hr continuous IV infusion for children. Intravenous administration is preferred for all patients because total dose given may be more accurately controlled.

What are adverse effects of deferoxamine therapy?

These primarily occur with rapid intravenous injection and include flushing, erythema, urticaria, hypotension, shock, and seizures.

What is the appropriate duration for deferoxamine therapy?

Treatment is continued until serum iron levels are within normal limits and the patient has resolution of clinical symptoms and signs. Treatment duration is typically 6 to 12 hours. Some patients produce vin-rosé–colored urine during chelation with deferoxamine. When this color resolves, therapy may be discontinued. The vin-rosé–colored urine is not an absolute marker for presence of toxicity.

Salicylate Toxicity

What is the mechanism for salicylate-induced toxicity?

1. The agent acts centrally to stimulate the respiratory center.
2. Skeletal muscle metabolism is increased, raising the demand for oxygen and elevating production of carbon dioxide, resulting in hyperventilation and further respiratory alkalosis.
3. The agent interferes with central and peripheral glucose metabolism and utilization.

How is salicylate poisoning classified?

Acute or chronic

What acute levels of salicylate cause toxicity?

Acute intoxication—doses of 150 to 300 mg/kg typically cause mild to moderate symptoms.

Doses >300 mg/kg produce severe toxicity, and doses >500 mg/kg may be lethal.

What chronic levels of salicylate cause chronic toxicity?

Chronic intoxication—typically >100 mg/kg per day for more than 2 to 3 days

What is the clinical presentation in acute salicylate toxicity?

Dehydration, hearing loss, tinnitus, tachypnea, nausea, vomiting, elevated PT, alterations in platelet function, electrolyte loss, and proteinuria

What is the usual acid–base abnormality in salicylate toxicity?

Older children and adults typically present with mixed acid–base states, as seen in respiratory alkalosis, elevated anion gap metabolic acidosis, and alkalemia.

What is the clinical presentation in chronic salicylate toxicity?

Same as acute toxicity but may also include pulmonary edema, CNS manifestations (e.g., agitation, confusion, blunted mental status, seizures, and coma), elevated LFTs, and kidney failure

When should salicylate levels be measured?

Levels should not be obtained sooner than 6 hours after ingestion because they may be falsely low. Salicylate levels may escalate for approximately 24 hours, depending on the amount and type of product ingested. If SR products are ingested, peak salicylate levels may be prolonged to 10 to 60 hours after ingestion. Repeated salicylate levels obtained 4 to 6 hours after the original level may be useful to monitor or document the status of the blood concentration.

Is there a treatment nomogram for salicylate toxicity?

Yes, the Dome nomogram. First, though, the patient's clinical presentation should be used to determine the severity of toxicity and subsequent treatment.

When is the Dome nomogram not an appropriate tool?

1. When the salicylate is taken over several hours or days
2. When the salicylate is enteric-coated or there is ingestion of a SR product
3. When the product has oil of wintergreen, which causes quick absorption
4. When patients have kidney dysfunction
5. When the time of ingestion is unclear
6. When there is acidemia

What is the treatment for salicylate toxicity?

Stabilization of the patient, then gastric decontamination, fluid therapy, intravenous sodium bicarbonate, possible extracorporeal elimination, treatment of seizure, and treatment of coagulopathy as needed

What type of gastric decontamination is used in salicylate toxicity?

A variety may be used, including gastric lavage alone or with activated charcoal, activated charcoal alone, or whole bowel irrigation

Why is sodium bicarbonate used in the treatment of salicylate toxicity?

As the blood becomes more alkalinized, salicylate moves into the ionized form and penetration into all tissues is reduced. Sodium bicarbonate also enhances salicylate elimination through alkalinization of the urine to trap and remove drug in ionized form.

How much sodium bicarbonate is used in the treatment of salicylate toxicity?

1 to 2 mEq/kg per liter of intravenous solution. D5W is recommended for solution to keep the intravenous fluid from being hypertonic. Serum pH of 7.55 should not be exceeded. If the clinician is attempting to create alkalotic urine, then urine pH should be >7.5.

What are adverse effects of treatment with sodium bicarbonate?	Hypernatremia, increasing alkalosis in patients with respiratory alkalosis, hypokalemia, and fluid overload
When should bicarbonate therapy be stopped in salicylate toxicity?	When salicylate levels reach 35 to 40 mg/dL and when the patient's clinical status improves and signs and symptoms resolve
When is extracorporeal elimination appropriate in salicylate toxicity?	When standard management is ineffective, there is evident damage in vital organs, the patient is at an extreme of age, or the liver or kidney cannot clear the drug

Miscellaneous

What is the primary symptom of arsenic poisoning?	Hemorrhagic gastroenteritis
What are the primary symptoms of acute lead poisoning (high level)?	Acute encephalopathy, seizure, coma, and death
What are the primary symptoms of mercury ingestion?	Gastroenteritis, nephritic syndrome and acute renal failure, cardiovascular collapse and death
What are the symptoms of acute mercury inhalation?	Pneumonitis, noncardiogenic pulmonary edema, CNS symptoms, and polyneuropathy
What are antidotes (adult dose) for the following? **Opiates**	Naloxone, initial dose of 2 mg unless the patient has a history of chronic narcotic use, in which case starting dose is 0.4 mg, which is titrated accordingly. Larger doses may precipitate severe withdrawal.
Methanol or ethylene glycol	Ethanol—loading dose, 10 mL/kg (10% solution), then continuous infusion of 0.15 mL/kg/hr

Anticholinergic agents	Physostigmine, 1 to 2 mg intravenously over 5 minutes
Organophosphates or carbamate	Atropine, 2 mg intravenously; may be repeated to dehydrate pulmonary secretions
INH and hydralazine	Pyridoxine gram/gram. Give an equivalent amount of pyridoxine to the estimated amount of hydralazine or INH ingested. If unknown then administer 5 g pyridoxine or repeat as needed to control seizure.
Alpha-adrenergic blockers	Phentolamine
Beta-adrenergic blockers	Glucagon 5 to 10 mg intravenously, then 2 to 10 mg/hr
TCAs	Bicarbonate 1 to 2 mmol/kg
Digitalis	Digibind (mg of digoxin ingested/0.6 = number of vials)
Benzodiazepines	Flumazenil, 0.2 mg intravenously; if no effect after 30 seconds, then 0.3 mg is administered intravenously; if no effect after 30 seconds, then 0.5 mg is administered intravenously every minute to a total dose of 3 mg. Seizures may occur during therapy.
Calcium channel blockers	Calcium chloride 1 g

BITES AND OTHER TOXINS

Should a totally occlusive band be applied following a reptile bite?	Although it is shown in the movies, total occlusion should be avoided. This usually leads to further tissue necrosis of the limb and bite site in addition to the local tissue damage caused by the bite itself.
Should suction be applied following a reptile bite?	It looks good in the movies, but the amount of venom that is extracted by this method is minimal and likely of no consequence.

What is the annual mortality rate for snakebites in the United States?	<1%. The eastern and western diamondback rattlesnakes are responsible for most of the deaths.
What snakes are responsible for large numbers of deaths?	Cobras (Asia and Africa), carpet- and saw-scaled vipers (Middle East and Africa), Russell's viper (Middle East and Asia), African vipers, and lancehead pit vipers (Central and South America)
Bites from which spiders may be lethal?	Brown or fiddler spiders and widow spiders are the most common. Others include the hobo spider (Pacific Northwest) and sac spiders.
What is the major injury of the brown spider bites?	Local tissue necrosis due to vascular thrombosis. Injury to the local nerve and secondary infection may occur. Rarely, hemolytic anemia, hemoglobinuria, and death occur.
What are the symptoms of widow spider bites?	Painful cramps at the bite site that spread to the body; salivation, diaphoresis, nausea, vomiting, headache, paresthesias, rhabdomyolysis, renal failure, respiratory arrest, and death
What is the usual sign of a fire ant bite?	A sterile pustule preceded by a wheal-and-flare reaction. Anaphylaxis occurs in 1% to 2% of people.
What is the incidence of immediate-type hypersensitivity to bee stings?	0.4% to 4.0%
Are all scorpions in the United States potentially lethal?	No. There are 40 different scorpions in the United States but only the bark scorpion (*Centruroides sculpturatus* or *C. exilicauda*), found in the southwestern United States and northern Mexico, is lethal. The rest just cause localized reactions with pain.

What common products may help treat stings of marine creature?	Vinegar, baking soda, rubbing alcohol, papain, fresh lemon or lime juice, and ammonia. Topical steroids, antihistamines, and lidocaine preparations may also help. Fresh water and perfumes should be avoided.
Eating which fish may cause ciguatera poisoning?	75% of cases involve barracuda, snapper, jack, and grouper.
What are the symptoms of ciguatera poisoning?	GI: pain, nausea, vomiting, diarrhea; neurologic: paresthesias, tongue and throat numbness, dysesthesias, tremor, fasciculations, etc.
What are the symptoms of scromboid?	Histamine-related: flushing, a sensation of warmth without fever, pruritus, conjunctival hyperemia, urticaria, angioneurotic edema, bronchospasm, and many others

FOOD-BORNE DISEASE

How common is food-borne disease?	Common. There are estimated to be 75 million cases of diarrhea annually in the United States secondary to food-borne disease. These lead to 325,000 hospitalizations and 5000 deaths.
What are the most common food-borne pathogens?	*Salmonella, Campylobacter, Shigella,* and *Cryptosporidium* account for 94% of the pathogens.
If nausea and vomiting are the presenting symptoms, what pathogens are common?	Bacterial are *Staphylococcus aureus* and *Bacillus cereus.* Viral are noroviruses.
What food-borne pathogens cause neurologic symptoms?	*Clostridium botulinum,* ciguatera toxin, scombroid, other shellfish, and mushrooms, *Listeria monocytogenes, Vibrio vulnificus, Toxoplasma gondii,* and hepatitis A.

ELECTRICAL INJURY

How common are deaths caused by electrical injury?

Approximately 1000 deaths per year are caused by electrical current, and 200 deaths per year are caused by lightning strikes; also, 5% of admissions to burn units are from electrical injuries.

What factors determine the extent of electrical injury?

Duration of contact, alternating current (tetanic contraction does not allow release of the contact), pathway through the body (what is in between), and resistance to the flow of electricity (lowered by moisture)

What renal injuries occur after an electrical injury?

1. Direct injury to the kidney secondary to electrical injury
2. Hypotensive injury
3. Renal tubular damage from myoglobin and hemoglobin secondary to muscle necrosis and hemolysis
4. Rapid volume loss into the destroyed or injured tissue

What other complications may occur in electrical injury?

Swelling may result in compartment syndrome, metabolic acidosis may result from lactate production, and infection may result from inadequately débrided tissue.

What are late neurologic sequelae of electrical injury?

Visual disturbances, peripheral neuropathy, incomplete transection of the spinal cord, reflex sympathetic dystrophies, late convulsive disorders, and intractable headaches

What does acute management of electrical injury entail?

1. Removal of the victim from the contact without touching the victim directly (unless power is definitely terminated)
2. ACLS (there is high risk for cardiac arrhythmias)
3. Rapid fluid and electrolyte replacement (standard formulas estimating replacement based on surface burn are inaccurate because of the extensive internal injury)
4. Wound management
5. Administration of tetanus toxoid and antibiotics

DROWNING

What is the mechanism of injury in drowning?	In "dry" drowning, laryngospasm develops and the victim dies of hypoxia caused by mechanical obstruction of airflow. In "wet" drowning, water reaches the alveoli and directly interferes with oxygen exchange or damages alveoli and causes ARDS.
Does water temperature affect prognosis in drowning?	Yes. Hypothermia induced by cold water slows metabolic rate and may induce a protective mechanism against hypoxia. Patients should be rewarmed per hypothermia protocol in addition to receiving respiratory support. The presence of hypothermia should lead to longer resuscitative efforts (i.e., the patient is not dead until he or she is warm and dead).
What is the acute management of drowning?	Victims should be removed from the water as soon as possible and given ACLS, with particular attention to airway and breathing. If any trauma is suspected, the patient's head and neck should be immediately stabilized. ACLS may be started in the water if immediate removal is impossible. A low threshold for endotracheal intubation is indicated. The patient should be placed on a cardiac monitor as soon as possible.
Should abdominal thrust be administered in the field?	Current ACLS recommendations are that abdominal thrust is not indicated except to remove a foreign body from the airway or to clear the airway if the patient does not ventilate with standard basic cardiac life support procedures.
What is a potential downside to the abdominal thrust?	The thrust may lead to aspiration of gastric contents and further alveolar damage.

What else should be done acutely in drowning cases?	Drowning often follows an inciting event such as head trauma, cardiac arrhythmia, myocardial infarction, alcohol intoxication, or drug use. These events should be treated accordingly during resuscitative efforts.
What laboratory abnormalities are common in drowning cases?	Hypoxia dominates over hypercapnia. The victim is often acidotic. Both hypoxia and acidosis may depress cardiac function. Blood chemistries are usually normal.
What are poor prognostic indicators in drowning cases?	Prolonged submersion, severe metabolic acidosis (pH <7.1), asystole, fixed and dilated pupils, and low Glasgow Coma Scale score (<5)

ALCOHOL

How much of a problem is alcohol consumption in the United States?	The average American intake is two drinks per day, and two thirds of Americans drink alcohol. Alcohol use, both acute and chronic, is responsible for 10% of all deaths, and 50% of fatal accidents and trauma cases are alcohol-related.
What are the four phases of alcoholism?	1. Prealcoholic syndrome 2. Prodrome (marked by guilt, sneaking drinks, and blackouts) 3. Addiction 4. Chronic health decline
What predisposes a person to alcoholism?	There is growing evidence for a genetic cause of susceptibility to alcohol abuse, although environmental pressures also play a role. A strong family history of alcohol abuse should lead to a higher index of suspicion.
What are clues to the diagnosis of alcoholism?	The patient becomes suspicious, notes periods of amnesia, disruption of personal life, a downward career drift, gastritis, diarrhea, myopathy, and tremor.

How is the diagnosis of alcoholism made?

1. EtOH level >150 mg/dL without intoxication is a positive indicator.
2. The **CAGE** questions have an 80% sensitivity.

What are the CAGE questions?

Have you ever tried to **C**ut down on drinking?

Have you ever felt **A**nnoyed by criticism about your drinking?

Have you ever had **G**uilty feelings about drinking?

Have you ever taken an **E**ye opener in the morning?

What are common laboratory abnormalities in alcoholism?

LFTs include elevated gamma-glutamyltranspeptidase, AST/ALT ratio >2:1, or isolated elevated AST.

MCV may be elevated with normal or low hematocrit.

PT may be prolonged.

A decreased BUN may signify chronic malnutrition.

What is alcohol withdrawal?

A state of physical and psychological distress created by a decline in the steady-state alcohol level that a person is accustomed to. A chronic alcoholic may "withdraw" long before the EtOH level reaches 0 mg/dL.

What influences the rate of alcohol metabolism?

The rate of metabolism is influenced by the chronicity of use, amount consumed acutely, and presence of metabolic disorders (e.g., liver disease) or other drugs (e.g., benzodiazepines).

How long after cessation of drinking is alcohol withdrawal seen?

Acute abstinence usually leads to symptoms within 7 days (often 48 to 72 hours).

What are signs of alcohol withdrawal?

Mild withdrawal presents with autonomic excitability (e.g., tachycardia, hypertension, and low-grade fever) and increasing agitation, often with tremor and confusion. In patients with severe withdrawal, autonomic instability and respiratory distress, agitation, and seizures may develop.

What is delirium tremens (DTs)?

Delirium tremens signifies severe withdrawal and has both a physical component (tremors and seizures) and a hallucinatory component. This is a life-threatening condition.

How is risk for alcohol withdrawal treated?

Any patient with a history of withdrawal or heavy drinking should receive benzodiazepine prophylaxis and careful monitoring.

What is the treatment for alcohol withdrawal?

If liver function is normal, the patient should receive chlordiazepoxide HCl (Librium), either by mouth or intravenously in a tapering fashion. A good starting dose is 50 mg every 4 hours the first day, then every 6 hours, then the dose is halved and the interval is tapered. If liver disease is present, 1 to 2 mg of lorazepam is used as a starting dose. The patient must be monitored for excessive sedation and the dose adjusted accordingly.

DRUGS OF ABUSE

What are the signs of chronic drug use?

Development of psychiatric problems such as depression or paranoia may signal abuse problems. As the addiction grows, antisocial behavior in the form of lying, manipulation, and failure to meet personal and business obligations becomes more prominent. Casual users may hide their use indefinitely.

What are the effects of cannabinoids?

Acutely, the effects mimic those of severe alcohol intoxication with depression.

Intoxication with cannabinoids can precipitate a severe depressive state. Physical examination may show conjunctival erythema and tachycardia. Angina may develop even hours after use. Chronic bronchitis may develop as well. Gynecomastia and infertility may result and the immune system may be depressed.

What are some of the cannabinoid withdrawal symptoms?

Withdrawal is marked by tremor, nystagmus, gastrointestinal distress, and sleep disturbance.

Are there any legal uses for cannabinoids?

Cannabinoids are potent antiemetics and can be used for control of intractable nausea in cancer patients in some states. They may also be used to stimulate appetite in some patients (in the form of tetrahydrocannabinol, or THC).

What are the effects of opiates?

Opiates cause CNS depression through several different receptors. Common findings include lethargy, somnolence, miosis, and respiratory and cardiac depression. Intravenous preparations may cause more rapid and profound effects than oral use. Abuse may develop from illegal street use or medical use of prescribed drugs.

Do opiates cause significant withdrawal?

Yes. Factors influencing severity include the drug half-life, dose, and chronicity of use.

What are signs of opiate withdrawal?

The opposite effects of intoxication, including nausea, diarrhea, lacrimation, rhinorrhea, myoclonus, insomnia, and piloerection

How soon after discontinuation of opiate use is withdrawal seen?

Drugs with short half-lives, namely morphine and heroin, may lead to withdrawal within 8 to 16 hours of last use.

What is the treatment for opiate withdrawal?

Treatment consists of observed, controlled administration of long-acting agents such as methadone. Clonidine (0.1 to 0.3 mg two to four times daily) may counteract some of the physical symptoms. A mild withdrawal syndrome consisting of autonomic dysfunction and sleep disturbance may persist for up to 6 months and interfere with long-term abstinence.

What are the dangers of intravenous drug use?

The most obvious is transmission of infectious diseases including hepatitis B and C and HIV because of shared needles.

Endocarditis of the tricuspid valve is seen almost exclusively in this group, and causative agents include normal skin flora (*Staphylococcus*) and unusual organisms such as *Pseudomonas*. Osteomyelitis may also develop, often in vertebral bodies. Intravenous drug abuse should be suspected in patients with sternoclavicular osteomyelitis, often a result of injecting into the jugular or subclavian veins. Injection of contaminated material may also lead to painful local phlebitis.

Are barbiturates similar in action to opiates?

Yes. Both act as CNS depressants. Prescriptions for barbiturates, except to treat seizure disorders, have declined. Because these are usually long-acting agents, withdrawal signs take longer to appear and are generally less severe.

What are the symptoms of withdrawal of anxiolytics such as benzodiazepines?

These cross-react with EtOH, which is why they are used to treat alcohol withdrawal. Abuse of anxiolytics is not uncommon; they are often prescribed inappropriately to treat "anxiety" and "nerves." Withdrawal symptoms are similar to those of alcohol withdrawal but do not appear for many days because anxiolytics are longer-acting agents.

What are the effects of sniffing glue?

Hydrocarbon-based commercial products such as glue and paint thinner can cause CNS depression and feelings of euphoria. They are often used by younger persons and may create long-term-memory and cognitive deficits. Prolonged exposure may lead to life-threatening CNS and respiratory depression.

Why is cocaine abuse dangerous?

Because it creates a high sympathetic discharge, cocaine use increases myocardial oxygen demands and may induce myocardial ischemia. It also induces coronary and peripheral vasospasm, which can cause a myocardial infarction or stroke. This effect may occur up to several days after cocaine use. Hyperpyrexia and malignant hypertension may also occur.

What is the treatment for cocaine-induced myocardial infarction?

Other than avoiding beta blockers, the key is to open the blood vessel with PCI or thrombolysis.

Why are beta blockers avoided in cocaine-induced myocardial infarction?

The theoretical concern of blocking the beta receptor and leaving unopposed alpha activity, which can cause vasospasm.

What other medication should be used for the treatment of cocaine overdose?

Intravenous diazepam at 0.5 mg/kg over 8 hours

What is "crack lung"?

ARDS-like damage, often unilateral, seen acutely after smoking cocaine

What is "crashing"?

Cocaine products produce a rapid, intense euphoric state, which may occur as quickly as 8 to 10 seconds after smoking "crack." This is followed by an abrupt drop in mood. Alcohol is often used to modulate this reaction.

What class of street drugs are amphetamines part of?

Potent metabolic stimulants. Milder forms are legally available and are often used as weight control aids.

What are the symptoms of amphetamine overdose?	Overdose causes tachycardia, anxiety, and agitation. A synthetic methamphetamine known as "ice" has gained popularity. Overdose may lead to hyperpyrexia, dilated pupils, tachypnea, rhabdomyolysis, hypertensive crisis, seizures, and cardiac arrhythmias.
What is the treatment of amphetamine overdose?	Treatment should be directed at the manifestations and include control of seizures with benzodiazepines and blood pressure control with labetalol or nifedipine.
What is the "street" name for MDMA (3,4-methylenedioxy-N-methylamphetamine)?	Ecstasy
What class or classes of street drugs does MDMA fall into?	It has properties of amphetamines and hallucinogenic properties of mescaline.
What are some of the toxic effects of MDMA?	As with other stimulants, there have been reports of hyperpyrexia, rhabdomyolysis, intravascular coagulopathy and hepatic necrosis, arrhythmias, and drug-related accidents or suicide.
What are the effects of "acid"?	LSD, or acid, causes hyperpyrexia, tachycardia, tremor, hypertension, pupillary dilatation, labile moods, and visual hallucinations. There are no reports of deaths directly attributable to the physiologic effects of LSD.
What is a "bad trip"?	LSD can provoke a prolonged panic episode lasting up to 24 hours. Supportive care consisting of "talking down" the patient and small doses of anxiolytic drugs may help.
What is "angel dust"?	Phencyclidine, or PCP
What are the effects of PCP?	PCP produces a state of intense agitation and analgesia. It has been described as causing acts of superhuman strength

(e.g., ripping off handcuffs), but the effect is more due to the analgesia than enhanced muscle strength. It may cause horizontal or vertical nystagmus, hyperacusis, and diaphoresis. Feelings of estrangement and distorted images of self develop. Overdose may lead to coma, which is treated with gastric lavage and acidification of urine.

Can drug use be confused with psychiatric disorders?

Yes. Cocaine may induce a state of paranoid delusions. Also, chronic cocaine use can unmask schizoform disorders. PCP use may appear to be an acute schizophrenic break.

ABBREVIATIONS

ACA	Anterior cerebral artery
AD	Alzheimer's disease
ADC	AIDS dementia complex
AIDS	Acquired immunodeficiency syndrome
AMS	Altered mental status
BPPV	Benign paroxysmal positional vertigo
BUN	Blood urea nitrogen
CBC	Complete blood count
CIDP	Chronic inflammatory demyelinating polyneuropathy

CJD	Creutzfeldt-Jakob disease
CNS	Central nervous system
c/s	Cycles per second (Hz)
CSF	Cerebrospinal fluid
CT	Computed tomography
EEG	Electroencephalogram
EMG	Electromyogram
ESR	Erythrocyte sedimentation rate
GBS	Guillain-Barré syndrome
GCS	Glasgow Coma Scale
GTC	Generalized tonic–clonic seizure
HIV	Human immunodeficiency virus
HSV	Herpes simplex virus
ICP	Intracranial pressure
JME	Juvenile myoclonic epilepsy
LEMS	Lambert–Eaton myasthenic syndrome
LP	Lumbar puncture
MCA	Middle cerebral artery
MG	Myasthenia gravis
MRA	Magnetic resonance arteriography
MRI	Magnetic resonance imaging
MS	Multiple sclerosis
NPO	Nil per os (nothing by mouth)
NSAID	Nonsteroidal anti-inflammatory drug
PCA	Posterior cerebral artery
PD	Parkinson's disease
PICA	Posterior inferior cerebellar artery
PML	Progressive multifocal leukoencephalopathy
RAS	Reticular activating system
SAH	Subarachnoid hemorrhage
SDH	Subdural hematoma
SE	Status epilepticus
TB	Tuberculosis
TEE	Transesophageal echocardiogram
TIA	Transient ischemic attack
TLE	Temporal lobe epilepsy
t-PA	Tissue plasminogen activator
TTE	Transthoracic echocardiogram
WBC	White blood cell

ALTERED MENTAL STATUS

What three things should be evaluated immediately in a patient with AMS?	Oxygenation, perfusion (i.e., blood pressure and pulse), and glucose level

What treatment should be given for an impaired level of consciousness of unknown etiology?	Oxygen, naloxone (opiate antagonist), and glucose. If alcoholism is suspected, thiamine should be given with the glucose.
What is the most common cause of toxic–metabolic encephalopathy in the hospital?	Drugs
List three other general medical conditions that may cause toxic-metabolic encephalopathy.	1. Infection: CNS or systemic infections 2. Organ failure: hepatic or renal 3. Electrolyte imbalance: hypoglycemia, hyperglycemia, hyponatremia, hypercalcemia

COMA AND BRAIN DEATH

What is coma?	An unarousable state of unconsciousness
What therapy should be given in the emergency department, before the cause of coma is established?	Glucose, thiamine, and naloxone.
If the brainstem is not intact, what causes of coma should be considered?	The primary consideration is that of a stroke syndrome (hemorrhage or ischemia) or pressure on the brainstem (herniation).
If the brainstem is intact, what causes of coma should be considered?	Stroke syndromes can still be considered, but it is more likely that the cause is toxic–metabolic encephalopathy, seizure, trauma, or infection, all things that can diffusely scramble cortical activity bilaterally.
What lab tests should be considered?	Blood chemistry, toxicology screen (including alcohol, aspirin and acetaminophen levels), ABG, CBC, and blood culture
What procedures should be considered in comatose patients?	Head CT and lumbar puncture initially. MR should be considered.

Coma suggests dysfunction of which brain structures?

Either the midbrain RAS, which "wakes up the cortex," or both cerebral cortices

Which bedside tests help establish whether coma results from dysfunction of the RAS or from bihemispheric dysfunction?

Cranial nerve reflex actions, particularly those of the eye movements and the pupillary light response

With regard to examination of the cranial nerves, what is seen with bihemispheric dysfunction?

These reflexes should be intact and symmetric.

With regard to examination of the cranial nerves, what is seen with midbrain damage?

The normal reflexes or symmetry of the reflexes is lost because the neurologic pathways that mediate these reflexes are located very close to the RAS.

What are four bedside tests of cranial nerve function that are useful in a comatose patient?

1. Pupillary light reflex
2. Corneal response
3. Vestibulo-ocular reflex (caloric response)
4. "Doll's eyes" (oculocephalic response)

What is the vestibulo-ocular reflex (or cold water calorics test)?

Instillation of ice-cold water against the tympanic membrane.

How is the vestibulo-ocular reflex performed?

The patient's head should be 30 degrees above supine and looking straight ahead. Approximately 100 mL of ice-cold water should be instilled into the ear canal for 1 to 2 minutes (a butterfly tubing from which the needle has been removed is helpful when placed on the end of a 30-mL syringe).

What is seen with vestibulo-ocular testing?

The normal tendency is for the eyes to conjugately deviate toward the side of the cold water instillation. The mnemonic COWS (**C**old–**O**pposite, **W**arm–**S**ame) is a popular way of remembering the direction of *nystagmus,* not the direction of eye deviation.

What does the presence of COWS indicate?

Is proof that the patient has an intact connection between the cortex and the brainstem

How much time should elapse before the second ear is tested?

Approximately 5 minutes should elapse before the test is attempted in the other ear. In some circumstances, the patient may display nystagmus with the fast component in the direction opposite to the instilled ear.

What are doll's eyes?

A less confusing term for this is the "oculocephalic reflex" or the "cervico-ocular reflex."

How is this tested?

With the patient's eyes open, the patient's head is briskly nodded back and forth (e.g., from left to right and back).

How does this test work?

Movement activates the same pathways as cold water instillation does in the vestibulo-ocular reflex, partly through causing movement of the endolymphatic fluid in the inner ear (as with cold calorics) and partly through activating proprioceptive receptors in the neck that feed position information to the vestibular system.

What is looked for during this testing?

The "active" part of the reflex is the turning of the eyes away from the direction of head turning, so that eye movement appears to lag behind head movement. The active reflex should not be confused with the passive return of the eyes to midgaze position after the head rotation is complete and there is no more stimulation to the system. Eye movements should be symmetric and conjugate, with equal excursion distances in both eyes.

What does posturing indicate?

Posturing usually indicates that the cortex is disconnected from the brainstem.

What does decorticate posturing indicate?

In decorticate posturing, the brainstem is probably mostly intact.

What does decerebrate posturing indicate?

Decerebrate posturing implies a worse injury and prognosis and indicates not only hemispheric dysfunction but also dysfunction of the rostral brainstem.

What is the physiologic basis of decorticate posturing?

Decorticate posturing indicates dysfunction above the midbrain's red nucleus.

What is the physiologic basis of decerebrate posturing?

Decerebrate posturing indicates a lesion of the brainstem between the red nucleus and the vestibular nuclei at the pontomedullary junction.

What breathing patterns are characteristic in a comatose patient and may assist in localization of the lesion?

From rostral to caudal (i.e., top to bottom):

Cheyne-Stokes, central neurogenic hyperventilation, apneustic breathing, and ataxic breathing.

What does Cheyne-Stokes breathing indicate?

May indicate a metabolic abnormality or disconnection of the cerebral cortex from the diencephalon or brainstem

Where is the lesion if central neurogenic breathing is seen?

Irritation to the midbrain

Where is the lesion if apneustic breathing is noted?

A lesion at the level of the pons

Where is the lesion if ataxic breathing is noted?

Ataxic breathing originates from the medulla, suggesting that all higher portions of the CNS above the medulla are dysfunctional.

What factors may confound the brain-death evaluation?

Barbiturates, drug overdose or sedation, neuromuscular blocking agents, anticholinergics (e.g., atropine), and hypothermia (body temperature $<32.2°C$)

What findings must be documented on the brain-death examination?	No posturing or withdrawal to torso, head, or appendicular noxious stimulation, absent pupillary light response, absent corneal response, absent oculocephalic and vestibulo-ocular reflexes, and absent gag or cough. Absence of spontaneous respiration must also be demonstrated.
What is an apnea test, and how is it performed?	To rule out the presence of spontaneous respirations, the patient is initially ventilated to a state of hyperoxia (Po_2 >200 mm Hg) and Pco_2 <40 mm Hg. The ventilator rate is lowered to 1 breath per minute (or continuous positive airway pressure of 10 mm Hg). Arterial blood gases are checked every 5 minutes until the Pco_2 is >60 mm Hg or Pco_2 rises >20 mm Hg. Spontaneous ventilation during this time is evidence that the brain is not dead.

BRAIN TRAUMA

What are the 3 components of the Glasgow Coma Scale?	1. Eye responsiveness 2. Verbal responsiveness 3. Motor responsiveness
How is the GCS scored?	Scores range from 3 (no responses) to 15 (normal). See Table 14–1.
What are the three signs of Cushing's triad of increased ICP?	Hypertension, bradycardia, respiratory irregularity
What are the typical symptoms seen in postconcussive syndrome?	Headache, dizziness, psychologic disorders, cognitive impairment
Which vessel is most often implicated in traumatic epidural hematoma?	Middle meningeal artery
What is the classic CT finding of an epidural hematoma?	Convex ("lens-shaped") hyperdensity that respects suture lines

Table 14–1. **Glasgow Coma Scale Scoring**

Category	Points for a Given Response
Eye opening	4 – Spontaneously opens eyes 3 – Opens eyes to speech 2 – Opens eyes to painful stimuli 1 – No eye opening
Verbal response	5 – Fully oriented 4 – Not fully oriented 3 – Verbalizes, but not normally conversant 2 – Vocalized unintelligible sounds 1 – No vocalization
Motor response	6 – Obeys verbal command to move 5 – Localizes to painful stimuli 4 – Withdraws arm from stimulus 3 – Stimulus causes flexion posturing 2 – Stimulus causes extension posturing 1 – No response

Which vessels are often implicated in SDH?	Bridging veins between inner and outer meningeal membranes
What is the classic CT finding of a SDH?	Concave ("crescent-shaped") hyperdensity that does not respect suture lines
What is diffuse axonal injury?	Disruption of cerebral or brainstem white matter tracts secondary to acceleration/deceleration injury, often from motor vehicle accidents
How is diffuse axonal injury diagnosed?	MRI is much more sensitive than CT
What is cerebral herniation?	The intracranial compartment is divided into two parts by the tentorium, an invagination of dura mater that is fairly rigid and has a circular opening, or notch, in its center, through which the brainstem passes. When pressure increases in the supratentorial compartment, in which the cerebral hemispheres lie, the brain may

be displaced or herniated through the tentorial notch, which causes pressure on the brainstem.

How can pupillary size changes indicate cerebral herniation is occurring?

If pressure increases enough in the supratentorial compartment, the brainstem may be forced further down into the infratentorial space, which can stretch the ipsilateral oculomotor nerve and cause the pupil to dilate. Additionally, as the uncus (the most medial part of the temporal lobe) swells into the tentorial opening, it may compress the third nerve on that side, "blowing" that pupil. On rare occasions, though, pupillary dilation may occur contralateral to the side of the pressure-inducing lesion.

Name five ways to manage elevated ICP.

1. Elevate the patient's head of bed above 30 degrees.
2. Hyperventilate to keep P_{CO_2} 25 to 30 mm Hg.
3. Administer 25% Mannitol (0.5 mg/kg) for osmotic diuresis.
4. Remove CSF by ventriculostomy.
5. Barbiturate/other general anesthetic-induced coma.

DEMENTIA

What is the most common cause of dementia?

The neurodegenerative diseases are the most common cause of dementia. AD accounts for approximately 50% to 60% of all dementia. The incidence of AD increases with age and is present in 30% to 50% of persons above 85 years of age.

What are some of the other causes of dementia?

PD, Huntington's disease, Pick's disease, progressive supranuclear palsy, and dementia with Lewy bodies (DLB)

How often are dementias reversible?

Rarely (<5%)

What are the reversible dementias?

Reversible dementias include dementia secondary to an infection of the CNS (such as neurosyphilis), metabolic and nutritional dementias (vitamin B12 deficiency), inflammatory dementias (vasculitis involving cerebral blood vessels), dementia caused by a structural defect impinging on the brain (a subdural hematoma or tumor), normal-pressure hydrocephalus, and endocrine-related dementia (hypothyroidism).

When should an EEG be obtained in the evaluation of the demented patient?

When onset of dementia is fairly rapid (over months) and when the patient complains of, or is noticed to have, multifocal myoclonic jerks. These symptoms may be a result of the prion disease Creutzfeldt-Jakob disease. The classic EEG findings include periodic epileptiform discharges.

What should the clinician look for when reviewing the neuroimaging of a demented patient?

Large ventricles (that are enlarged out of proportion to whatever cortical atrophy might be present), which could suggest the presence of normal-pressure hydrocephalus; evidence of previous strokes, which could yield a diagnosis of a vascular dementia; and evidence to rule out existing reversible traumatic sequelae, such as a subdural hematoma, or a surgically remedial lesion, such as a neoplasm

When should an LP be considered in the evaluation of dementia?

When chronic meningitis or an inflammatory disease affecting the brain is suspected to be the cause (e.g., in the immunosuppressed patient). Also, in the patient with suspected normal pressure hydrocephalus, a high-volume LP (in which at least 30 mL of CSF is removed) may cause the patient to improve acutely, thus helping to establish the diagnosis.

ALZHEIMER'S DISEASE

Name a gene polymorphism that is associated with AD.	Three different variants of the apolipoprotein E gene exist on chromosome 19 (E2, E3, and E4). E4 is associated with an increased risk of dementia. However, many people with apo E4 never develop dementia, whereas many people without apo E4 do.
Should apo E be used for screening or diagnosis?	Screening relatives of patients with AD with apo E should probably be discouraged. Its role as a diagnostic tool is unclear and is less important than the dementia workup above.
How is AD managed?	There is no cure for AD, although anticholinesterase drugs (tacrine, donepezil, rivastigmine, galantamine) and one NMDA receptor antagonist (memantine) are approved for use in the disease (see Table 14–2). By increasing cholinergic activity in some patients with AD, some improvement in memory function may be elicited. Antipsychotic medications may help control some of the behavioral problems (e.g., agitation) that may develop in patients with AD.

Table 14–2. **Cognition-Enhancing Medications**

Medication	Class	Dose	Common Side Effects
Donepezil	Cholinesterase inhibitor	5–10 mg qd	Nausea, vomiting, fatigue, dizziness
Rivastigmine	Cholinesterase inhibitor	3–6 mg bid	Same as above
Galantamine	Cholinesterase inhibitor	8–12 mg bid or 16–24 mg qd (extended release)	Same as above
Memantine	NMDA receptor antagonist	10 mg bid	Dizziness, confusion, agitation, headache

VASCULAR DEMENTIA

How common are vascular dementias?	They are the second most common type of dementia after the degenerative dementias and often occur concomitantly with degenerative dementias. Pure vascular dementias, however, are relatively rare in patients without a known history of clinical stroke.

OTHER DEMENTIAS

What is the clinical triad of normal-pressure hydrocephalus?	Gait apraxia (a specific form of ataxia), urinary incontinence, and dementia
How is the diagnosis of NPH established?	Marked improvement in gait after high-volume lumbar puncture (>30 mL of CSF)
What is the main serious risk of a large-volume LP?	Subdural hematoma
What features distinguish dementia with Lewy bodies from AD?	Mental status fluctuations, parkinsonian features, and frequent visual hallucinations often are seen in dementia with Lewy bodies.

ENDOCRINE ABNORMALITIES AND VITAMIN DEFICIENCIES

What vitamin deficiency, which is often found in alcoholics, can result in an acute neurologic syndrome when glucose is administered to deficient patients?	Thiamine (vitamin B1)
What vitamin deficiency causes subacute combined degeneration?	Vitamin B12 (cyanocobalamin)
What are the neurologic sequelae of pyridoxine (vitamin B6) deficiency?	Both excess and deficiency of vitamin B6 can cause neuropathy. The deficient state tends to cause a mixed sensorimotor neuropathy. In neonates, deficiency may cause seizures.

What is the purpose of folate supplementation?	Because of the increased risk of neonatal neural tube defects
What is the purpose of vitamin K supplementation?	Phenytoin, carbamazepine, phenobarbital, and primidone can cause a deficiency of vitamin K–dependent clotting factors in the neonate.
When should vitamin K be given?	Women on these drugs should take 20 mg/day of vitamin K1 (phytonadione) during the last few weeks of pregnancy. Neonates should be given vitamin K1 at birth.
What are the neurologic manifestations of vitamin E deficiency?	Decreased cerebellar coordination, peripheral neuropathy, night blindness, and eye movement abnormalities
Calcifications seen on head CT in the basal ganglia, dentate nuclei of the cerebellum, and the cerebellar cortex suggest what potential endocrine abnormality?	Hypoparathyroidism. Other neurologic effects of hypoparathyroidism result from hypocalcemia and include tetany, cramps, seizures, and paresthesias.
Which is associated with seizures and coma, hypoglycemia or hyperglycemia?	Both
Too rapid correction of hyponatremia can cause what neurologic condition?	Osmotic myelinolysis or central pontine myelinolysis

HEADACHE AND FACIAL PAIN

What are four important causes of an organic headache syndrome?	CNS infection, elevated ICP, SAH, and CNS tumor
Which is more common, functional or organic headache?	Functional headache occurs in 95% of headache patients.

ORGANIC HEADACHE

Who are susceptible to pseudotumor cerebri?	Primarily young obese women
How is the diagnosis of pseudotumor cerebri made?	Elevated opening CSF pressure (>20 cm H_2O) but no mass lesion seen on imaging studies

VASCULAR HEADACHE

What is *common* migraine?	Migraine headache with neither aura nor transient neurologic deficit
What are three types of prescription drugs used to abort the headache of a migraine attack?	Triptans, mixed analgesics (such as Fiorinal), and ergotamine derivatives (see Table 14–3)
Why is the amount of ergotamine that a patient may take limited to 10 mg per week?	To avoid the risk of "ergotism" with higher doses
What is ergotism?	Excessive vascular contraction, resulting in symptomatic peripheral vascular ischemia or symptomatic coronary artery constriction
What are three contraindications to ergotamine use?	Symptomatic coronary artery disease, peripheral vascular disease, or complicated migraine

Table 14–3. Triptans

Generic Name	Formulation and Dosage
Sumatriptan	Subcutaneous injection (6 mg), nasal spray (5, 20 mg), oral tablet (25, 50, 100 mg)
Rizatriptan	Oral tablets and rapidly dissolving tablet (5, 10 mg)
Zolmitriptan	Oral tablet (2.5, 5 mg), oral disintegrating tablet (2.5, 5 mg), nasal spray (5 mg)
Naratriptan	Oral tablet (1, 2.5 mg)
Almotriptan	Oral tablet (6.2, 12.5 mg)
Frovatriptan	Oral tablet (2.5 mg)
Eletriptan	Oral tablet (20, 40 mg)

How are triptans administered?

All may be administered orally, and other preparations include nasal spray, subcutaneous injection, or orally disintegrating tablet.

What five prophylactic drug therapies prevent or reduce the frequency of migraine?

1. Beta-adrenergic blockers such as propranolol
2. Calcium-channel blockers such as verapamil
3. Tricyclic antidepressants such as amitriptyline
4. Valproic acid
5. Topiramate

What is a cluster headache?

Clustered attacks of severe, unilateral, orbital headache with nasal congestion and lacrimation

Which gender is most affected by cluster headache?

Men

Distinguish the behavior of a patient with cluster headache.

The patient with cluster headache paces.

TENSION-TYPE HEADACHE

What two types of drugs are useful for treating tension headache?

1. Tricyclic antidepressants, such as amitriptyline
2. Analgesics, especially NSAIDs

FACIAL PAIN

What is an important laboratory finding frequently seen in patients with temporal arteritis?

Elevated ESR

Why is temporal arteritis a relative emergency?

If not treated, it may result in blindness.

What is the treatment for trigeminal neuralgia?

Anticonvulsants such as carbamazepine, gabapentin, or phenytoin or tricyclic antidepressants

What surgical procedures are used in patients with trigeminal neuralgia who fail medical management?	Microvascular decompression, stereotactic "gamma knife" surgery, and chemical ablation of the trigeminal sensory ganglion
Where does temporomandibular joint pain occur?	In front of the ear

OTHER HEAD PAINS

How is post-LP headache prevented?	By using a small-bore needle. Keeping the patient supine may also help.
What is definitive therapy for post-LP headache?	A "blood patch." Sterile blood is removed from the patient and injected into the LP site (but not into the dural space), where it presumably patches the leak in the dura.

BACK PAIN

What findings on neurologic examination support back pain of neurologic origin?	Weakness and sensory loss related to a specific nerve root associated with an absent deep tendon reflex. For example, weakness of plantarflexion with sensory loss in the S1 dermatome associated with an absent ankle jerk would be consistent with an S1 radiculopathy.
What two complaints should be urgently evaluated in a patient with back pain?	Leg weakness and urinary or bowel incontinence.

Table 14–4.   Common Radiculopathies

Spinal Cord Level	Pain	Weakness	Sensory Deficit	Hyporeflexia
1	Lateral forearm/ index finger	Biceps/ infras- pinatus	Deltoid	Biceps
2 C6		Biceps	Shoulder to thumb	Biceps and brachioradialis
3 C7	Scapula/axilla		Lateral hand	Triceps
4 L5	Buttocks/ thigh	Great toe dorsiflexion		None
5 S1	Buttocks/ posterior leg	Ankle plantar flexion	Posterolateral calf and foot	

What do leg weakness and incontinence suggest?	These suggest that spinal cord compression may be present.
In Table 14–4 on the prior page, fill in the open cells of the table.	
Row 1	C5
Row 2	Trapezius to thumb
Row 3	Triceps
Row 4	Skin and dorsum of foot
Row 5	Ankle
What is neurogenic claudication?	Precipitation of symptoms of lumbar stenosis during ambulation, presumably because of ischemia of lumbosacral roots

VERTIGO AND DIZZINESS

What symptoms help distinguish light-headedness attributable to presyncope from disequilibrium?	Presyncope may have transient autonomic symptoms (e.g., tachycardia, diaphoresis, nausea).
Where is the anatomic defect that causes peripheral vertigo?	Vestibular apparatus and vestibular nerve
Where is the anatomic defect that causes central vertigo?	Vestibular nucleus and pathways in the brainstem
What are the three most common peripheral causes of vertigo?	1. BPPV 2. Labyrinthitis (also called vestibular neuronitis) 3. Ménière's disease
How is the Dix–Halpike maneuver performed?	The sitting patient quickly lies supine and drops his or her head 30 degrees down and over the end of the exam table. Lateral rotation of the head stimulates the posterior semicircular canal of the ear that is toward the floor. After a short latency, horizontal or rotatory nystagmus and/or vertigo may be produced.

What are three classic symptoms of Ménière's syndrome?	1. Unilateral tinnitus 2. Unilateral deafness 3. Paroxysmal vertigo
List the two most common causes of central vertigo.	1. Vertebrobasilar TIA or stroke 2. Brainstem tumor

PERIPHERAL NEUROPATHY, NUMBNESS, AND TINGLING

What is the most common cause of mononeuritis multiplex?	Systemic vasculitis (e.g., polyarteritis nodosa)
What is the most common inherited neuropathy?	Charcot–Marie–Tooth disease (hereditary sensorimotor neuropathy type 1)
What is the initial treatment for carpal tunnel syndrome?	If the case is mild, treatment is usually with NSAIDs and a wrist splint.
What is the indication for surgery for carpal tunnel syndrome?	If initial treatment fails or there is associated denervation seen on the EMG
What are examples of common demyelinating neuropathies?	Charcot–Marie–Tooth disease and uremia
What are examples of axonal neuropathies?	Alcohol and chemotherapeutic agents (e.g., vincristine)
What is an example of a common cause of a mixed neuropathy?	Diabetes

GUILLAIN-BARRÉ SYNDROME AND OTHER NEUROMUSCULAR DISEASES

What is the Miller Fisher variant of GBS?	Ophthalmoplegia, ataxia, areflexia
What laboratory evidence supports the diagnosis of GBS?	CSF shows protein >55 mg/dL without a significant pleocytosis (i.e., albuminocytologic dissociation). EMG is normal initially but eventually shows findings of demyelination.

What is CIDP?	Chronic inflammatory demyelinating polyneuropathy, a recurrent form of GBS
How does CIDP differ from GBS?	CIDP is characterized by frequent relapses, whereas GBS is usually monophasic.
How is CIDP treated?	High dose prednisone or other immuno-suppressants more often than plasma exchange or intravenous immunoglobulin
What is myasthenia gravis?	A disease characterized by neuromuscular transmission defect, producing weakness
What causes the defect in neuromuscular transmission?	Autoantibodies against postsynaptic skeletal muscle nicotinic acetylcholine receptors
What clinical features are classic of MG?	Fatigable weakness of skeletal muscles
Which muscles are most frequently involved?	Eyelid and extraocular muscles, causing ptosis and fluctuating diplopia
What tests are useful in diagnosing MG?	1. EMG/NCS 2. ACh receptor antibody titer 3. Edrophonium (Tensilon) test
What radiograph is important to obtain in a patient with MG?	Chest CT looking for a thymoma
What are three types of therapy?	1. Anticholinesterase [e.g., pyridostigmine (Mestinon)] 2. Immunosuppressants [e.g., prednisone, azathioprine (Imuran), mycophenolate mofetil (CellCept)] 3. Immunomodulation with plasma exchange or intravenous immunoglobulin
List 10 medications that should be avoided in patients with MG.	Azithromycin, aminoglycosides, clindamycin Procainamide, beta blockers, lidocaine, IV magnesium Chloroquine Phenytoin, lithium

PARKINSON'S DISEASE

What is the difference between PD and parkinsonism?	PD is an idiopathic disorder that is responsive to L-dopa. Parkinsonism has similar features to PD but is secondary to another cause and is often not responsive to L-dopa.
Why is carbidopa included with the L-dopa?	Carbidopa prevents the peripheral catabolism of L-dopa to dopamine. L-dopa can penetrate the blood–brain barrier, but dopamine cannot. Once in the brain, L-dopa is used to synthesize dopamine, which alleviates the symptoms of PD.

For the following medications, list their mode of action:

Benztropine, trihexyphenidyl	Muscarinic anticholinergic
Amantadine	Stimulates release of dopamine; glutamate antagonist
Levodopa	Precursor to dopamine
Carbidopa	Dopa decarboxylase inhibitor
Pramipexole, ropinirole	Dopamine agonist
Selegiline, rasagiline	Monoamine oxidase-B inhibitor
Entacapone, tolcapone	Catechol-*O*-methyl transferase inhibitor

Name five medications to avoid in PD.	Typical antipsychotics, metoclopramide, prochlorperazine, reserpine, MAOIs

STROKE AND SUBARACHNOID HEMORRHAGE

What risk factors are associated with a first stroke?	Hypertension, diabetes, smoking, and advancing age. Hypercholesterolemia has not been shown definitively to be a stroke risk factor, although treatment for hypercholesterolemia has been shown to reduce risk of stroke recurrence.

What can be done for secondary stroke prevention?

Having had one stroke increases the risk of having another. Aspirin and other antiplatelet agents decrease the annual risk of repeat stroke by approximately 25% to 30%. For patients with carotid stenosis of >70% who are symptomatic (e.g., with TIAs or a history of stroke), and certain asymptomatic patients with tight carotid stenoses, consider carotid endarterectomy.

How is stroke prevented in the patient with atrial fibrillation or another cardioembolic source of stroke?

In appropriate patients (consider risk of falling), anticoagulation with warfarin is the most effective treatment and may lessen the risk of cardioembolic stroke in such patients by 60% to 80%.

What is the role of heparin in stroke?

The use of heparin in acute stroke is controversial, but it may be useful for strokes that appear to be actively progressing (stroke in progress), particularly if progressive thrombosis of the basilar artery is suspected. Heparin may also lower the risk of an imminent repeat cardioembolic event after a primary cardioembolic event has occurred, and it may be helpful in patients with "crescendo TIAs" or in selected arterial dissections.

What is a potential complication of heparin therapy in an acute stroke?

Conversion of an uncomplicated ischemic stroke into a devastating hemorrhagic stroke

What are the major criteria for administering IV t-PA?

Ischemic stroke (no hemorrhage on CT). No history of hemorrhagic illness, current warfarin, heparin, or enoxaparin, or recent history of stroke, head trauma, lumbar puncture, or surgery. No uncontrollable hypertension and adequate platelet count. Onset time <3 hours.

When a patient is thought to clinically have had a stroke, what initial ancillary test should be performed immediately?

CT of the brain should be performed to distinguish the cause of the perceived stroke as being either ischemic or hemorrhagic. Ischemic stroke may take more than 24 hours to manifest on CT, so CT is expected to be normal initially.

What is the initial management of the patient with ischemic stroke who is not a candidate for t-PA?

Administration of aspirin, 325 mg

Permissive hypertension

Avoidance of hypoglycemia, hyperglycemia, overhydration, and dehydration

Electrocardiographic monitoring to check for arrhythmias, left ventricular and atrial hypertrophy or enlargement, and old or new myocardial infarction

Why is permissive hypertension acceptable?

Because hypotension may increase the area of infarction.

What other therapies are important prior to discharging the stroke patient?

Swallow evaluation, physical therapy, and occupational therapy consultations

When is the risk of herniation after a stroke the greatest?

2 to 5 days after the stroke, when the edema around the infarcted area is maximal

What are the advantages of MRI over CT for acute stroke?

MRI has better resolution than CT and may show a small stroke that is not evident on CT. It is superior for imaging the posterior fossa and allows performance of MRA to evaluate cerebral blood vessels noninvasively.

What are the disadvantages of MRI compared with CT in the setting of an acute stroke?

MRI is inferior to CT in detecting acute bleeding and requires an extended period of time (approximately 30 minutes to 1 hour), during which the patient cannot be observed closely.

What techniques are used to evaluate the status of the blood vessels to the brain?

Carotid ultrasound and Doppler can image the carotid arteries in the neck.

MRA and CT angiography can image either intracranial blood vessels or extracranial arteries.

Table 14–5. Aphasia

	Syndrome	Fluency	Comprehension	Repetition
1	Broca's		(+)	(+)
2	Wernicke's		(−)	(−)
3	Conduction	(+)		(−)
4	Transcortical motor		(+)	(+)
5	Transcortical sensory	(+)	(−)	

(−) = impaired (+) = preserved

Conventional angiography is the "gold standard," but it is invasive and carries risks.

In addition to an electrocardiogram, what other cardiac workup should be considered in the patient with a new stroke?

TTE and TEE can help determine whether a cardioembolism was likely to have been the source of stroke. TEE is more sensitive for detecting left atrial thrombi and cardiac vegetations, but it is costly and invasive.

For Table 14–5 above, fill in the open cells with regard to the neurologic exam features:

    Row 1 — Impaired

    Row 2 — Preserved

    Row 3 — Preserved

    Row 4 — Impaired

    Row 5 — Preserved

After the diagnosis of SAH is made, what additional study is essential?

Angiography, to look for a ruptured aneurysm (the most common source of SAH)

If an aneurysm is found, what can be done to prevent rebleeding?

Surgical clipping or endovascular coiling of the aneurysm

Table 14–6. ILAE Seizure Classification

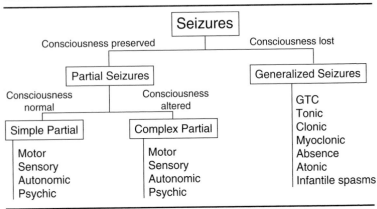

SEIZURES

DEFINITIONS

What is epilepsy?

A continuing tendency toward spontaneous recurrent seizures as a result of some persistent pathologic process affecting the brain. The latter criterion excludes patients with provoked seizures, who have an otherwise normal brain. The International League Against Epilepsy has classified epilepsy syndromes according to the predominant type of seizure, EEG findings, age of onset, interictal abnormalities, and natural history.

What is the prevalence of seizures and epilepsy?

Approximately 10% of the population may experience a seizure at some time of life, but only 3% of people develop epilepsy.

What is the most common generalized epilepsy syndrome arising in childhood?

Childhood absence epilepsy is an idiopathic generalized epilepsy syndrome in which absence seizures begin in early childhood and usually abate by late adolescence. (The syndrome is caused by an inherited abnormality of neurotransmission involving the thalamus and cortex.

The EEG characteristically shows generalized 3 c/s spike-and-wave activity in between and during seizures. MRI is normal.)

What is the most common generalized epilepsy syndrome arising in adolescence or early adulthood?

Juvenile myoclonic epilepsy is an idiopathic generalized epilepsy syndrome in which brief generalized myoclonic jerks and convulsions begin in late adolescence and persist throughout life. (It is inherited as an autosomal dominant trait, but the pathologic abnormality is not known. The interictal EEG shows characteristic generalized multiple spike-and-wave activity in between seizures and occasionally with myoclonic jerks. MRI is normal.)

What is the most common epilepsy syndrome of adults?

TLE is a symptomatic partial epilepsy syndrome in which complex partial seizures begin in late adolescence or early adulthood and more or less persist throughout life. It is usually associated with mesial temporal sclerosis, but the etiology is not known. (The interictal EEG demonstrates spikes originating from the temporal lobe. MRI may show atrophy and sclerosis of mesial temporal structures.)

What EEG findings suggest pseudoseizure?

A normal EEG

DIAGNOSTIC TESTS

What is the most sensitive and specific method for determining that a spell is a seizure?

Simultaneous video and EEG monitoring during a spell. However, during simple partial seizures, the EEG is usually normal.

What is the most sensitive neuroimaging study in the evaluation of epilepsy?

MRI defines brain anatomy with greater detail and often identifies subtle abnormalities that are not seen on CT.

Table 14–7. Antiepileptic Medications

"Traditional" AEDs	"Newer" AEDs
Carbamazepine	Felbamate
Clonazepam	Gabapentin
Clorazepate	Lamotrigine
Diazepam	Levetiracetam
Ethosuximide	Oxcarbazepine
Phenobarbital	Pregabalin
Phenytoin	Tiagabine
Primidone	Topiramate
Valproic Acid	Zonisamide

TREATMENT

Which drugs have the broadest spectrum of antiseizure activity?	Valproic acid, lamotrigine, and topiramate
In Table 14–8, fill in the open cells with regard to medication side effects.	
Row 1	Leukopenia, hyponatremia from SIADH, rare aplastic anemia or hepatitis
Row 5	Sedation, depression
Row 6	Gingival hyperplasia, hirsutism, coarse features, cerebellar ataxia, osteoporosis
Row 8	Weight gain, alopecia, neural tube defects, thrombocytopenia, tremor

Table 14–8. Important Side Effects of Selected AEDs

	Medication	Adverse Effect
1	Carbamazepine	
2	Ethosuximide	Nausea, headache, blood dyscrasias
3	Felbamate	Aplastic anemia, hepatitis
4	Lamotrigine	Rash (Stevens-Johnson), especially with valproic acid
5	Phenobarbital	
6	Phenytoin	
7	Topiramate	Cognitive impairment, nephrolithiasis, glaucoma, weight loss
8	Valproic acid	

Table 14–9.   Monitoring AED Blood Levels

Medication	Therapeutic Range (μg/mL)
Phenytoin	10–20
Valproic acid	50–100
Carbamazepine	4–12
Phenobarbital	15–40

What is the risk of seizure recurrence in patients withdrawn from medications?

Risk of seizure recurrence remains 20% to 70%, even for patients who are good candidates for drug withdrawal.

Table 14–9 shows the common therapeutic levels.

STATUS EPILEPTICUS

What is status epilepticus?

30 minutes of continuous seizure activity or intermittent seizures without return to baseline level of consciousness

How long should a seizure continue before intervention is started?

About 5 minutes. If seizure activity continues for more than 5 or 10 minutes, it is unlikely to stop spontaneously.

When does brain injury become an issue with a seizure?

After about 30 minutes of seizure activity; but keep in mind it takes time for emergency medical help to arrive and begin medication, so intervention must start early.

What is the most common etiology of status epilepticus?

Anticonvulsant noncompliance

How is nonconvulsive status epilepticus diagnosed?

By EEG

What are some commonly used drugs in the treatment of status epilepticus?

Lorazepam, diazepam, phenytoin, fosphenytoin, phenobarbital, midazolam, and propofol

PARANEOPLASTIC SYNDROMES

What are four neurologic autoimmune-related paraneoplastic syndromes?	Encephalomyelitis, peripheral neuropathy, cerebellar degeneration, and LEMS
What are the most common cancers that result in a paraneoplastic syndrome?	Lung cancer (small cell), ovarian cancer, and breast cancer
How is LEMS distinguished from myasthenia gravis?	By EMG. The response to repetitive nerve stimulation in patients with myasthenia gravis usually becomes progressively weaker, whereas in LEMS patients it grows stronger.

CNS INFECTIONS[1]

MENINGITIS

What is the incidence of bacterial meningitis?	>3 cases per 100,000 population. *Neisseria meningitidis* and *Streptococcus pneumoniae* are the most common offending pathogens.
What is the mortality rate for bacterial meningitis?	Overall mortality rate is >10%.
What is the incidence of viral meningitis?	Exact incidence is unknown because it is underreported and difficult to make an exact diagnosis. One study reported >10 cases per 100,000 person-years.
What are normal measurements for CSF for the following: **Opening pressure?**	50 to 195 mm H_2O (equivalent to <18 cm of CSF)

---

[1] In collaboration with V. Shami, N. Thielman, and C. Sable.

WBCs/PMNs?	WBCs <5/PMNs <1
CSF glucose:blood?	0.6
CSF protein?	15 to 40 mg/dL
What is the treatment for bacterial meningitis?	If bacterial meningitis is suspected, the patient should be treated with antibiotics immediately.

TUBERCULOUS MENINGITIS

What organism usually causes tuberculous meningitis?	*Mycobacterium tuberculosis* and, rarely, *Mycobacterium bovis*
How long does it take to culture *Mycobacterium*?	Up to 1 month. As much CSF as possible must be submitted to the laboratory because there are usually very few tubercle bacilli.
What is the prognosis of tuberculous meningitis?	Even with appropriate treatment, 10% to 30% of patients die. Coma at the time of presentation is the most significant predictor of a poor outcome.
What are the pathologic findings seen in tuberculous meningitis?	Exudate in the subarachnoid space, especially at the base of the brain involving adjacent brain (causing basal meningoencephalitis), cranial nerves (causing cranial neuropathies), arteries (causing stroke), or obstruction of basal cisterns (causing hydrocephalus)
What is the natural history of untreated tuberculous meningitis?	Confusion progressing to stupor and coma, with cranial nerve palsies, elevated intracerebral pressure, decerebrate posturing, and death in 1 to 2 months

ENCEPHALITIS

What is the most common cause of identifiable encephalitis?	HSV (HSV-1 in adults and HSV-2 in neonates)

Are there seasons or geographic areas of increased risk for herpes encephalitis?	No
What can be checked in the serum to evaluate for viral encephalitis?	Serum antibodies may be helpful for some pathogens, but both acute and convalescent (taken 1–3 weeks later) specimens are required. Checking IgM in serum or CSF may be helpful in some cases but is not definitive.
Are any polymerase chain reaction tests available for viral encephalitis?	Available for HSV and VZV encephalitis

What do the following diagnostic tests show in encephalitis?

CT scan (of the head with contrast)	Often shows enhancement in the region of the brain involved. In HSV encephalitis, the temporal lobes are most commonly involved. *Listeria monocytogenes* causes a rhombencephalitis (involvement of the brainstem), and focal enhancement in the region of the brainstem may be seen on CT.
EEG	May demonstrate focal abnormalities in the temporal lobe region (periodic lateralized epileptiform discharges or PLEDS)
MRI of the head	More sensitive than CT and more likely to reveal abnormalities early in the disease process. MRI is also more sensitive for *Listeria* rhombencephalitis due to improved visualization of the brainstem. The combination of CT, EEG, and MRI reveals 99% of cases of HSV encephalitis.
What are the common gross pathologic changes seen in encephalitis?	Hemorrhagic necrosis of frontal and temporal lobes

What microscopic pathologic changes are seen in HSV encephalitis?	Necrosis and inflammation with eosinophilic intranuclear inclusion bodies (Cowdry type A)
What is the treatment for HSV encephalitis?	High-dose intravenous acyclovir for 14 to 21 days (relapses occur with shorter courses)

BRAIN ABSCESS

What is the incidence of brain abscess?	<1 in 10,000 hospital admissions
What are the demographics of brain abscesses?	It is more common in men, with a median age of incidence of 30 to 45 years.
What is cerebritis?	Area of low density seen on CT or altered signal on MRI with an area of ring enhancement that does not decay on delayed scans. This is the early stage of a brain abscess before it develops into a capsule.
What pathogens cause brain abscess in immunocompetent persons?	Streptococci, bacteroides and *Prevotella,* Enterobacteriaceae, *Staphylococcus aureus,* fungi, *S. pneumoniae,* and *Haemophilus influenzae*
What pathogens cause brain abscess in immunocompromised persons (i.e., persons with defects in cell-mediated immunity)?	*Toxoplasma gondii, Nocardia, Listeria,* and *M. tuberculosis* in addition to those listed for persons who are immunocompetent
What is the most common cause of a focal CNS lesion in patients with AIDS?	*T. gondii.* Empiric therapy for toxoplasmosis is given if the IgG is positive and CT and MRI findings are compatible.
When should a brain biopsy be considered?	For patients who fail to respond to empiric therapy or have unusual features

What is the most common cause of a focal CNS lesion in immunocompromised patients other than AIDS patients?

There is no single predominant cause of a focal CNS lesion, and an early brain biopsy is required.

When is medical therapy alone appropriate for brain abscess?

Cerebritis (hemorrhage may result with biopsy)

Underlying condition that greatly increases surgical risk

Abscess that is deep or in a dominant location

Multiple abscesses, especially if remote from each other

Abscess <2.5 cm

Early abscess improvement (in many cases cerebritis)

Concomitant meningitis or ependymitis

What factors indicate a poor prognosis in brain abscess?

Delayed diagnosis

Poor localization

Multiple, deep, or loculated abscesses

Ventricular rupture

Coma

Fungal abscess

Inappropriate antibiotics

PRION DISEASE

What is a prion?

Small, infectious proteinaceous particle

What laboratory test can aid in the diagnosis of CJD?

Elevated 14-3-3 protein levels in the CSF

What is the prognosis for CJD?

Invariably fatal

HIV AND THE NERVOUS SYSTEM

What are three CNS diseases caused specifically by HIV?

HIV meningitis, vacuolar myelopathy, ADC

HIV MENINGITIS

What are the clinical characteristics of primary HIV meningitis?	Indistinguishable from any other aseptic meningitis

AIDS DEMENTIA COMPLEX

What are typical CSF findings in ADC?	Mild CSF lymphocytosis, increased protein, and sometimes oligoclonal bands
What do imaging studies in ADC demonstrate?	Cerebral atrophy, ventricular dilation, and subcortical white matter disease (suggesting demyelination)

HIV VACUOLAR MYELOPATHY

What is the prevalence of HIV vacuolar myelopathy?	It is found at autopsy in approximately 25% of AIDS patients.
What other HIV neurologic disease is comorbid with vacuolar myelopathy?	ADC
What is the major differential diagnosis of vacuolar myelopathy?	Cervical stenosis and vitamin B12 myelopathy, which also affect corticospinal and posterior columns
Is the course of vitamin B12 myelopathy different from vacuolar myelopathy?	Vacuolar myelopathy usually has earlier incontinence and fewer sensory abnormalities.

PERIPHERAL NERVOUS SYSTEM COMPLICATIONS OF HIV

How common is peripheral nerve disease in patients with AIDS?	Approximately 50% of patients have disease of peripheral nerves at autopsy.

SOLITARY BRAIN LESIONS AND HIV

What is the differential diagnosis for a solitary brain lesion seen on MRI in AIDS?	Toxoplasmosis, primary CNS lymphoma, and brain abscess

MULTIPLE SCLEROSIS

What are the demographics of MS?	Approximately 65% of those with MS are white women, who typically present between the ages of 20 and 40 years.

What is seen in the CSF examination of patients with MS with regard to:

    Electrophoresis?

In approximately 90% of cases, the CSF contains oligoclonal bands unique to the CSF (i.e., they are not found in blood).

    White blood cells?

There may occasionally be a slightly elevated leukocyte count (<25), which tends to be lymphocytic.

    Protein?

Mildly elevated protein occurs in approximately 25% of cases.

What in the CSF can be used as an indicator of an acute exacerbation?

Myelin basic protein can be a good indicator of an acute exacerbation, but it is present for only approximately 2 to 3 days after an exacerbation occurs.

How often does the MRI show demyelination in patients with MS?

In approximately 90% of patients with MS.

What is Lhermitte's sign?

Trunk and limb paresthesias induced by neck flexion

What is Uthoff's phenomenon?

Worsening neurologic deficits precipitated by elevated temperatures

What treatment may provide symptomatic relief for patients with an acute exacerbation of MS?

High-dose methylprednisolone at the time of the acute attack. A common dose and schedule is to give 1000 mg daily for 3 to 5 days, followed by a 2- to 3-week prednisone taper.

What outpatient regimen is often used for MS patients having an acute attack, even though there is only anecdotal evidence of its efficacy?

Oral prednisone tapers

After 10 years, how many MS patients are ambulatory rather than wheelchair bound?

At 10 years, approximately two thirds are ambulatory.

Chapter 15 Pharmacology

ABBREVIATIONS
ALLERGY AND IMMUNOLOGY
CARDIOLOGY
DERMATOLOGY
ENDOCRINOLOGY
GASTROENTEROLOGY
HEMATOLOGY
Immunizations

INFECTIOUS DISEASES
NEPHROLOGY
NEUROLOGY
ONCOLOGY
PREGNANCY
PULMONOLOGY
PSYCHIATRY
RHEUMATOLOGY

ABBREVIATIONS

ACE	Angiotensin-converting enzyme
ACTH	Adrenocorticotropic hormone
ARB	Angiotensin II receptor blocker
cGMP	Cyclic guanine monophosphate
CNS	Central nervous system
COPD	Chronic obstructive pulmonary disease
CR	Controlled-release
CYP 3 4A	Cytochrome P-450 enzyme 3 4A
DMARD	Disease-modifying antirheumatic agent
EPS	Extrapyramidal side effects
H2RA	Histamine-2 receptor antagonist
HIT	Heparin induced thrombocytopenia
HMG-CoA	Hydroxymethyl glutaryl coenzyme A
INR	International normalized ratio
IVP	Intravenous push
LDL	Low-density lipoprotein
LFT	Liver function test
MDI	Metered dose inhaler
MIC	Minimum inhibitory concentration
MSSA	Methicillin-susceptible *Staphylococcus aureus*
NHL	Non-Hodgkin's lymphomas
NSAID	Nonsteroidal anti-inflammatory drug
PE	Pulmonary embolism
PEA	Pulseless electrical activity

655

PPV	Polyvalent pneumococcal vaccine
SSRI	Selective serotonin reuptake inhibitor
TFTs	Thyroid function tests
TZDs	Thiazolidinediones
VT/VF	Ventricular tachycardia/ventricular fibrillation
VTE	Venous thromboembolism

ALLERGY AND IMMUNOLOGY

An anaphylactic reaction is most likely to be observed over what time period following drug administration?

Within as little as 30 minutes and almost always within 2 hours.

After a patient recovers from anaphylaxis, is there a value in observing them for a longer period of time?

Yes, following recovery, the reaction can recur 6 to 8 hours following exposure.

Should patients with a penicillin allergy be advised to also avoid the use of cephalosporins?

If the patient experienced only mild cutaneous eruptions, the incidence of a serious reaction to cephalosporins is relatively low and these agents may be used.

What medications have been associated with the development of serum sickness reactions?

Sulfonamides, cephalosporins (especially cefaclor), minocycline, hydantoins, and penicillins.

Does the development of "red-man syndrome" following vancomycin administration require discontinuation of the drug?

No, this is a pseudoallergic reaction and it is most likely due to fast rate of infusion of the drug. Usually slowing the infusion rate is all that is needed.

What causes red-man syndrome?

Release of histamine as well as other mediators from cutaneous mast cells

Is it necessary to pretreat patients with a shellfish allergy with steroids prior to receiving contrast media?

Although routinely done in clinical practice, pretreatment of these patients is not necessary.

What causes the contrast reaction?	Iodine allergies reflect primarily the hyperosmolarity of the contrast agent with resultant non-IgE mediated mast cell degranulation.
What are shellfish allergies usually due to?	Although shellfish may be rich in iodine, the reaction to shellfish is usually caused by IgE antibodies to the proteins in the fish and not the iodine.
Which class of medications that contain a sulfa moiety is often associated with an allergic reaction?	Most allergic reactions occur from sulfa-containing antimicrobial agents.
Can a person with a known reaction to sulfamethoxazole be administered furosemide?	Yes. While both contain sulfa moieties, the configuration of the sulfa component on the benzene ring is very different and the likelihood of a reaction is more theoretical than factual.
What other sulfa-containing medications are also unlikely to cause reactions?	This also holds true for medications such as celecoxib, oral sulfonylureas, and sumatriptan.
What is the mechanism of action of calcineurin inhibitors (cyclosporine, tacrolimus)?	These agents inhibit T-cell proliferation by inhibiting the production of IL-2 and other cytokines by T cells.
When is the most appropriate time to draw blood levels for the calcineurin inhibitors?	The blood levels for these agents should be ordered at a trough. Levels should be drawn $\frac{1}{2}$ hour prior to the next dose.
What are the most common adverse effects associated with the calcineurin inhibitors?	Hypertension, nephrotoxicity, hyperkalemia, hypomagnesemia, and neurotoxicity
What is the mechanism of action of mycophenolate mofetil?	Mycophenolate mofetil works through noncompetitive binding to inosine monophosphate dehydrogenase (IM-PDH). The inhibition of this enzyme reduces lymphocyte proliferation.

What are the risks of administering azathioprine in combination with allopurinol?

Azathioprine is an inactive compound that is converted to 6-mercaptopurine (6-MP). The 6-MP is metabolized primarily by xanthine oxidase. Since allopurinol inhibits xanthine oxidase, the bioavailability of 6-MP and azathioprine can be increased by as much as fourfold, increasing the risk of bone marrow suppression and pancytopenia.

CARDIOLOGY

What is the dose of amiodarone for a patient with pulseless VT/VF?

300 mg IVP

What is the appropriate dose of vasopressin in pulseless VT/VF, PEA, and asystole?

40 units administered IVP

What medications should be avoided in patients receiving a continuous infusion of dobutamine?

Those medications with negative inotropic activity. Some of these are verapamil, diltiazem, procainamide, and beta-adrenergic blocking agents.

What is the risk of using nitroprusside in patients with acute myocardial infarction?

May worsen ischemic injury through vasodilatation of nondiseased vessels diverting blood from regions supplied by stenotic vessels (coronary steal syndrome) and reflex tachycardia.

Which vasopressor may be preferentially used in septic patients with arrhythmic disturbances?

Phenylephrine, owing to its effect of reflex bradycardia. Vasopressin also has a relatively neutral impact on arrhythmias.

Should HMG-CoA reductase inhibitors (statins) be discontinued when the hepatic transaminases increase to above three times the upper limit of normal?

Not necessarily. It depends on the dose of the statin and whether or not other LFT abnormalities coexist, such as elevated total bilirubin. In the majority of cases (70%), transaminase elevations will resolve spontaneously without intervention.

Do patients taking HMG-CoA reductase inhibitors (statins) metabolized through the CYP 3A4 enzyme system (atorvastatin, simvastatin, lovastatin) have to avoid the consumption of grapefruit juice?

Yes and no. Inhibition of CYP3A4 results in increased level of medications that are metabolized through this pathway, possibly increasing the risk of adverse effects. However, to be clinically significant, patients would have to consume >1 quart of grapefruit juice daily. Therefore a daily glass of grapefruit juice along with these agents is unlikely to cause any harm.

What is the most appropriate alternative agent to prescribe in a patient who developed angioedema with ACE inhibitors?

Angiotensin receptor blocker (ARB). Although both classes of agents can cause this reaction, the mechanism between the two is different and ARBs can be utilized.

What side effects of hydralazine therapy contribute to ineffective and unpredictable blood pressure control in patients?

Reflex tachycardia, increased renin activity, and fluid retention can result from the stimulation of sympathetic outflow secondary to hydralazine's potent vasodilation.

What hypoglycemic symptom is not masked by beta blockers?

Sweating

When is the onset of the antihypertensive effect of a clonidine patch?

2 to 3 days in which overlapping with oral clonidine is required when transitioning from oral to transdermal clonidine to prevent rebound hypertension.

What additional effect of furosemide that occurs prior to diuretic effects may provide relief to patients with pulmonary edema?

Furosemide causes direct vasodilation, resulting in a rapid decrease in blood pressure.

When should serum digoxin concentrations be drawn to avoid misinterpretation of falsely elevated levels?

Levels are most reliable if drawn just before the next dose and no sooner than 6 to 8 hours after the last dose because of slow digoxin distribution between the blood and tissues.

How should warfarin dosing be empirically adjusted when amiodarone therapy is started?

The warfarin dose should be decreased by half when amiodarone is started, with close monitoring of the INR owing to amiodarone's inhibition of warfarin metabolism.

Above what cumulative dose of doxorubicin is there a higher risk of irreversible myocardial toxicity and heart failure?

450 to 550 mg/m^2

DERMATOLOGY

What amount and duration of use should high-potency topical steroids be limited to?

No more than 50 g/week for up to 2 weeks of use

What kind of hyperpigmentation may result from chronic amiodarone therapy?

Blue-gray discoloration occurs in 1% to 3% of patients on chronic amiodarone therapy. It may take up to a year or more after discontinuation to resolve. Sunlight can exacerbate this.

For which fungal skin infection should topical antifungal treatment not be used alone?

Tinea capitis treatment with topical antifungals should also include an oral antifungal agent owing to reduced absorption of topical formulations. In particular, ketoconazole shampoo should not be used because it is ineffective against scalp ringworm.

What topical preparations for the treatment of lice and scabies should not be used in patients with ragweed or chrysanthemum allergies?

Pyrethrin (Rid, A-200) and permethrin (Elimite, Nix)

How soon after varicella zoster exposure is the varicella vaccine effective for postexposure prophylaxis?

It should be administered within 3 days of exposure to varicella zoster.

What topical antibiotic causes more frequent allergic contact dermatitis than others?

Neomycin causes hypersensitivity reactions in 4% to 6% of patients.

When does phenytoin-induced skin eruption usually occur during treatment?

This usually occurs 7 to 21 days after initiation and almost always within the first 2 months of therapy.

If a phenytoin-induced skin eruptions occur, should the drug be stopped?

Yes, these reactions may proceed to fatal reactions, like toxic epidermal necrolysis.

How can warfarin-induced tissue necrosis be managed?

Discontinuation of warfarin with vitamin K reversal and the use of heparin

What drug can be used to minimize tissue injury from extravasation of sympathomimetic agents?

Phentolamine

ENDOCRINOLOGY

What sulfonylureas are associated with the longest duration of hypoglycemia?

Chlorpropamide and glyburide

Which insulin should not be mixed with any other kind of insulin due to its acidic pH?

Insulin glargine (Lantus)

When should patients on repaglinide or nateglinide be told to skip a dose?

When a meal is skipped, doses of meglitinide should be skipped too.

How much time should pass after initiating or changing the dose of TZDs before assessing the full effect?

Up to 3 to 4 months may be needed for the full effect TZDs.

How much weight gain may be seen with the TZDs?

Mild weight gain of 1.2 to 3.5 kg may be seen with rosiglitazone, and mild to moderate weight gain of 2 to 8 kg may be seen with pioglitazone

What drugs may be used in central diabetes insipidus secondary to their antidiuretic effects?

Chlorpropamide and carbamazepine

What corticosteroid may be administered prior to an ACTH stimulation test due to lack of interference with the cortisol assay?

Dexamethasone

When should TFTs be monitored after adjusting thyroid replacement medications?

6 to 8 weeks after dose adjustments until a maintenance dose is achieved

What effects on thyroid function does interferon alpha-2B for hepatitis C infection have?

Both hypothyroidism and hyperthyroidism may be observed, and in most patients these abnormalities are transient, requiring treatment if symptomatic.

What treatment for hyperthyroidism should not be given before radioactive iodine (RAI) treatment?

Iodides such as Lugol's solution should not be used because they cause decreased uptake of RAI by the thyroid gland. Thioamides should be stopped 3 days prior to RAI.

GASTROENTEROLOGY

What are five risk factors for NSAID-induced ulcers?

Age over 60 years, previous upper GI bleeding, concomitant corticosteroid therapy, concomitant anticoagulant therapy, high-dose and multiple NSAID use

What is the most common hematologic effect of the H2RAs?

Thrombocytopenia. It is reversible once the drug is discontinued.

What specific medications fall in the class of phenothiazines?

Include chlorpromazine, prochlorperazine, promethazine, and thiethylperazine

What are the concerns that limit the use of droperidol?

QT prolongation and torsades de pointes (black-box warning). The drug should be reserved for use after failure of other treatment options.

What is the appropriate dose of loperamide for the management of acute diarrhea?

The initial dose is 4 mg, followed by 2 mg after each loose stool up to a maximum of 16 mg/day.

In what clinical situations should the use of antidiarrheals be avoided?

In the setting of *Clostridium difficile* and bacterial enteritis caused by *Escherichia coli*, *Shigella*, or *Salmonella*.

HEMATOLOGY

What is the appropriate dose of vitamin B12 for the treatment of B12 deficiency?

100 μg IM daily for 1 week, weekly for 1 month, then monthly thereafter for maintenance

What are the vitamin K–dependent clotting factors and their respective half-lives?

They are factors II, VII, IX, X, and their half-lives are approximately 60, 6, 24, and 25 to 60 hours respectively.

What is the most prothrombotic substance in the body?

Tissue factor

What is the mechanism of action of fondaparinux?

Selectively inhibits antithrombin III that potentiates the neutralization of factor Xa, thus inhibiting thrombin and subsequent thrombus formation

What is the dosing of fondaparinux for the treatment of PE?

5 mg for patients <50 kg, 7.5 mg for patients 50 to 100 kg, and 10 mg for patients >100 kg

What is the appropriate first-line therapy in patients with von Willebrand disease type I?

A trial of desmopressin that works to stimulate endothelial cell release of von Willebrand factor and factor VIII

What is the likelihood of cross-reactivity with a low-molecular-weight heparin in a patient with documented HIT?

Approximately 97%; these drugs should not be used in the setting of HIT.

Name six drugs that have been associated with thrombocytopenia.

Abciximab, ticlopidine, linezolid, heparin, isotretinoin, H2Ras, and trimethoprim

What is the most appropriate course of action in a patient with an INR of 5 who is not actively bleeding or in need of an emergent procedure?

Hold the warfarin and allow the INR to fall on its own. Reversing with vitamin K can lead to delays in reanticoagulation.

Can the anticoagulant effect of enoxaparin be reversed?

Yes, partially. Protamine can be administered at a dose of 1 mg for every 1 mg of enoxaparin, and 60% to 75% reversibility may be achieved.

What patients are at highest risk for the development of a serious adverse effect with protamine?

Patients taking protamine-containing insulin, vasectomized or infertile males, and those with sensitivity to fish. These patients have a higher risk of developing antiprotamine antibodies and subsequently there is an adverse effect upon protamine administration.

IMMUNIZATIONS

What is the dosing schedule for the hepatitis B vaccine?

The dosing is 0.5 mL administered IM at 2, 4, and 6 months of age.

How many pneumococcal bacteria does the pneumococcal polysaccharide vaccine (PPV) protect against?

23

What are six indications for the administration of the PPV vaccine?

Patients over the age of 65, patients with heart disease, lung disease, sick cell disease, diabetes, or kidney failure

How is the pneumococcal vaccine administered?

0.5 mL given either IM or SQ

What is the appropriate dose of live attenuated influenza vaccine in adults?

This vaccine is given intranasally and is administered by spraying the vaccine into each nostril.

What are the most common adverse effects associated with the influenza vaccine administered IM?

Injection-site tenderness and low-grade fever that can begin as early as 6 to 12 hours following the vaccine and may last for 1 to 2 days

What is a rare adverse effect of the influenza vaccine?

Cases of Guillain-Barré syndrome have been reported.

What vaccine should be made readily available for college freshmen?

The meningococcal vaccine

INFECTIOUS DISEASES

What is one laboratory calculation that should be performed before prescribing the vast majority of antimicrobial agents?

Calculate the patient's creatinine clearance prior to prescribing any antibiotic.

Do vancomycin levels need to be monitored when the drug is administered orally for the treatment of *Clostridium difficile*?

No. Oral vancomycin exhibits a local effect in the GI tract and is not absorbed.

What antifungal drug and fluoroquinolone should not be used for urinary tract infections due to lack of urinary penetration?

Anidulafungin and moxifloxacin are not effective agents for urinary tract infections.

What is the most appropriate antibiotic to prescribe for gram negative coverage in a patient who is anaphylactic to penicillin?

Aztreonam

What are two common problems associated with the use of linezolid?

Linezolid is not a bactericidal agent; it is a static drug. Additionally, the drug requires monitoring of platelet counts due to the risk of thrombocytopenia.

When should nitrofurantoin use be avoided for the treatment of urinary tract infections caused by *E. coli*?

Patients with CrCl < 30 mL/min due to decreased ability to concentrate in the urine. Should also be avoided in elderly patients due to the risk of developing pulmonary fibrosis.

What are the most common causative organisms for infective endocarditis?

They include streptococci, staphylococci, and enterococci.

What is the recommended antibiotic and treatment duration for left-sided endocarditis due to MSSA?

Nafcillin 2 g every 4 hours for a treatment period of 4 to 6 weeks

What is the appropriate dose of gentamicin for synergy in the treatment of endocarditis?

1 mg/kg every 8 hours provided the patient has normal renal function

What are the difficulties in treating a patient with enterococcal endocarditis?

No single agent is bactericidal against this organism. Usually penicillin has high MICs and intrinsic resistance occurs with all cephalosporins. Therefore, combination therapy with a cell wall active agent along with an aminoglycoside is necessary.

NEPHROLOGY

In patients with hyperphosphatemia, when should calcium carbonate be taken to enhance its dissolution in the stomach?

With or directly before meals (calcium carbonate is more soluble at a lower gastric pH)

What calcium-containing product should not be used as a phosphate binder in patients with renal failure?

Calcium citrate should not be used because it increases the risk of aluminum toxicity by increasing gastric absorption of aluminum.

How frequently should darbepoetin dosages be adjusted in the treatment of anemia of chronic kidney disease?

No more than every 6 weeks

Which intravenous iron products do not require a test dose before treatment?

Iron sucrose and sodium ferric gluconate

What antihypertensive drug–drug interaction is often used in transplant patients to achieve desired cyclosporine levels with lower cyclosporine doses?

Diltiazem is often used because it inhibits the hepatic elimination of cyclosporine and allows lower doses of cyclosporine to be used.

What side effects may result from accumulation of the active metabolite of meperidine, normeperidine, in patients with renal impairment?

Neurotoxic side effects such as tremors, myoclonus, and seizures are particular risks associated with use of meperidine in patients with compromised renal function.

When does acute tubular necrosis from aminoglycoside therapy typically occur?

Usually after 7 to 10 days of therapy

What is the advantage of extended-release and transdermal forms of oxybutynin over immediate-release forms?

They have similar efficacy but transdermal and oral extended-release products have fewer anticholinergic side effects, such as dry mouth and constipation, but with added costs.

NEUROLOGY

When should serum concentrations of antiepileptic drugs be obtained?

In general, samples should be drawn before the morning dose and after four or five half-lives after initiation or dosage change.

What second-generation anticonvulsant is known to cause a skin rash for which the patient should seek immediate medical attention?

Lamotrigine, especially with rapid dose escalation. Phenytoin, carbamazepine, and phenobarbital are all first-generation anticonvulsants that also may cause a rash.

What cardiovascular effects may occur with rapid intravenous administration of phenytoin?

Hypotension, bradycardia, and cardiac dysrhythmias, including ventricular fibrillation, are effects most likely due to the propylene glycol diluent of the IV formulation.

What anticonvulsants are also FDA-approved for migraine prophylaxis?

Divalproex or valproic acid and topiramate

How long after dosing initiation of carbamazepine might a patient be at risk for loss of seizure control secondary to carbamazepine's induction of its own metabolism?

Autoinduction of carbamazepine's metabolism begins 3 to 5 days after dosing and is complete in about 1 month.

At what total phenytoin serum concentration do many patients have nystagmus?

Total phenytoin levels >20 μg/mL. Ataxia and diplopia frequently occur with levels >30 μg/mL and seizures and coma at concentrations >40 μg/mL.

What are two ways to overcome the slow onset of sustained-release carbidopa-levodopa (Sinemet CR) to improve morning immobility in patients with Parkinson's disease?

Supplement morning sustained-release carbidopa-levodopa with an immediate-release product

Give sustained-release carbidopa-levodopa to be taken 1 hour before arising

What medication used to control motor fluctuations in Parkinson's disease is also beneficial in the treatment of restless legs syndrome?

Ropinirole

What CNS side effects may occur with metronidazole at high doses (>1.5 g)?

Peripheral neuropathy and seizures are potential side effects.

ONCOLOGY

What is the most concerning adverse effect associated with the use of cisplatin?

Nephrotoxicity. Cisplatin is directly toxic to the renal tubules.

What should be done to minimize the adverse event with cisplatin?

Hydration. Patients should be administered 1 to 2 L of 0.9% normal saline pre- and postadministration; lower doses of the drug should be used in patients with renal insufficiency.

In what types of cancers does aldesleukin have a role?

Aldesleukin (interleukin-2, IL-2) is indicated for renal cell cancer and melanoma.

How does aldesleukin work?

The drug stimulates the growth, differentiation, and proliferation of activated T cells. IL-2 also generates lymphokine-activated killer-cell activity and stimulates the immune system against tumor cells.

What chemotherapeutic agents are most commonly implicated in the development of mucositis?

Mucositis is most commonly associated with 5-FU, methotrexate, and doxorubicin.

What medications are available that fall into the antiestrogen class for the treatment of breast cancer?

The available agents include aminoglutethimide, anastrazole, exemestane, fulvestrant, letrozole, megestrol acetate, tamoxifen, and toremifene.

What is the appropriate dose of filgrastim (G-CSF) in patients with neutropenia secondary to chemotherapy?

5 μg/kg/day with the exception of peripheral blood stem cell mobilization, where the recommended dose is 10 μg/kg/day.

At what point should platelet transfusions be considered in a patient with chemotherapy-induced thrombocytopenia?

When platelet counts drop below 20,000/mm³, there is increased risk for intracranial hemorrhage. Platelet transfusions are usually indicated when the platelet count drops to <10,000/mm³, or possibly sooner if the patient experiences signs or symptoms of hemorrhage.

PREGNANCY

What are the pharmaco-kinetic properties that make a drug more likely to cross the placenta and cause potential harm to the fetus?

Those that have low molecular weight (usually <1000 Da) and are highly lipophilic, un-ionized drugs

What are pharmacokinetic properties that make a drug less likely to cross into breast milk?

Drugs that have low lipid solubility, high molecular weight, and are ionized or highly protein-binding are less likely to cross into breast milk.

What does each FDA drug class mean during pregnancy?

    Class A

No documented fetal risk

    Class B

Animal studies suggest risk, but this has not been confirmed in human studies.

    Class C

No controlled human studies, but animal studies demonstrate adverse fetal effects. Use only if the benefit outweighs the risk.

    Class D

There is evidence in humans of adverse fetal effects. Use only in life-threatening cases.

    Class X

Documented adverse fetal effects in humans. These drugs are contraindicated.

Are loop diuretics acceptable to use in pregnant women?

They are class C agents. Other methods to control volume in patients should be tried first.

Are loop diuretics acceptable to use in breast-feeding women?

Yes. However, these agents will often reduce milk production.

Can ACE inhibitors be prescribed for women who are pregnant?

No. They fall into a class C group for the first trimester and class D for the second and third trimesters.

Can ACE inhibitors be prescribed for women who are breast-feeding?

ACE inhibitors are regarded by the American Academy of Pediatrics to be compatible with breast-feeding. Enalapril and captopril are secreted in lesser amounts in breast milk compared to others, but all are considered acceptable.

In which pregnancy category are the statin agents listed?

Statins are listed in pregnancy category X and should not be used.

What about statin use during breast-feeding?

It is unknown but possibly unsafe to use.

Can warfarin be used for treatment of VTE or PE in pregnancy?

Warfarin should be avoided due to the potential for fetal bleeding, stippled epiphyses, malformations of the nose, or CNS abnormalities (class X).

What antithrombotic agents can be used for prophylaxis or treatment of VTE or PE in pregnancy?

Low-molecular-weight heparins are the preferred agent, but unfractionated heparin may also be used in these conditions.

What medications may be recommended for the management of migraine or tension headaches during pregnancy?

Acetaminophen is the preferred agent. Nonsteroidal anti-inflammatory agents may be acceptable early in pregnancy but are contraindicated after 37 weeks of gestation.

What antimicrobials are considered safe to use for the treatment of urinary tract infections in pregnancy?

Ampicillin, amoxicillin, cephalexin, and nitrofurantoin are considered safe.

What types of vaccinations should be avoided during pregnancy?

Any vaccine that is a live virus should be avoided during the course of the pregnancy.

Should hypothyroidism be treated during pregnancy?

Absolutely. Untreated hypothyroidism can result in significant cognitive and other neurologic deficits in the fetus. There is also an increased risk of preeclampsia, low birth weight, and premature birth.

What medication can be prescribed to increase milk supply in a patient with declining serum prolactin concentrations?

Metoclopramide 10 mg three times a day for 7 to 14 days

PULMONOLOGY

What class of medications should be administered first to treat an acute asthma exacerbation?

Inhaled short acting beta-2 receptor agonist by nebulizer or MDI every 20 minutes

How do anticholinergic agents work in the setting of COPD?

The anticholinergic agents produce bronchodilation by competitively inhibiting cholinergic receptors in the bronchial smooth muscle.

What is the appropriate dose of anticholinergic agents for the management of COPD?

Ipratropium: 2 puffs four times daily; tiotropium: 1 capsule inhaled once daily

What are the most likely pathogens in uncomplicated acute exacerbations of COPD?

Haemophilus influenzae, Moraxella catarrhalis, Streptococcus pneumoniae, and *Haemophilus parainfluenzae*

What is the description and when is the most likely time course for a patient to experience an ACE inhibitor–induced cough?

Nonproductive, persistent, and paroxysmal. The cough may be observed as early as 3 days following initiation of therapy or may not occur for up to 1 year.

If the patient has an ACE inhibitor–induced cough, how long does it take to resolve?

It will usually dissipate within 4 days but may take up to 4 weeks.

What is the proposed mechanism ACE inhibitor–induced cough?	Inhibition in the breakdown of bradykinin and substance P. These substances then facilitate inflammation and stimulate lung irritation.
What are four medications that can induce pneumonitis and/or fibrosis?	Some of the agents are bleomycin, amiodarone, carmustine, and busulfan.
What is the mechanism of action of bosentan?	It acts on both the ET-A and ET-B receptors in the endothelium and vascular smooth muscle. Levels of endothelin 1 are elevated in pulmonary hypertension and can promote fibrosis, cell proliferation, and tissue remodeling.
What is the appropriate dose of bosentan for treatment of pulmonary hypertension?	62.5 mg twice daily for 4 weeks, then increase to 125 mg twice daily
What is the mechanism of action of sildenafil for the treatment of pulmonary hypertension?	Sildenafil citrate is an inhibitor of cGMP-specific phosphodiesterase type-5 (PDE5) in smooth muscle, resulting in relaxation and vasodilation. In pulmonary hypertension, this leads to vasodilation of the pulmonary vascular bed.

PSYCHIATRY

What SSRI does not require tapering?	Fluoxetine may be stopped abruptly because it has a long half-life of 60 hours and will clear the body after 2 weeks without major risk of withdrawal side effects.
What drug-drug interaction occurs between the antimicrobial linezolid and SSRIs?	Concomitant use of linezolid and SSRIs may increase the risk of serotonin syndrome. The literature supports discontinuation of the serotonergic agent 2 weeks before starting linezolid.
At what dose of bupropion do patients have an increased seizure risk?	The risk is dose-dependent, with increased risk at daily doses >450 mg. Bupropion is contraindicated in patients

with a history of seizures, bulimia or anorexia secondary to increased seizure risk.

What considerations should be taken when using antidepressants to treat anxiety disorders?

For the first weeks of treatment, SSRIs may need to be overlapped with benzodiazepines due to a lag time of 2 to 4 weeks for effectiveness and the occurrence of initial increased agitation and anxiety within a week of SSRI initiation.

Which antipsychotic drugs are available as long-acting depot preparations that can assist with patient compliance?

Two conventional antipsychotics available are haloperidol given every 28 days and fluphenazine given as fluphenazine decanoate every 2 to 4 weeks or fluphenazine enanthate every 1 to 2 weeks. Risperidone is the only second-generation antipsychotic available as a long-acting injection given every 2 weeks, but it has a 3-week lag time to full effect, requiring 3 weeks of concurrent oral antipsychotics.

What atypical antipsychotics are associated with weight gain?

Olanzapine and clozapine have the highest incidence of weight gain followed by quetiapine. This is usually most significant during the first 12 weeks of treatment, with a 3- to 15-lb weight gain.

Which atypical antipsychotics cause the least weight gain?

Ziprasidone and aripiprazole have a low tendency to promote weight gain.

What drugs may cause an increase in lithium levels?

NSAIDs, ACE inhibitors, and diuretics (thiazide-like diuretics having the greatest impact)

RHEUMATOLOGY

How often should intra-articular depot corticosteroids be given for rheumatoid arthritis joint pain?

Injections should be given no more than once every 3 months in the same joint.

Why are intra-articular injections limited?

Because too many injections may accelerate joint destruction

When are liver biopsies indicated during methotrexate (MTX) therapy?

For patients with suspected or known liver disease, a history of hepatitis, or jaundice, and for patients with persistent LFT abnormalities during or after MTX therapy

What FDA class, with regard to pregnancy, is leflunomide?

Class X. It is also unsafe during lactation.

What medication is recommended for childbearing women to enhance the elimination of leflunomide?

Cholestyramine given 8 g three times a day for 11 days is recommended for all childbearing women stopping leflunomide, since up to 2 years may be required to reach undetectable levels of the active metabolite.

What medication must be used in combination with infliximab for rheumatoid arthritis and why?

Methotrexate to minimize the formation of antibodies to infliximab

What warning regarding infection risk do the DMARDs adalimumab, etanercept, and infliximab have?

Patients are at risk for tuberculosis (TB) infection, and use is cautioned in patients with a history of TB or who are predisposed to infection.

What dose of hydralazine is associated with drug-induced lupus?

Daily dosages of >200 mg or a cumulative dose of 1 g

When is colchicine most effective during an acute gout attack?

Use within the first 12 to 24 hours of an attack is most effective because effectiveness decreases as duration of inflammation increases.

What class of antihypertensive drugs increases the risk of Stevens-Johnson syndrome when given with allopurinol?

ACE inhibitors

ABBREVIATIONS

ADHD	Attention-deficit/hyperactivity disorder
ANC	Absolute neutrophil count
APAP	Acetaminophen
ASA	Aspirin
AVH	Auditory and/or visual hallucinations
B-52	Benadryl 50 mg, haloperidol 5 mg, lorazepam 2 mg
BAL	Blood alcohol level
BPAD	Bipolar affective disorder
BPD	Borderline personality disorder
CBC	Complete blood count

CBT	Cognitive behavioral therapy
CBZ	Carbamazepine
CHF	Congestive heart failure
CNS	Central nervous system
CK	Creatine phosphokinase
CSF	Cerebrospinal fluid
CT	Computed tomography
CVA	Cerebrovascular accident
DBT	Dialectical behavioral therapy
DTs	Delirium tremens
ECT	Electroconvulsive therapy
EEG	Electroencephalogram
EPS	Extrapyramidal symptoms
GAD	Generalized anxiety disorder
GMC	General medical condition
HCG	Human chorionic gonadotropin
HI	Homicidal ideation
HIV	Human immunodeficiency virus
LFT	Liver function test
LOC	Loss of consciousness
MAOI	Monoamine oxidase inhibitor
MDD	Major depressive disorder
MDE	Major depressive episode
MMPI	Minnesota Multiphasic Personality Inventory
MMSE	Mini-Mental State Exam
MRI	Magnetic resonance imaging
NMS	Neuroleptic malignant syndrome
NPH	Normal-pressure hydrocephalus
OCD	Obsessive compulsive disorder
PTSD	Posttraumatic stress disorder
RPR	Rapid plasmin reagin
SA	Suicide attempt
SI	Suicidal ideation
SNRI	Serotonin-norepinephrine reuptake inhibitor
SSRI	Selective serotonin reuptake inhibitor
TCA	Tricyclic antidepressant
TD	Tardive dyskinesia
TFT	Thyroid function test
TLE	Temporal lobe epilepsy
UA	Urinalysis
UDS	Urine Drug Screen
VPA	Valproic acid
5-2-1	Haloperidol 5 mg, lorazepam 2 mg, benztropine 1 mg

PSYCHIATRIC ASSESSMENT

What should be included in a psychiatric history?

Information regarding onset, duration, temporal features, intensity, progression, and alleviating and exacerbating conditions of psychiatric symptoms. A thorough history must include a general medical history and review of systems, past psychiatric and medical histories, developmental and family history, social history including substance abuse, neurological history, current medications, and allergies. Owing to the nature of psychiatric illness, outside informants should be used whenever possible.

What is a mental status examination?

A detailed description of appearance, behavior and psychomotor activity, speech and language, mood (the patient's expression of his internal emotional state, usually a quote), affect (the examiner's description of the patient's emotional state), thought process, thought content, perceptual disturbances (i.e., hallucinations, delusions), insight, judgment, estimated intelligence (usually based on the history, vocabulary, and use of language), and neuropsychiatric and cognitive function (MMSE)

In performing the Mini-Mental State Exam (MMSE):[1]

    What questions can be asked to test orientation?

The date, day, month, season, year, floor, hospital, town, county, and state (*10 points*)

    What is a common way to test the patient's attention and ability to calculate?

Serial 7s—subtract 7 from 100 serially; stop after 5 answers. (*5 points*)

Alternatively, have the patient spell "world" backwards.

---

[1]From Folstein MF, Folstein SE, McHugh PR. "Mini-mental state." A practical method for grading the cognitive state of patients for the clinician. *J Psychiatr Res* 1975; 12(3):189–198.

How can short-term memory be tested?	Give the patient the names of three unrelated objects and make sure they register (*3 points*); 5 minutes later ask the patient to recall them. (*3 points*)
In what ways can language and language comprehension be tested?	Ask the patient to name a pen and a watch by sight. (*2 points*)
	Ask the patient to repeat, "No ifs, ands, or buts." (*1 point*)
	Give written ("Close your eyes") (*1 point*) and verbal (three-stage) commands for the patient to follow. (*3 points*)
	Ask the patient to write a sentence. (*1 point*)
How is spatial ability tested?	Ask the patient to copy two intersecting pentagons. (*1 point*)
How is the overall test scored?	The scores from the patient's correct answers are summed and compared to the total possible points. (*30*)
When can false-positive results occur on a mental state exam?	Poor effort, "pseudodementia" (i.e., dementia of depression)
When can false-negative results occur on a mental state exam?	Highly educated or intelligent individuals with early dementia and patients with right hemisphere lesions
What is the role of the physical examination in evaluating patients with psychiatric disorders?	Without exception, a thorough physical and neurologic examination is required for a complete psychiatric assessment. The brain is the substrate of behavior and can be affected by a myriad of medical illnesses.
What medical illnesses in the following categories can present with psychiatric problems?	
Neurologic	CVA, head trauma, epilepsy (especially complex partial), narcolepsy, NPH, Parkinson's disease, multiple sclerosis,

	Huntington's disease, and dementia [Alzheimer's type, vascular, Lewy body, Pick's disease (frontotemporal)]
Endocrine	Hypo- or hyperthyroidism, adrenal and parathyroid conditions, hypo- or hyperglycemia, hypopituitarism, pheochromocytoma, and gonadotrophic hormone
Metabolic	Fluid and electrolyte imbalance, hepatic encephalopathy, uremia, porphyria, Wilson's disease, hypoxia, hypotension, and hypertensive encephalopathy
Toxic	Intoxication or withdrawal from alcohol or drugs of abuse, side effects of prescription or over-the-counter drugs, herbals or natural "health" supplements, and exposure to environmental toxins
Nutritional	Deficiencies of vitamin B12, thiamine, nicotinic acid, or trace metals; malnutrition and dehydration
Infectious	AIDS, neurosyphilis, encephalitis, meningitis, brain abscess, viral hepatitis, infectious mononucleosis, tuberculosis, Lyme disease, and systemic bacterial or viral infections
Autoimmune	CNS vasculitis due to systemic lupus erythematosus or other autoimmune/rheumatologic diseases
Neoplastic	CNS primary or metastatic tumors, endocrine tumors, and pancreatic carcinoma
What common laboratory tests are ordered for psychiatric problems?	CBC, basic chemistries, LFTs, TFTs, HCG, RPR, B12, folate, UA, toxicology screens (APAP, ASA, UDS, BAL, etc.), therapeutic drug concentrations, occasionally CSF studies, head CT or MRI, EEG, and electrocardiogram

How many axes are there in the multiaxial categories?	5 – Axis I to axis V
For each category, describe the multiaxial category:	
Axis I	Clinical psychiatric disorders
Axis II	Personality disorders and specific developmental disorders
Axis III	Existing medical, surgical, or neurologic conditions
Axis IV	Psychosocial and environmental stressors
Axis V	Global assessment of functioning, reflecting the current or most recent highest level of functioning (social, occupational, psychological) on a scale from 1 (grossly impaired: danger of hurting self or others) to 100 (superior function)

MOOD DISORDERS

What illnesses are comprised by the mood disorders?	Major depression, dysthymic disorder, bipolar disorder, and cyclothymic disorder

MAJOR DEPRESSION

What is major depression?	A significant disturbance of mood and neurovegetative function (i.e., appetite, sleep, energy, libido, and concentration), which is persistent for a minimum of 2 weeks and not caused by the direct physiologic effects of a general medical condition or substance abuse
What is the prevalence of major depression?	Lifetime, 15%; 10% to 25% for women and 5% to 10% for men. The incidence of major depression is 10% in primary care patients, 15% in medical inpatients, and even higher for elderly patients.

What is the risk for relapse after one episode of major depression?　50%

What is the risk for relapse after three episodes of major depression?　80%

What are risk factors for major depression?　Female gender (up to twofold greater prevalence), environmental stress (e.g., loss of a spouse, unemployment), and genetics. First-degree relatives have a 1.5 to 3 times greater chance of development of major depression than the general population.

What are symptoms and signs of major depression?　Persistent presence of depressed mood, diminished interest (anhedonia), significant weight loss or weight gain reflecting appetite disturbance, insomnia or hypersomnia, psychomotor agitation or retardation, decreased energy, excessive guilt, feelings of worthlessness, inability to concentrate, impaired memory, and suicidal ideation. Anxiety, somatic complaints, or psychotic symptoms may be associated.

For each of the potential aspects of major depression below, list the features of each:

Psychotic　Delusions and hallucinations are present along with symptoms of major depression.

Catatonic features　Immobility or excessive, purposeless motor activity, mutism, posturing, echolalia or echopraxia

Melancholic　Loss of pleasure, lack of reactivity to usually pleasurable stimuli, mood worse in the morning, early-morning awakening, marked psychomotor retardation, anorexia, and excessive guilt

Atypical	Mood reactivity, hypersomnia, leaden paralysis, weight gain, rejection sensitivity
Postpartum	Depression within 4 weeks of delivery
Seasonal pattern	Depression generally in the fall or winter
What laboratory findings are associated with major depression?	About 10% of hospitalized depressed patients have a diagnosis of hypothyroidism.
What is the differential diagnosis of major depression?	Mood disorder resulting from a general medical condition, substance-induced mood disorder, dysthymic disorder, dementia, ADHD, bipolar depressed, adjustment disorder with depressed mood, and schizoaffective disorder
What percentage of individuals with a single episode of major depression will eventually develop bipolar disorder?	5% to 10%
What are the reasons to hospitalize someone with major depression?	Suicidality, psychotic depression, or inability to care for self (e.g., malnutrition)
What is the treatment for major depression?	Antidepressant medications (e.g., SSRIs, SNRIs, TCAs, MAOIs) or benzodiazepines for short-term treatment of anxiety symptoms; augmentation with lithium, thyroid hormone, or buspirone; individual psychotherapy; ECT
How well do antidepressants work?	More than 50% of patients with major depression will recover fully when an adequate dose of an antidepressant is used for an adequate duration of time (at least 6 weeks).
Why are SSRIs first-line treatments for depressive disorder illnesses?	Efficacy and tolerability

What are some of the side effects of SSRIs?

Most troubling side effects include gastrointestinal and sexual dysfunction

Why are TCAs infrequently used to treat depression when they are as effective as SSRIs?

TCAs have multiple side effects (anticholinergic, antihistaminergic, cardiac) and a low threshold for toxicity; an overdose on a 1-week supply can be deadly.

Why are MAOIs infrequently used?

One must follow strict dietary restrictions and avoid tyramine-containing foods as well as serotonergic and sympathomimetic medications. Additionally, MAOIs can cause severe orthostasis.

What can happen if MAOIs are used in combination with tyramine-containing foods or with serotonergic or sympathomimetic medications?

An adrenergic crisis (hypertension, fever, tachycardia, arrhythmia) may occur.

What advantage does the MAOI transdermal patch selegiline offer?

At the lowest dosage, no dietary modification is required.

What medications are SNRIs?

Venlafaxine and duloxetine

How does buspirone work?

Buspirone is a $5-HT_{1A}$ partial agonist. It increases dopamine and norepinephrine in the CNS.

How does bupropion differ from SSRIs?

It rarely induces sexual dysfunction and may be used as an adjunct in SSRI-induced sexual dysfunction.

What side effect is most worrisome with bupropion immediate release?

Seizures (especially in patients with anorexia); but this risk is comparable to that of SSRIs when administered in a sustained-release preparation.

How does mirtazapine work?

It is an alpha-1 adrenergic antagonist (which increases serotonin and norepinephrine at the synapse), potent histaminergic H_1 receptor antagonist (somnolence and weight gain), and a $5-HT_2$ and $5-HT_3$ receptor antagonist.

How does trazodone work?	It inhibits serotonin reuptake, antagonizes alpha-1 adrenergic receptors, and has antihistaminergic activity. It is usually used as a treatment for insomnia in lower than therapeutic doses (i.e., 100 mg vs. 400 mg).
What side effect of trazodone is rare, but requires immediate medical attention?	Priapism (especially in older men with vascular disease)
What are the primary indications for ECT?	Failure of several antidepressant trials, severe depression with psychotic features, high risk of suicide, and previous good response to ECT
What are the contraindications to ECT?	Increased intracranial pressure is the only absolute contraindication; however, other high risk medical conditions (i.e., recent myocardial infarction or CVA) must be thoroughly reviewed.
What is the response rate for ECT?	70% to 90%, thus making it the most effective treatment for major depression
What are the primary side effects of ECT?	Memory loss and delirium
What is the prognosis for major depression?	Up to 15% of patients die by suicide; 50% of patients will have a second episode.

DYSTHYMIC DISORDER

What is dysthymic disorder?	A chronic illness characterized by depressed mood more days than not for at least 2 years.
How does dysthymic disorder present?	Two or more neurovegetative symptoms including poor appetite or overeating, sleep disturbance, decreased sexual interest, decreased energy, low self-esteem, and poor concentration. It may present with irritability in adolescents. No major depressive episode is present during the first 2 years.

What is the prevalence of dysthymic disorder?

Lifetime, 6%

What are risk factors for dysthymic disorder?

Adolescence and family history of mood disorders; there are no gender differences for incidence rates.

What is the differential diagnosis for dysthymic disorder?

Major depression, minor depressive disorder, mood disorder caused by a general medical condition, substance-induced mood disorder, and personality disorder

What is the treatment for dysthymic disorder?

Antidepressants, cognitive therapy, and insight-oriented (psychoanalytic) psychotherapy

How common is double depression, and what is it?

40% of patients with MDD also meet criteria for dysthymic disorder (double depression).

What percentage of patients with dysthymic disorder experience onset of symptoms before age 25 years?

50%; 20% of patients with dysthymic disorder progress to MDD, 15% to bipolar II, and <5% to bipolar I.

BIPOLAR DISORDER (MANIC-DEPRESSIVE ILLNESS)

What is bipolar disorder?

A chronic, remitting mood disorder characterized by periods of mania, depression, or mixed mood episodes. It may be associated with psychotic symptoms.

What is a manic episode?

A distinct period of persistently and abnormally elevated, irritable, or expansive mood lasting at least 1 week; the episode causes marked impairment.

What is a hypomanic episode?

A distinct period of persistently elevated, irritable, or expansive mood lasting at least 4 days; it is not severe enough to cause marked impairment, and there is no psychosis.

What are some of the features of a manic or hypomanic episode?	Inflated self-esteem or grandiosity, decreased sleep (rested after 3 hours), pressured speech, racing thoughts, distractibility, psychomotor agitation, and enhanced libido or unrestrained buying sprees
What drugs are associated with manic-like episodes?	Amphetamines, baclofen, bromide, bromocriptine, caffeine, captopril, cimetidine, cocaine, corticosteroids, cyclosporine, disulfiram, hallucinogens, hydralazine, isoniazid, levodopa, methylphenidate, metrizamide, opiates and opioids, procarbazine, and procyclidine
What is a mixed mood episode?	Features of both major depression and mania are present for at least 1 week. Also known as dysphoric mania, a mixed mood episode is thought to be a rapid alteration of mania and depression and places one at a higher risk of suicide.
What is the prevalence of bipolar disorder?	Lifetime, 1% to 2% Type I has a 0.4% to 1.6% lifetime prevalence Type II has a 0.5% lifetime prevalence
What is the difference between bipolar type I and type II?	Patients with bipolar type I have at least had one manic or mixed episode; a depressive episode is not necessary. Patients with bipolar type II have had at least one depressive and one hypomanic episode without having a manic or mixed episode.
What gender differences exist in bipolar disorder?	The incidence is equivalent among males and females; however, some studies suggest that a rapid-cycling bipolar course is more common in women.
What does it mean for one to be bipolar with rapid cycling?	At least four episodes of a mood disturbance (depressive, mixed, manic, or hypomanic) in the past year

What is the average age of onset for bipolar disorder?

19 years; new-onset bipolar disorder is uncommon after the fifth decade of life.

What are risk factors for bipolar disorder?

First-degree relatives of bipolar patients have increased rates of mood disorders. Twin and adoption studies support a strong genetic influence. Varied stressors often serve as environmental triggers for mood episodes.

What is the differential diagnosis for bipolar disorder?

Mood disorder caused by a general medical condition, substance-induced mood disorder, cyclothymia, personality disorders (especially borderline), schizophrenia, and schizoaffective disorder

What is the treatment for bipolar disorder?

Consider hospitalization for acute mania, severe depression, and associated psychosis; mood stabilizers (e.g., lithium, lamotrigine, and VPA), benzodiazepines, and antipsychotic medications for acute mania and psychosis; ECT for severe, intractable mania; and psychotherapy.

Which mediations should be avoided and why?

Antidepressants are avoided because they commonly precipitate mania.

Which medications are indicated for acute mania?

Lithium, valproic acid, and atypical antipsychotics

What are the side effects and toxicities associated with lithium?

Lithium is generally nontoxic below 1.2 mEq/L; however, sedation, poor memory and concentration, fine hand tremor, nausea, diarrhea, polyuria, polydipsia, psoriasis, and weight gain may all be signs of minor toxicity. For severe toxicity (i.e., delirium, arrhythmia, acute renal failure, etc.) dialysis is needed.

What is lithium's effect on suicide?

Randomized studies have shown a powerful preventive effect on suicide.

What is the teratogenicity associated with lithium?

Ebstein's anomaly, a malformation of the tricuspid valve, is associated with lithium use in the first trimester.

Which anticonvulsant is likely to be more effective than lithium in treating mixed and rapid-cycling bipolar states?	Valproic acid
What are the toxic effects of valproic acid?	Mild and transient elevations of AST and ALT and possible fatal hepatotoxicity, hemorrhagic pancreatitis, thrombocytopenia, aplastic anemia; thus, monitor LFTs and CBC.
What are the teratogenic effects associated with valproic acid?	Neural tube defects and neonatal liver disease
What is the most serious side effect of lamotrigine?	A rash, which may lead to Stevens-Johnson syndrome
What other medications can be used for bipolar disorder?	Carbamazepine, oxcarbazepine, topiramate, and gabapentin
Does the frequency of mood disturbances change with age, and how does this affect treatment?	Each episode makes an additional future episode more likely (kindling theory); the subsequent episodes may be longer in duration and less likely to respond to medication.
What is the prognosis for bipolar disorder?	Rule of thirds: One third develop a chronic, unremitting course. One third continue to have intermittent episodes. One third have remission with treatment. Up to 15% of patients die by suicide.
What comorbid conditions exist in conjunction with bipolar disorder?	Substance abuse: 60% lifetime prevalence Anxiety disorders: 50% lifetime prevalence Attention deficit hyperactivity disorder Cluster B personality disorders (especially borderline) Eating disorders

CYCLOTHYMIC DISORDER

What is cyclothymic disorder?

A chronic mood disturbance lasting at least 2 years and characterized by fluctuating periods of depressive symptoms (which do not meet criteria for major depression) and hypomanic symptoms

What is the prevalence of cyclothymic disorder?

Lifetime, 1%

What are risk factors for cyclothymic disorder?

First-degree relatives have an increased incidence of mood disorders, especially bipolar I. There is an increased family history of substance abuse.

What are symptoms and signs of cyclothymic disorder?

Chronic, persistent presence of mood disturbance with features of hypomania and depression. Substance abuse is common; 5% to 10% have substance dependence.

What is the average age of onset for cyclothymic disorder?

Teens or early twenties; 33% develop a major mood disorder, primarily bipolar II.

What is the differential diagnosis for cyclothymic disorder?

Mood disorder caused by a general medical condition, substance-induced mood disorder, rapid-cycling bipolar disorder, borderline personality disorder, and ADHD.

What is the treatment for cyclothymic disorder?

Mood stabilizers (e.g., lithium, lamotrigine, VPA, and CBZ) and antimanic drugs; not antidepressants because they may induce manic or hypomanic episodes in 40% to 50% of cyclothymic patients; and psychotherapy

COGNITIVE DISORDERS

DELIRIUM

What is delirium?

A potentially reversible cognitive disturbance caused by a general medical condition that typically develops acutely and fluctuates over time

What percent of medically ill hospitalized patients exhibit delirium?	10% to 30%; the percentage is higher in surgical and cardiac intensive care units.

For each system, name the major causes of delirium:

Cardiovascular?	Heart failure, arrhythmias, hypotension
Endocrine?	Dysfunction of the pituitary, thyroid, parathyroid, adrenal, or pancreas
Gastrointestinal?	Hepatic encephalopathy, impaction in the elderly
Infectious?	Sepsis, urinary tract infection
Neurologic?	Epilepsy, postictal states, concussions, meningitis or encephalitis, brain tumor, etc.
Pulmonary?	Carbon dioxide narcosis, hypoxia
Renal?	Uremic encephalopathy

For each of the following, name what can be associated with delirium:

Metabolic?	Electrolyte imbalance
Nutritional deficiency?	Thiamine, B12, folic acid
Drugs?	Anticholinergic agents, opiates, sedatives, steroids, etc.
Poisons?	Heavy metals, carbon monoxide
Surgical?	Postoperative states
What are the risk factors for the development of delirium?	Elderly, history of brain damage, having cardiac surgery, burn injury, and sleep deprivation
What is the treatment for delirium?	The primary goal is to treat the underlying cause.

How can the psychosis associated with delirium be treated?	Minimize medications if possible. However, haloperidol is often used to treat the agitated, delirious patient; off-label use of atypical antipsychotics is also done. Of note, antipsychotics are associated with prolongation of the QTc, leading to arrhythmias.

DEMENTIA

What is dementia?	Chronic and continuing cognitive decline involving deficits in memory and one additional impairment (aphasia, apraxia, agnosia, or executive dysfunction)
What is the prevalence of dementia in those over 65 years of age?	1.5%
What is the prevalence of dementia in those over 85 years of age?	16% to 25%
What disorders may cause dementia?	Alzheimer's disease, Parkinson's disease, Huntington's disease, Pick's disease, Lewy body disease, vascular disease [e.g., multi-infarct dementia or small vessel (Binswanger's) dementia], drugs (e.g., chronic alcoholic dementia/thiamine deficiency), head trauma, normal-pressure hydrocephalus, intracranial masses, thyroid disease, neurosyphilis, B12 deficiency, AIDS, chronic sleep apnea, lupus, and severe depression (dementia of depression)
What is the treatment for dementia?	For reversible causes (although they are evident in less than 15% of cases): psychosocial interventions (e.g., patient safety, legal issues, finances); behavioral interventions (e.g., wandering, psychosis, agitation); medications (e.g., cognitive enhancers)

What are the cognitive enhancers?	Cholinesterase inhibitors—donepezil, rivastigmine, and galantamine
	N-methyl-D-aspartate receptor antagonist—memantine
What are the FDA indications for cognitive enhancers?	Alzheimer's disease, vascular dementia
How do the cognitive enhancers work?	None of these medications stop the progression of cognitive decline; rather, they may slow the rate of decline by up to a year.

PSYCHOTIC DISORDERS

What are psychotic symptoms?	Delusions, hallucinations, disorganized speech (e.g., incoherence, marked loosening of associations, neologisms), and grossly disorganized or catatonic behavior. Symptoms may be described as impairment in reality testing.
What psychiatric diseases can present with psychotic symptoms?	Delirium, dementia, mood disorders, substance use disorders, schizophrenia, and the schizophrenia-like disorders [e.g., schizophreniform disorder, brief psychotic disorder, schizoaffective disorder, delusional disorder, and shared psychotic disorder (folie à deux)]

SCHIZOPHRENIA

What is schizophrenia?	A chronic, relapsing-remitting psychotic illness of at least 6 months' duration that includes at least 1 month of two or more active phase symptoms. Impairment in social and occupational functioning is a key feature.
What are the active-phase symptoms of schizophrenia?	"Positive symptoms" (e.g., delusions, hallucinations), disorganized speech, grossly disorganized or catatonic behavior, and "negative" symptoms (e.g., affective flattening, paucity of thought and speech, and lack of motivation)

What are the subtypes of schizophrenia?

Paranoid, disorganized, catatonic, undifferentiated, and residual

What is the annual incidence of schizophrenia?

0.5 to 5.0 per 10,000; prevalence, 1 in 100

What gender differences exist in schizophrenia?

Although the prevalence is equal in men and women, men tend to be afflicted earlier than women; the peak age of onset for men is between 10 and 25 years of age, whereas for women it is between 25 and 35 years. Men also are more likely to be impaired by negative symptoms.

What are risk factors for schizophrenia?

Genetic predisposition—twin studies show 45% to 50% monozygotic concordance compared with 10% to 15% dizygotic concordance. First-degree relatives have a 5- to 10-fold increased risk. Birth during early winter months and spring, obstetric complications, lower socioeconomic status, and immigration have all been associated.

What features have a good prognosis?

Late or acute onset, an obvious precipitant, good premorbid functioning, married, strong support system, positive symptoms, mood disorder component, family history of mood disorders

What features have a poor prognosis?

Young or insidious onset, no precipitant, poor premorbid functioning, unmarried, poor support, negative symptoms, withdrawn behavior, many relapses

What is the differential diagnosis of schizophrenia with regard to medical conditions?

Psychotic disorder due to a general medical condition (e.g., AIDS, B12 deficiency, CNS tumor, CVA, herpes encephalitis, lupus, neurosyphilis, porphyria, Wilson's disease); substance-induced psychotic disorder; epilepsy (especially TLE); delirium; dementia

What is the differential diagnosis of schizophrenia with regard to psychiatric conditions?

Mood disorder with psychotic features, schizoaffective disorder, schizophreniform disorder, brief psychotic disorder, delusional disorder, and cluster A personality disorder

What is the treatment for schizophrenia?

Antipsychotic medications (e.g., typical or atypical neuroleptics) and behavioral and group therapies; consider hospitalization.

How do typical antipsychotics work?

These agents antagonize dopamine D_2 receptors.

What side effects are seen with typical high-potency antipsychotics?

Dystonia, akathisia, and parkinsonian symptoms (e.g., haloperidol, fluphenazine)

What side effects are seen with typical low-potency antipsychotics?

Sedation, hypotension, weight gain, and anticholinergic symptoms (e.g., chlorpromazine)

Are the side effects of TD and NMS related to drug potency?

TD and NMS are unrelated to the neuroleptic's potency.

How do atypical antipsychotics work?

These agents antagonize dopamine D_2 as well as serotonin $5\text{-}HT_2$ receptors.

What advantages do atypical antipsychotics have over typical antipsychotics?

Reduced EPS and better effectiveness in treating negative symptoms

What disadvantages exist?

They are more costly and linked to hyperglycemia and diabetes; certain atypicals are also linked to weight gain and hyperlipidemia. The FDA warns of an increased mortality risk in elderly dementia patients on atypical antipsychotics.

What are the atypical agents?

Clozapine, olanzapine, quetiapine, risperidone, paliperidone, ziprasidone, and aripiprazole

Which atypical is most effective for treatment-resistant psychotic patients?

Clozapine—prevents relapse, improves negative symptoms, reduces aggression, and it may decrease the risk of suicide in patients with schizophrenia

Why is clozapine used infrequently?

Side effects, including agranulocytosis (granulocytes $<500/mm^3$) in 1% of patients; weekly monitoring of the ANC is required.

Which atypical can be given every 2 weeks in depot formulation?

Risperidone (as Risperdal Consta)

How is aripiprazole unique?

It is a partial agonist at D_2 and $5\text{-}HT_{1A}$ receptors and a potent antagonist at $5\text{-}HT_{2A}$ receptors.

What adjuvant therapies can be considered for treatment resistant schizophrenia?

Dual antipsychotic therapy, lithium, ECT, antidepressants, buspirone, anticonvulsants (CBZ, VPA), benzodiazepines, and beta blockers

What percentage of schizophrenics will have disabling residual symptoms and impaired social functioning?

25% to 50%; in fact, only about 20% have a good outcome.

What other problems are associated with schizophrenia?

Suicide; over 50% of schizophrenics attempt suicide and 10% to 15% succeed.

At least 75% of schizophrenics smoke cigarettes, 30% to 50% are alcoholics, 15% to 25% are cannabis users, and $<10\%$ are cocaine users.

Schizophrenics have an increased rate of violence, especially in those who experience paranoia.

Around 50% of the homeless probably have schizophrenia.

SCHIZOPHRENIFORM DISORDER

What is schizophreniform disorder?

Essential features (risk factors, signs/symptoms, differential, and treatment) are the same as those of schizophrenia except (1) total duration of the illness is at least 1 month but less than 6 months and (2) impaired social and occupational functioning is not required for diagnosis. When the diagnosis is made without waiting for recovery, it should be qualified as "provisional."

What is the prevalence of schizophreniform disorder?

Lifetime, 1 in 500

What is the prognosis for schizophreniform disorder?

Prognosis is better with short duration of illness. 60% to 80% will progress to schizophrenia or schizoaffective disorder. There is a high suicide risk.

BRIEF PSYCHOTIC DISORDER

What is a brief psychotic disorder?

Sudden onset of one or more of the following psychotic symptoms: delusions, hallucinations, disorganized speech, or disorganized or catatonic behavior. Duration is at least 1 day but less than 1 month with ultimate return to premorbid functioning.

What is the prevalence of brief psychotic disorder?

Unknown, but it is considered rare.

What are risk factors for brief psychotic disorder?

Catastrophic stressors, young adulthood, and associated premorbid personality disorders

What is the differential diagnosis for brief psychotic disorder?

Factitious disorder, malingering, psychotic disorder resulting from a general medical condition, substance-induced psychosis, delirium, epilepsy, dissociative identity disorder, borderline personality disorder, and schizotypal personality disorder

What is the treatment for brief psychotic disorder?

Hospitalization, antipsychotic medications, benzodiazepines (for 2 to 3 weeks), and psychotherapy

What is the prognosis for brief psychotic disorder?

50% of patients who are first classified as having brief psychotic disorder are later diagnosed with schizophrenia or other chronic psychiatric syndromes. However, European studies have reported a good prognosis, with 50% to 80% of patients having no further major psychiatric ailments.

SCHIZOAFFECTIVE DISORDER

What is schizoaffective disorder?

An illness with features of both schizophrenia and mood disorders characterized by an uninterrupted period of illness during which, at some point, there is a major depressive, manic, or mixed episode concurrent with psychotic symptoms consistent with schizophrenia. In addition, there is a period of at least 2 weeks that consists of delusions or hallucinations in the absence of mood symptoms.

What are the subtypes of schizoaffective disorder?

Bipolar and depressive

What is the prevalence of schizoaffective disorder?

Lifetime, 0.5% to 0.8%

What gender differences exist in schizoaffective disorder?

There is a lower prevalence in men than in women. As in schizophrenia, the age of onset for women is later than for men.

What are risk factors for schizoaffective disorder?

Genetics and female gender. There is increased risk for schizophrenia among the relatives of probands with schizoaffective disorder.

What are symptoms and signs of schizoaffective disorder?	The presence of symptoms consistent with mania, major depression, or a mixed mood state concurrent with psychotic symptoms consistent with schizophrenia. Furthermore, one must have additional psychotic symptoms without the mood syndrome.
What is the differential diagnosis of schizoaffective disorder?	Psychotic disorder resulting from a general medical condition, delirium, dementia, substance-induced psychotic disorder, delusional disorder, and mood disorder with psychotic features
What is the treatment for schizoaffective disorder?	Hospitalization, antipsychotic medications, mood stabilizers, antidepressants, and group psychotherapy; ECT can be considered.
What is the prognosis for schizoaffective disorder?	In general, prognosis ranges between that of patients with schizophrenia and those with mood disorders. Those with predominantly affective symptoms have a better prognosis than those with predominantly schizophrenic symptoms.

DELUSIONAL DISORDER

What is delusional disorder?	An illness characterized by the presence of one or more nonbizarre delusions for at least 1 month. Delusions may be erotomanic, grandiose, jealous, persecutory, somatic, mixed, or unspecified.
What is the prevalence of delusional disorder?	0.025% to 0.03%
What gender differences exist in delusional disorder?	There are slightly more female patients than male. Men are more likely to have paranoid delusions or delusions of infidelity, whereas women are more likely to have erotomanic delusions.

What are risk factors for delusional disorder?

Midlife, recent immigration, low socioeconomic status, family history, personality features (e.g., atypical interpersonal sensitivity), sensory impairment, and social isolation

What are signs and symptoms of delusional disorder?

One or more nonbizarre delusions for at least 1 month. Tactile and olfactory hallucinations may be present, but there are no other symptoms of schizophrenia.

What is the differential diagnosis of delusional disorder?

Delirium, dementia, malingering, factitious disorder, psychotic disorder caused by a general medical condition, substance-induced psychotic disorder, schizophrenia, mood disorders with psychotic features, shared psychotic disorder, OCD, somatoform disorders, paranoid personality disorder

What is the treatment for delusional disorder?

Generally difficult to treat owing to the patient's poor insight and compliance with treatment. Hospitalization if the patient is agitated, antipsychotic medications, psychotherapy, and family therapy

SHARED PSYCHOTIC DISORDER (FOLIE À DEUX)

What is a shared psychotic disorder?

A delusion that develops in one person (the secondary case) who is involved in a close relationship with another person (the primary case) who has a preexisting delusion. Usually, the primary case is dominant in the relationship and chronically ill (e.g., schizophrenia). The secondary case is typically more gullible and passive. The relationship may involve more than two people and has been reported in families (folie à famille).

What is the incidence of shared psychotic disorder?

Rare. It may be more common in women.

What are risk factors for shared psychotic disorder?	Affected individuals often have a family history of schizophrenia. A genetic predisposition has also been suggested. Old age, low intelligence, cerebrovascular disease, and alcohol abuse are often involved factors.
What is the differential diagnosis of shared psychotic disorder?	Malingering, factitious disorder, psychotic disorder caused by a general medical condition, substance-induced psychotic disorder, schizophrenia, mood disorders with psychotic features, delusional disorder, OCD, somatoform disorders, paranoid personality disorder, delirium, and dementia
What is the treatment for shared psychotic disorder?	Separation from the primary case may be all that is necessary for the secondary case to give up the delusional belief. Family therapy with nondelusional members of the family and antipsychotic medications may be necessary. Treatment of the psychiatric disorder afflicting the primary case is necessary.

ANXIETY DISORDERS

What illnesses are comprised by the anxiety disorders?	Panic disorder with and without agoraphobia, specific phobia, social phobia, obsessive-compulsive disorder, posttraumatic stress disorder, acute stress disorder, and generalized anxiety disorder
What is the lifetime prevalence of pathologic anxiety?	25%, thus making anxiety disorders the most prevalent psychiatric disorders in the population
What medical conditions are commonly associated with anxiety?	Endocrine: diabetes, thyroid or parathyroid disease, pheochromocytoma Drug-related: caffeine, steroids, sympathomimetics, thyroid hormone, or withdrawal from alcohol, sedatives, or narcotics

Metabolic: electrolyte abnormalities, acidosis

Neurologic: seizures (e.g., TLE), vestibular dysfunction

Respiratory: causes of hypoxia (e.g., COPD, CHF)

PANIC DISORDER

What is panic disorder?	Recurrent, unexpected panic attacks with or without agoraphobia; one panic attack must be followed by at least 1 month of fear about having further attacks, worry about the consequences of an attack, or change in behavior related to the attack.
What is a panic attack?	The sudden development of a discrete period of intense fear or discomfort
What are some of the signs and symptoms of a panic attack?	Tachycardia, palpitations, sweating, trembling, shortness of breath, choking sensation, chest pain or tightness, abdominal discomfort, dizziness, derealization or depersonalization, fear of losing control or dying, paresthesias, or chills or hot flushes
What is agoraphobia?	Anxiety of being in places where escape is difficult or impossible (e.g., public, crowded places). The fear is usually associated with having a panic attack in an unprotected place.
What is the prevalence of panic disorder?	Lifetime, 1.5% to 3.5%
What is the usual duration and course of symptoms of panic disorder?	Attacks usually begin with a 10-minute period of escalating symptoms and last 20 to 30 minutes.
What is the differential diagnosis for panic disorder?	Anxiety disorder caused by a general medical condition and substance-induced anxiety disorder

What is the treatment for panic disorder?	Antidepressants, benzodiazepines (e.g., alprazolam, clonazepam, and lorazepam), and cognitive therapies
What advantage do benzodiazepines have in treating panic disorder?	Benzodiazepines have the most rapid onset of action, usually within the first week. They can also be used effectively on an as-needed basis.
What disadvantage do benzodiazepines have in treating panic disorder?	Potential for abuse, dependence, withdrawal effects, and cognitive impairment (especially in the elderly); patients should not drive or operate dangerous equipment while taking benzodiazepines.

SPECIFIC PHOBIA (SIMPLE PHOBIA)

What is specific phobia?	A persistent, unreasonable fear brought about by the presence or anticipation of a specific object or situation (e.g., animals, blood, heights, enclosed spaces, etc.)
What is the lifetime prevalence of specific phobia?	10%
What is the treatment for specific phobia?	Exposure-based interventions (utilizing CBT) are the mainstay of treatment. Benzodiazepines used on an as-needed basis can limit anxiety and facilitate exposure.

SOCIAL PHOBIA (SOCIAL ANXIETY DISORDER)

What is social phobia?	A persistent, unreasonable fear of social or performance situations where the individual is exposed to possible scrutiny and is afraid of acting in a way that is embarrassing
What is the lifetime prevalence of social phobia?	3% to 15%
What is the treatment for social phobia?	SSRIs, MAOIs, beta blockers, benzodiazepines, and CBT, including exposure interventions and role playing

OBSESSIVE-COMPULSIVE DISORDER

What is OCD?	An illness characterized by recurrent obsessions or compulsions that cause significant distress or impairment in functioning
What are obsessions?	Persistent and recurrent images, impulses, or thoughts that are not merely excessive worries about real-life problems but rather intrusive and inappropriate
What are compulsions?	Repetitive behaviors (e.g., hand washing, checking) or mental acts (e.g., praying, counting) that a person feels compelled to perform in order to reduce anxiety or prevent an imagined dreaded event or situation
What is the prevalence of OCD?	Lifetime, 2% to 3%
What are risk factors for OCD?	Studies show a higher rate of concordance for monozygotic than dizygotic twins; 35% of first-degree relatives of patients are also afflicted with the disorder.
What are symptoms and signs of OCD?	Generally, gradual onset of obsessions or compulsions, usually in late teens or early twenties. The patient generally has insight into the irrationality of the illness. Skin problems may be present owing to excessive washing.
What is the differential diagnosis of OCD?	Anxiety disorder caused by a general medical condition, substance-induced anxiety disorder, body dysmorphic disorder, major depressive episode, hypochondriasis, specific phobia, and tic disorders
What is the treatment for OCD?	High-dose SSRIs; clomipramine; MAOIs; augmentation with lithium, VPA, or CBZ; buspirone; benzodiazepines; and cognitive behavioral therapy

POSTTRAUMATIC STRESS DISORDER

What is PTSD?	Characteristic symptoms that develop after a person is exposed to a traumatic event involving actual or threatened death or serious injury to self or others and the person's response involved horror, helplessness, or intense fear
What is the prevalence of PTSD?	Lifetime, 8%; for those injured in combat, the prevalence is 20%
What are risk factors for PTSD?	Exposure to considerable conflict or unrest; suffering a life-threatening accident or assault
What are symptoms and signs of PTSD?	Greater than 1 month of persistent reexperiencing of the traumatic event through recurrent and intrusive images, thoughts, or perceptions; recurrent distressing dreams of the event; flashbacks; avoidance of stimuli associated with the trauma; and hyperarousal and hypervigilance, including difficulty sleeping, irritability, difficulty concentrating, hypervigilance, and exaggerated startle response
What is the differential diagnosis of PTSD?	Head injury from sustained trauma, substance-related disorders, adjustment disorder, acute stress disorder, OCD, malingering, factitious disorder, dissociative disorders, and borderline personality disorder
How does acute stress disorder differ from PTSD?	For acute stress disorder, symptoms occur within 4 weeks of the traumatic event and last no more than 4 weeks.
What is the treatment for PTSD?	Mainstays of treatment are SSRIs, TCAs, MAOIs, and buspirone. Other treatments include lithium, VPA, CBZ, clonidine, propranolol, benzodiazepines, antipsychotics, and psychotherapy (e.g., individual, CBT, or group).

GENERALIZED ANXIETY DISORDER

What is generalized anxiety disorder?	Excessive worry and anxiety over a number of activities or situations occurring for a period of at least 6 months
What are symptoms and signs of generalized anxiety disorder?	Anxiety associated with restlessness, easy fatigability, difficulty concentrating, irritability, muscle tension, or disturbed sleep
What is the prevalence of GAD?	Lifetime, 5%; women are twice as likely to be affected.
What is the differential diagnosis for generalized anxiety disorder?	Anxiety disorder resulting from a general medical condition, substance-induced anxiety disorder, mood disorder with anxious features, adjustment disorder, ADHD, hypochondriasis, somatization disorder, and personality disorders
What is the treatment for generalized anxiety disorder?	SSRIs, SNRIs, TCAs, MAOIs, buspirone, beta blockers, benzodiazepines, CBT, and anxiety management skills (e.g., relaxation techniques)

ADJUSTMENT DISORDERS

What is an adjustment disorder?	Development of clinically significant behavioral or emotional symptoms in excess of what would normally be expected within 3 months of an identifiable stressor.
What is the natural history of the illness?	The condition resolves within 6 months of the stressor being terminated.
What are the different types of adjustment disorders?	Adjustment disorder with depressed mood, anxiety, mixed anxiety and depressed mood, disturbance of conduct, mixed disturbance of emotions and conduct, and unspecified

What is the prevalence of adjustment disorder?	2% to 10%; women are diagnosed twice as often as men; nearly 50% of patients with specific medical problems or stressors have been diagnosed with an adjustment disorder.
What is the differential diagnosis of adjustment disorder?	Personality disorders, mood disorders, anxiety disorders (e.g., PTSD, acute stress disorder), substance-related disorders, bereavement, and nonpathologic response to stress
What is the treatment for adjustment disorder?	Psychotherapy primarily; may augment with SSRIs for traumatic grief, low-dose antipsychotic medications if there are signs of decompensation, and short-term use of benzodiazepines for anxiety

SUBSTANCE-RELATED DISORDERS

What is substance dependence?	A pathologic pattern of substance use manifest by the development of tolerance, withdrawal, and inability to decrease the amount of usage despite repeated attempts. A large amount of time is spent obtaining the substance, or an individual gives up social, occupational, or recreational activities to obtain or use the substance.
What is substance abuse?	A pathologic pattern of substance use characterized by recurrent substance-related legal problems, recurrent substance use in situations that are physically hazardous, and failure to fulfill personal, occupational, and educational responsibility as a result of substance use.
What is the lifetime prevalence for alcohol dependence (alcoholism)?	10% in women, 20% in men
What is the lifetime prevalence for alcohol abuse?	5% in women, 10% in men

What is the "CAGE" questionnaire?

C: Have you felt you should cut down on drinking?

A: Are you annoyed by people criticizing drinking?

G: Have you felt guilty about drinking?

E: Have you ever had an eye-opener in the morning?

Each letter is scored either 0 or 1; a score of 2 or more is clinically significant.

What are the stages of behavioral change?

Precontemplation, contemplation, preparation, action, maintenance, relapse

What is the most common cause for failure of alcoholism treatment?

Failure to adequately diagnosis and treat comorbid psychiatric disorders in these dual-diagnosis patients

What pharmacologic treatments are there for alcoholism?

Disulfiram, naltrexone, and acamprosate

EATING DISORDERS

What is anorexia nervosa?

A condition resulting in refusal to eat normally and fear of gaining weight such that body weight is less than 85% of that expected for a given age and height. Furthermore, there is a disturbance in how one's weight or shape is experienced.

What are the subtypes of anorexia nervosa?

Restricting type and binge-eating/purging type

What is the prevalence of anorexia nervosa?

0.3% of young adult females are affected

What psychiatric disorders are often comorbid with anorexia nervosa?

Depression, social phobia, and OCD

What is the treatment for anorexia nervosa?

Hospitalization if needed to restore the patient's nutritional state; inpatient eating disorder programs using behavioral management and psychotherapy; CBT; family therapy; medications (e.g., fluoxetine, cyproheptadine)

What is bulimia nervosa?	A condition marked by recurrent episodes of binge eating as well as recurrent inappropriate compensatory behavior (e.g., self-induced vomiting, diuretics, laxatives, etc.) in order to prevent weight gain
What are the subtypes of bulimia nervosa?	Purging type and nonpurging type
What is the prevalence of bulimia nervosa?	1% to 3% of young adult females
What is the treatment for bulimia nervosa?	First-line treatment is CBT; use antidepressants to treat associated depression and anxiety.

SOMATOFORM DISORDERS

What are the somatoform disorders?	Somatization disorder, conversion disorder, pain disorder, hypochondriasis, and body dysmorphic disorder
What is somatization disorder?	A chronic disorder marked by multiple physical complaints that occur over several years and result in impairment and/or frequent use of medical services
What is conversion disorder?	There are symptoms or deficits affecting voluntary motor or sensory function suggesting a neurologic or general medical condition, but it is better explained by psychological factors.
What is pain disorder?	Pain at one or more sites is the primary focus; the pain causes clinically significant impairment, and psychological factors play an important role.
What is hypochondriasis?	Preoccupation with fears of having, or the belief that one has, a serious medical illness

| What is body dysmorphic disorder? | Preoccupation with an imagined defect in the way one looks or exaggerated concern about a minor physical anomaly |

FACTITIOUS DISORDERS

What is factitious disorder?	A condition marked by the intentional production of physical or psychological symptoms where the motivation for such behavior is to assume the sick role
What eponym refers to factitious disorder with predominantly physical signs and symptoms?	Münchhausen syndrome
What is Münchhausen syndrome by proxy?	Someone (usually a parent) intentionally produces physical signs or symptoms in another person (usually a child) who is under his or her care.
How does malingering differ from factitious disorder?	Malingerers have secondary gain (e.g., financial gain, evading criminal prosecution, avoiding work) for feigning physical or psychological symptoms.
How do somatization disorder and conversion disorder differ from factitious disorders?	The production of symptoms in somatization disorder and conversion disorder is not under voluntary control but rather the result of an unconscious conflict.

ATTENTION-DEFICIT/HYPERACTIVITY DISORDER

What are the symptoms of ADHD?	Inattention—the individual pays poor attention to detail, has difficulty sustaining attention, fails to listen when spoken to, loses things easily, and is distractible and forgetful
	Hyperactivity—the individual fidgets, is unable to sit still, feels "on the go," has difficulty playing quietly, talks excessively
	Impulsivity—blurts out answers, unable to wait his or her turn, interrupts others

What is the prevalence of ADHD?	3% to 5% in school-age children; unknown in adults, although the disorder is thought to persist into adolescence and adulthood in half of those affected
What gender differences exist in ADHD?	The male-to-female ratio is between 4:1 and 9:1
What are the risk factors for ADHD?	Evidence supports genetic factors; developmental factors and psychosocial factors may contribute.
What is the differential diagnosis of ADHD?	Anxiety disorders, mood disorders, learning disorders
What is the treatment for ADHD?	CNS stimulants: methylphenidate, d-enantiomer of methylphenidate, amphetamine salt and dextroamphetamine combinations Norepinephrine reuptake inhibitor: atomoxetine Psychosocial interventions: behavioral interventions, social skills groups

PERSONALITY DISORDERS

What is a personality disorder?	An enduring pattern of behavior and inner experience that deviates significantly from the expectations of an individual's culture. This pattern may be manifest in the individual's way of perceiving and interpreting self or others; range, intensity, lability, or appropriateness of affect; impulse control; or interpersonal functioning.
What percent of patients with an axis I diagnosis have comorbid personality disorders?	35%; of note, in the general population the prevalence of personality disorders is 10% to 20%.
When is the onset for personality disorders?	In adolescence; the patterns are of long standing.

What are the major categories of personality disorders?	Cluster A ("weird") Cluster B ("wild") Cluster C ("wimpy")
Give examples of cluster A behaviors and the personality disorders in the group.	Cluster A ("weird"): odd or eccentric; includes paranoid, schizoid, and schizotypal personality disorders
Give examples of cluster B behaviors and the personality disorders in the group.	Cluster B ("wild"): dramatic, emotional, or erratic; includes antisocial, borderline, histrionic, and narcissistic personality disorders
Give examples of cluster C behaviors and the personality disorders in the group.	Cluster C ("wimpy"): excessive fearfulness or anxiety; includes avoidant, dependent, and obsessive-compulsive personality disorders

URGENCIES AND EMERGENCIES

ACUTE PSYCHOSIS

What is acute psychosis?	The acute or subacute onset of psychotic symptoms
What are symptoms and signs of acute psychosis?	Delusions, hallucinations, disorganized speech (e.g., incoherence, loosening of associations, thought blocking), grossly disorganized behavior, and catatonic excitement or stupor
What diagnostic tests are ordered for the workup of acute psychosis?	Tests to rule out organic causes including CBC, basic chemistries, LFTs, TFTs, RPR, B12, folate, UA, toxicology screens (APAP, ASA, UDS, BAL, heavy metals, etc.), urine porphyrins, HIV, antinuclear antibody (ANA), ceruloplasmin, head CT or MRI, EEG, and occasionally CSF studies
What is the differential diagnosis for acute psychosis?	Psychotic disorder due to a general medical condition [e.g., AIDS, B12 deficiency, CNS tumor, CVA, herpes

encephalitis, endocrine disorders, iatrogenic (e.g., steroids), lupus, metabolic disarray, neurosyphilis, porphyria, toxic causes, Wilson's disease]; substance-induced psychotic disorder; epilepsy (especially TLE); delirium; dementia; primary psychotic disorder; primary mood disorder with psychotic features; and cluster A personality disorders

What is the treatment for acute psychosis?

Hospitalization, treatment of underlying cause (whether organic or psychiatric), antipsychotic medications, and benzodiazepines for acute agitation

NEUROLEPTIC MALIGNANT SYNDROME

What is NMS?

A life-threatening complication of antipsychotic medications that can occur at any time in treatment

What is the prevalence of NMS?

0.02% to 2.5% of patients exposed to dopamine receptor antagonists (e.g., antipsychotics)

What are risk factors for NMS?

Use of high-potency antipsychotic medications (e.g., haloperidol and fluphenazine) in high doses, particularly when the dosage is increased rapidly; higher number of intramuscular injections; and concurrent use of lithium

What are symptoms and signs of NMS?

Hyperthermia, severe muscular rigidity, autonomic instability including tachycardia, hypertension, tachypnea, and diaphoresis, as well as changes in level of consciousness

What laboratory tests are ordered for NMS?

CK (elevated in 50% of cases), aldolase, white blood cell count (leukocytosis), electrolytes, creatinine, LFTs, and urine myoglobin

What is the treatment for NMS?

Discontinue antipsychotic medications; transfer to the intensive care unit for supportive measures (e.g., hydration, cooling, hemodynamic monitoring); electrolyte balance; dialysis may be necessary given renal function; pharmacotherapy.

What pharmacologic interventions exist for NMS?

Dantrolene 2.5 mg/kg initial dose, then 2 mg/kg intravenously every 6 to 12 hours; avoid if LFTs are very abnormal

Bromocriptine: 2.5 mg orally every 6 hours, titrated to a maximum dose of 40 mg/day (divided qid)

Amantadine: 100 mg orally, titrated to 200 mg every 12 hours

Other treatments: clonazepam, carbamazepine, ECT

What is the prognosis for NMS?

10% to 20% mortality rate

ACUTE DYSTONIC REACTION

What is an acute dystonic reaction?

An extrapyramidal symptom consisting of intermittent and sustained muscle spasms of the head, neck, and trunk leading to involuntary movements. It is a direct result of treatment with antipsychotic medications and is now much less likely with atypical neuroleptics.

What are risk factors for an acute dystonic reaction?

Male gender, age younger than 30 years, and high dosages of potent typical antipsychotic medications

What are symptoms and signs of an acute dystonic reaction?

Opisthotonos, retrocollis, torticollis, oculogyric crisis, tongue protrusion, dysarthria, dysphonia, and dysphagia

What is the differential diagnosis of an acute dystonic reaction?

Tetanus and seizures

What is the treatment for an acute dystonic reaction?	Intramuscular benztropine 2 mg or diphenhydramine 50 mg; repeat in 15 minutes if not effective

ALCOHOL WITHDRAWAL AND DELIRIUM TREMENS

What is alcohol withdrawal?	A physiologic syndrome resulting from the cessation of prolonged and heavy alcohol use. The syndrome progresses soon after the cessation of alcohol use and may include grand mal seizures or DTs (alcohol withdrawal delirium).
What are the symptoms and signs of alcohol withdrawal in the first 6 to 8 hours?	Tremulousness
What are the symptoms and signs of alcohol withdrawal at 12 hours?	Seizures
What are the symptoms and signs of alcohol withdrawal at 72 hours to 1 week?	DTs (vivid visual or tactile hallucinations, profound disorientation, increased autonomic activity, fluctuating psychomotor activity)
What are the laboratory findings in alcohol dependence?	Elevated delta-glutamyl transferase (GGT), mean corpuscular volume (MCV), triglycerides, high-density lipoprotein (HDL), aspartate aminotransferase (AST) and alanine aminotransferase (ALT) (2:1 AST:ALT ratio)
What is the differential diagnosis for alcohol withdrawal?	Sedative or hypnotic withdrawal (including benzodiazepines)
What is the treatment for alcohol withdrawal?	Thiamine, folate, magnesium ("banana bag" or "rally pack"); detoxification with benzodiazepine taper given orally (preferred) or parenterally, depending on severity; benzodiazepines as needed for autonomic hyperactivity or agitation associated with delirium; and antipsychotic medications for delirium (but keep in mind that they lower the seizure threshold)

Which benzodiazepine is preferred in the setting of normal liver function and alcohol withdrawal?	A long-acting benzodiazepine such as chlordiazepoxide; however, chlordiazepoxide has erratic absorption intramuscularly so give it orally only.
Which benzodiazepine is preferred in the setting of abnormal liver function and alcohol withdrawal?	A benzodiazepine with no active metabolites such as lorazepam

SUICIDE

What is the epidemiologic makeup of suicide?	In the year 2000, suicide represented 1.2% of all deaths, thus averaging 80 suicides per day in the United States.
What is the prevalence of suicide?	In the year 2004, 11 per 100,000 in the United States (1 person every 16.2 minutes with 1 attempt every 39 seconds)
What major factors in the following categories affect suicide risk?	
Personal and social	Male gender
	Age older than 45 years; $\geq$85 is the highest-risk group
	Widowed, divorced, or separated marital status
	White or Native American
	Immigrant status
	Lone dweller or socially isolated
	Unemployed, retired, or having financial difficulties
Previous history	Family history of affective disorder, suicide, or alcoholism
	Previous history of an affective disorder, suicide attempt, or alcoholism
	Beginning psychiatric treatment or 6 months after discharge from treatment
	Impulsivity
Life stresses	Bereavement and separation
	Loss of job or house
	Incapacitating or terminal illness

Psychiatric illnesses	Depression
	Antisocial personality
	Alcohol or drug addiction
	Dementia, delirium, and organic brain syndromes

What symptoms are worrisome with regard to suicide risk?

Insomnia, weight loss, slowed speech, agitation, severe anxiety, listlessness, social withdrawal, loss of interest, hopelessness, feelings of worthlessness, and suicidal thoughts

What signs are worrisome with regard to suicide attempts?

When the patient takes precautions against discovery, takes preparatory action (e.g., procures means of suicide, makes warning statements, writes suicide notes, and gets personal affairs in order), and uses violent methods or lethal drugs

What is the prevalence of psychiatric illness among patients who commit suicide?

Greater than 90%

What psychiatric illnesses are predominant in suicidal patients?

Major depression, substance abuse, anxiety disorders, personality disorders (borderline, antisocial), and schizophrenia

What is the treatment for suicidality?

Hospitalization and treatment of underlying disorder

What medications have been shown to decrease the risk of suicide?

Lithium maintenance for bipolar patients; clozapine for schizophrenic patients

What percent of suicides occur in people who have tried suicide before?

50%

Of those who attempt suicide unsuccessfully, how many will make another attempt in the next 2 years?

15% to 35%

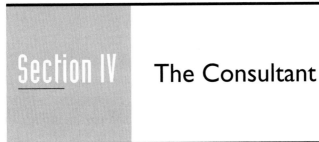

Section IV   The Consultant

The Consultant

ABBREVIATIONS

BUN	Blood urea nitrogen
CABG	Coronary artery bypass grafting
CAD	Coronary artery disease
CBC	Complete blood count
COPD	Chronic obstructive pulmonary disease
CRI	Cardiac risk index
CVD	Carotid vascular disease
DVT	Deep venous thrombosis
ECG	Electrocardiogram
FEV$_1$	Forced expiratory volume during the first second
FVC	Forced vital capacity
GI	Gastrointestinal
GU	Genitourinary
HF or CHF	Heart failure or congestive heart failure
HgbAlC	Glycosylated hemoglobin
H/O	History of
JVD	Jugular venous distension
MET	Metabolic equivalent
MI	Myocardial infarction
MRSA	Methicillin-resistant *Staphylococcus aureus*
NPO	Nil per os (nothing by mouth)

PFT	Pulmonary function test
PVD or PAD	Peripheral vascular disease or peripheral arterial disease
PVC	Premature ventricular contraction
VT	Ventricular tachycardia

ROLE OF THE MEDICAL CONSULTANT

What is the role of the medical consultant?	To provide expertise in medical areas of patient care, often when the patient's primary care team specializes in an area other than internal medicine
When should the consult be carried out?	Consults may be emergent, urgent, or elective. It is important to determine the nature of the consult and to respond appropriately. In general, a courteous and rapid response to any consult is appreciated by the primary team.
How broad are the recommendations generated by the consultant?	The recommendations are usually relatively narrow in scope and limited to those needed to answer the clinical question posed to the consultant. The consult recommendations are considered to be goal-directed. It is usually not helpful to point out obvious/standard medical issues (e.g., "avoid hypotension").
Are any peripheral recommendations appropriate?	Yes. Under some circumstances, it is appropriate to provide contingency plans. In a patient whose condition is changing or who may fail an initial therapeutic recommendation, it may be helpful to include a backup plan.
Should there be any other information included in the consult?	Sometimes it is appropriate to provide recent, concise articles from a journal that the primary team is unlikely to have been exposed to. This is never a substitute for direct communication with the primary team.

How are the consultant's recommendations reported?

The recommendations are recorded in writing in the patient's chart on the consult note. If the note is dictated the key points should still be written in the chart.

Whose responsibility is it to ultimately decide how and whether or not to carry out a consultant's recommendations?

The patient's primary care team. If the consultant feels that patient care is significantly compromised by failure to carry out the recommendations, it would be appropriate for the consultant to discuss them in person with the primary team. It is not appropriate to engage in "chart wars."

How long should the consulting team follow up the patient?

Each case varies, but generally the patient is followed up until the clinical questions at hand are resolved or until the consult team is no longer providing useful input. After signing off the case, the consultant should indicate willingness to become involved again if the patient's status changes.

PREOPERATIVE CLEARANCE OF THE SURGICAL PATIENT

Why is it important to perform preoperative evaluations on patients undergoing surgery?

To assess the patient's risk for cardiac and other adverse events, trying to ensure the best medical and surgical outcome with the lowest adverse event rate

What are the benefits of a preoperative evaluation?

Any existing medical problems can be treated before surgery to maximize the patient's chances of having an uneventful procedure and recovery. This is especially important before elective surgery because clearance is a process of weighing the need for surgery against the risk of surgery. A higher level of risk is tolerated when a patient needs emergency surgery than when the patient is undergoing an elective procedure.

What is the cardiac risk for patients undergoing high-risk procedures?

>5% risk of a cardiac event

What are examples of high-risk operations?

Emergency operations (major surgery)

Aortic or major suprapubic vascular surgeries

Prolonged surgical procedures with significant fluid shifts

What is the cardiac risk for patients undergoing intermediate-risk procedures?

Risk of a cardiac event between 1 and 5%

What are examples of intermediate-risk procedures?

Carotid or distal peripheral vascular surgeries

Head and neck

Intraperitoneal or intrathoracic surgeries

Orthopedic and prostate surgeries

What is the cardiac risk for patients undergoing low-risk procedures?

<1% risk of a cardiac event

What are examples of low-risk procedures?

Endoscopic procedures

Superficial procedures

Cataract surgery

Breast surgery

If a patient does suffer a perioperative MI, what is the relative increased risk of death?

About two to four times that over an MI not occurring in the perioperative period.

When in the surgical course is death most likely to occur?

During induction of anesthesia, 10%

During surgery, 35%

Within 48 hours of surgery, 55%

Other than specific medical illness, are there any general risk factors for patients undergoing surgery?

Yes. Age is a contributor to surgical risk. Patients below 65 years of age have a 1% mortality rate, whereas those above 65 years of age have a 5% mortality rate.

What important elements of a patient's history should be discussed with cardiac patients about to undergo surgery?

Previous MI, chest pain, dyspnea, syncope, dysrhythmias, history of rheumatic fever, and history of diabetes

What elements of the physical examination are especially important for cardiac patients about to undergo surgery?

Vital signs are important, as are JVD, bruits, slow carotid upstroke, a displaced point of maximal impulse (PMI), murmurs, S3 gallop, and rubs.

What is the Goldman scale?

Developed in 1977, the Goldman scale quantifies operative risk for MI based on several variables assessed by history, physical examination, and simple laboratory data.

What nine variables are associated with an increased risk of perioperative MI or death in Goldman's work, and what were their point values?

Table 17–1. Goldman Scale

Variable	Point Value
Third heart sound or JVD	11
MI within 6 months	10
Nonsinus rhythm	7
>5 PVCs per minute	7
Age >70 years	5
Emergency procedure	4
Hemodynamically significant aortic stenosis	3
Aortic, intra-abdominal, or intrathoracic surgery	3
Poor general health	3

Table 17–2. Preoperative Risk

How do the point values help determine preoperative risk?

Points	MI, Pulmonary Edema, VT	Death
0–5	0.7%	0.2%
6–12	5.0%	2.0%
13–25	11.0%	2.0%
>26	22.0%	56.0%

What other preoperative evaluation indices are there?	In addition to Goldman, Detsky (*Arch Int Med* 146:2131–2134:1986), L'Italien (*JACC* 1996;27:779), and Eagle (*J Am Coll Cardiol* 1996;27:779–86) have excellent risk indices.
What is the Cardiac Risk Index?[1]	History of: Ischemic heart disease Cerebrovascular disease: any H/O TIA or CVA. Diabetes mellitus: use of insulin Renal insufficiency: creatinine >2.0 mg/dL High-risk surgery: intrathoracic, intraabdominal, or suprapubic vascular
How is this index useful?	One point is assigned for each positive; scores >2 are higher-risk and warrant use of beta blockade.
What is "hemodynamically significant" aortic stenosis?	Indicators of significance (in the absence of echocardiography) are poor exercise tolerance, a history of syncope, HF, or angina, a late-peaking systolic murmur, delayed pulses, and absence of the aortic component of the second heart sound (A_2).
Dysrhythmia is more likely to result in complications of what nature?	Dysrhythmias are a marker for ischemic heart disease.
How much is risk increased for cardiovascular events for diabetic patients compared with their nondiabetic counterparts?	Two times for male diabetics and four times for female diabetics

---

[1] Lee TH. *Circulation* 1999;100:1043; Lindenauer PK. *NEJM* 2005;353:349.

Is hypertension a marker for an increased risk of cardiac complications?

By itself, no, although diastolic pressure greater than 110 mm Hg is sometimes considered a relative contraindication to elective surgery. When hypertension is a manifestation of other serious illness such as renal artery stenosis, hyperaldosteronism, or pheochromocytoma, the illness should be treated before the patient undergoes elective surgery.

What is the most important tool for assessing risk associated with surgery for cardiovascular patients?

The history and physical examination is the most important element of the evaluation.

Do patients with vascular disease (peripheral or cerebrovascular) have a higher rate of CAD?

Yes. One third of patients with PVD/CVD have no significant CAD (<50% stenosis). One third have moderate CAD (>50% stenosis). One third have severe CAD (>70% stenosis), with 5% to 10% being inoperable.

Can patients who have undergone CABG and are symptom-free then undergo other surgery?

Patients who have undergone CABG have an approximately 1% incidence of a cardiac event while undergoing surgery.

When is a preoperative ECG indicated?

1. A history of cardiac disease, or with history and physical examination findings that suggest cardiac disease (e.g., diabetes mellitus, atherosclerosis, hypertension, dysrhythmias, certain malignancies, collagen vascular diseases, and infectious diseases)
2. Undergoing intrathoracic, intra-abdominal, aortic, or emergency surgery
3. At risk for electrolyte abnormality
4. Any patient taking a potentially cardiotoxic medication
5. Any man above 45 years of age or any woman above age 50

When should preoperative chest films be obtained?

1. A history of cardiovascular disease (e.g., valvular disease, CHF, and coronary or cerebrovascular disease)
2. A history of pulmonary disease (e.g., asthma, COPD, occupational lung disease, and tobacco use)
3. A history of a malignancy
4. Age greater than 60 years
5. Symptoms and signs of an infection

What are the two most important risk factors for significant postoperative cardiac events?

Presence of heart failure and recent MI

What is a significant cardiac event?

Sudden death, MI, unstable angina, pulmonary edema, or serious dysrhythmia (e.g., such as VT or ventricular fibrillation)

What is the risk of a cardiac event occurring in a surgery patient without a cardiac history?

Approximately 0.5% (10 times less than in a patient with cardiac history)

How does the presence of unstable angina affect operative risk?

It has never been studied, but it seems logical that patients with unstable angina should not undergo *elective* surgery (except CABG). These patients should have the extent of their disease defined and should then receive appropriate medical therapy.

What is the risk that a patient who undergoes surgery and has had a prior MI will have another such cardiac event?

The risk depends on how recently the patient experienced the cardiac event and how large a stress the surgery causes (e.g., thoracic aneurysm more stressful than a cataract operation). In general, the risk of subsequent MI is approximately 5%. In the first 4 to 6 weeks after an MI, however, the risk is higher.

What is the *mortality rate* of surgical patients who have had a recent MI?

6% if MI was less than 3 months before surgery, 2% if MI was 3 to 6 months before surgery, and 1.5% if MI was >6 months before surgery

Is there anything that can be done to lower the perioperative risk in patients who have had a recent MI and need surgery?

Yes. Some evaluation for residual ischemia (and treating it if found) is helpful. Beta-blocker therapy has been shown to be helpful and should be considered in all high-risk patients.

Do high-risk patients benefit from the use of a pulmonary artery catheter?

Some high-risk patients may benefit, but there is also the risk of the line placement to be considered.

Do low-risk patients also benefit from perioperative beta-blocker use?

No. Using the CRI scale, patients with <2 points have a higher likelihood of harm with preoperative beta blockers.

What noninvasive cardiac tests are thought to be most predictive of ischemic complications in the perioperative period, and what are their approximate predictive values?

1. An exercise stress radionucleotide test (test of choice if patient can ambulate) has a negative predictive value (the test is negative and no cardiac complication occurs) of 93%.
2. The negative predictive value of a dipyridamole radionucleotide test (for those who cannot attain high workload on a treadmill) is >95%.
3. The negative predictive value of a dobutamine echocardiogram is 93% to 100%.

Can a stress test help predict risk in other ways?

Patients can be divided into functional class based on the maximal metabolic stress level they can achieve before stopping a treadmill test. The higher the functional class, the lower the perioperative risk.

How many METs achieved is a low functional class (i.e., higher risk)?

Patients who achieve only 1 to 3 METs are in the low-functional category.

How many METs achieved is a moderate functional class (i.e., moderate risk)?

Patients who achieve only 4 to 7 METs fall into the moderate category.

How many METs achieved is a high functional class (i.e., low risk)?

Patients who exercise to >7 METs are in the high-functioning category.

What types of routine activities are consistent with a high functional class?	>10 METs, equivalent to participation in strenuous sports like swimming, singles tennis, football, basketball, skiing
What types of routine activities are consistent with a moderate functional class?	4 to 10 METs (in increasing order): the ability to do light housework (dusting, dishes); climb a flight of stairs or a hill; walk at 4 mph; run a short distance; do heavy housework (lifting, moving furniture); participate in bowling, dancing, and doubles tennis
What types of routine activities are consistent with a low functional class?	1 to 4 METs: the ability for self-care (eating, dressing, using the toilet); walking indoors and around the house; walking a block or two on level ground at 2 to 3 mph
Do all patients with a *history of cardiac disease* require preoperative stress testing?	If the patient had surgical revascularization within 5 years, percutaneous revascularization within the previous 2 years, or cardiac testing within 2 years and has had no clinical deterioration or significant cardiac symptoms, more testing is not required.
Should patients who are NPO take blood pressure medication on the morning of surgery?	Yes, unless otherwise instructed. By not taking such previously prescribed treatment, the patient is predisposed to perioperative blood pressure variability and postoperative cardiac complications. The major risks of anesthesia are related to hypotension and rebound hypertension.
Does regional anesthesia reduce the rate of postoperative cardiac complications compared with that of general anesthesia?	Except in patients with HF, the type of anesthesia selected does not alter outcome with regard to cardiac status. However, regional anesthesia is often used in sicker patients undergoing surgery. The ultimate choice of anesthetic is appropriately left to the anesthesiologist.

PREOPERATIVE EVALUATION OF LUNG FUNCTION

What is the most important element of evaluation of pulmonary function?	Patient history and physical examination

List factors that predispose the patient to pulmonary complications.

Obesity, smoking, COPD, chronic bronchitis, type of surgery or incision, asthma, occupational lung disease, sleep apnea, neuromuscular disease, coma, nutritional depletion, acidosis, endotracheal intubation, hypotension, hypoxemia, and azotemia are all potential contributors to postoperative pulmonary complications.

Does a patient benefit from quitting smoking before surgery?

Yes.

How much time before surgery is needed to decrease pulmonary complications?

Patients who quit smoking 8 weeks before surgery have a statistically significant decrease in the number of pulmonary complications compared with those who do not, independent of functional status as assessed by PFTs.

How soon does mucociliary function improve after smoking cessation?

Improvement in lung function and mucociliary clearance is detectable in <1 month after quitting.

What other benefit occurs with smoking cessation?

Carboxyhemoglobin levels decrease quickly, thus improving oxygen delivery.

Which patients with predisposing characteristics for pulmonary complications should undergo PFTs?

This is a judgment call. Functional limitation such as difficulty with walking steps or distances should prompt further evaluation. Any patient with an abnormal lung examination (e.g., wheezing or rhonchi) may benefit from PFTs.

What other studies are useful for evaluation of pulmonary risk?

When indicated by the history and physical examination, chest radiographs, ECG, and arterial blood gases

What finding on PFTs is truly predictive of perioperative pulmonary complications?

None. FVC, FEV_1, maximum breathing capacity, maximum midexpiratory flow, and arterial blood gas findings have all failed to reliably predict pulmonary complications.

What PFT abnormality is prohibitive for surgery?

No degree of abnormality on PFT is considered prohibitive for *non-lung* surgery down to an FEV_1 of 450 mL (or generally an FEV_1 of 1000 mL for chest cases).

What are abnormal PFTs predictive of, or how are they helpful?

Patients with clusters of abnormalities on the PFT studies are more likely to suffer complications than those without underlying pulmonary conditions.

Are certain PFT findings prohibitive for patients undergoing lung resection?

Advanced age coupled with FEV_1 <2 L, maximum voluntary ventilation <50% predicted, or an abnormal ECG has been found to portend postoperative difficulties. In general, a patient should have a predicted postoperative FEV_1 of at least 800 mL. As is the case with non-lung surgery, the correlation between the degree of abnormality on PFTs and postoperative complications is poor (at least when predicted postoperative FEV_1 is >800 mL).

Does use of anesthesia (other than general anesthesia) decrease respiratory complications?

Yes and no. If the anesthesia is strictly local, as in a nerve block, the answer is yes. But with spinal anesthesia the answer is no.

Why is that?

Anesthesia itself is only a small contributor to pulmonary complications. Other factors such as the type of surgery (e.g., upper abdominal or thoracic), loss of hyperinflation by sighing, pain, and sedation all contribute to the development of pulmonary complications. These factors are present regardless of the type of anesthesia used.

PREOPERATIVE USE OF THE LABORATORY

Should every surgery patient have preoperative laboratory tests?

No. The indications for these are provided by the history and physical examination or by the type of surgery planned.

Is a chemistry profile a routine study before surgery?

This study is appropriate for most individuals, such as those above 60 years of age with hypertension, diabetes, or renal disease. Also, patients who take diuretics, bowel preparations, or nephrotoxic drugs should undergo a preoperative chemistry study.

Is a complete blood count profile a routine study before surgery?

The CBC can be reserved for patients undergoing procedures in which large blood losses are expected or who have indication on history and physical examination of anemia. Others who require a CBC include patients above 60 years of age.

In whom should coagulation studies be obtained?

Any patient actively bleeding or with a known or suspected bleeding disorder (including causes such as warfarin or aspirin therapy); also patients with liver disease or malabsorption.

ANTIBIOTIC PROPHYLAXIS BEFORE SURGERY

Are prophylactic antibiotics always indicated before surgery?

No. Antibiotics are indicated when infection would be particularly serious, when prosthetic or artificial material is to be implanted, or when the planned procedure is likely to give rise to infection.

All surgical procedures involve some risk of infection, so why not always use antibiotic prophylaxis?

Use of antibiotics is not without some risk, specifically the risks of toxicity, allergic reaction, superinfection, and the development of resistance.

Should the coverage provided by prophylactic antibiotics be broad or narrow?

The coverage should be focused—that is, directed at the most likely pathogens of potential infectious complication.

When would prophylactic antibiotics other than cefazolin be indicated?

1. When likely pathogens would not be well covered by cefazolin, as in colorectal surgery or appendectomy. Under these circumstances, providing

better protection against anaerobic organisms, including *Bacteroides fragilis*, would be necessary.

2. When the patient is allergic to beta-lactam antibiotics.
3. In cases of MRSA, which is susceptible to vancomycin.
4. When the patient has prosthetic material in place.

In preoperative cases, when should the antibiotic be given?

The antibiotic should be given just before the procedure to ensure that there are adequate drug levels throughout the surgery. In cases of major blood loss or prolonged operation, a second dose might be indicated.

Should antibiotics be continued postoperatively?

Not usually. An exception is when infectious complications are likely, as when there is accidental spillage of stool during an abdominal procedure. In such a case, antibiotics are no longer considered prophylaxis but rather therapeutic and necessary.

Are prophylactic antibiotics indicated for laparoscopic surgery?

The need for prophylaxis is determined by the type of procedure performed, not the method of surgery. The use of prophylactic antibiotics in laparoscopic surgery is less well studied than the use of prophylactic antibiotics in traditional surgical incisions, but currently recommendations are the same for both.

INDICATIONS AND REGIMEN FOR SUBACUTE BACTERIAL ENDOCARDITIS PROPHYLAXIS (REFER TO CHAPTER 3, "CARDIOLOGY")

In general terms, for which procedures should prophylaxis be given?

Procedures that are likely to produce bacteremia. Sterile procedures do not require specific prophylaxis. Each procedure should be evaluated individually.

DEEP VENOUS THROMBOSIS PROPHYLAXIS

What are the risk factors for DVT?

Age older than 40 years, surgery lasting more than 1 hour, previous DVT or pulmonary embolus, extensive tumor, hip or knee surgery, major trauma or fractures, and stroke. Other risk factors include MI, HF, obesity, immobility, postpartum state, and hypercoagulable state.

Do all surgical patients benefit from DVT prophylaxis?

Yes, but not necessarily pharmacologic prophylaxis. Patients at low risk of DVT can wear graduated compression stockings and undertake early ambulation as prophylactic measures.

Who are the patients at low risk for DVT?

Patients below 40 years of age who are undergoing procedures lasting <1 hour or patients who are pregnant

Which patients are at moderate DVT risk?

Patients include those above 40 years of age who are undergoing a procedure lasting >1 hour or who have medical conditions such as MI or HF. Postpartum patients have moderate risk of DVT.

What DVT prophylaxis is recommended for patients at moderate DVT risk?

Patients with a moderate risk of DVT often are given pharmacologic prophylaxis. Prophylaxis involves the methods used for low-risk patients plus one of the following: subcutaneous low-molecular-weight heparin, heparin (5000 U) twice per day, intravenous dextran, or external pneumatic compression devices.

Which patients are at high risk of DVT?

Patients above 40 years of age who are undergoing long procedures, often orthopedic, and might have a history of DVT, pulmonary embolism, stroke, or recent trauma

What DVT prophylaxis is appropriate for high-risk patients?	The best outcomes may occur when a heparin-based therapy or oral warfarin is combined with a nonpharmacologic intervention such as a pneumatic compression device. May also consider subcutaneous heparin three times daily. Other therapies used for these patients include warfarin or vena caval interruption (filter).
Why not use warfarin only in patients at high risk for DVT?	Warfarin is associated with a higher risk of bleeding complications (approximately 6%) than heparin (approximately 2%).
Is aspirin ever used as prophylaxis against DVT?	Aspirin is not as effective as the other methods discussed; therefore it is not recommended.
Why are dextrans rarely used as prophylaxis for DVT?	Dextrans have been associated with anaphylactic reactions, they are expensive, and they require intravenous administration.
What other methods of DVT prophylaxis are in development?	Fondaparinux has been shown to be beneficial in patients at moderate DVT risk. Hirudin is promising based on results of early trials. Murine monoclonal antibodies that bind the fibrinogen receptor on platelets are in development.

PERIOPERATIVE MANAGEMENT OF THE DIABETIC PATIENT

Why is the type of diabetes (i.e., type 1 or type 2) important to distinguish during the perioperative period?	Type 1 diabetic patients are prone to ketoacidosis, whereas type 2 diabetic patients generally are not. Both are subject to variations in glucose control perioperatively, given NPO status (hypoglycemia) and the stress of illness and surgery (hyperglycemia).
In general, how is the type 1 diabetic patient managed perioperatively?	While NPO, the patient is given intravenous glucose and insulin drips at 1 to 3 U/hr with titration (sliding scale) based on serum glucose levels.

How is the insulin-requiring type 2 diabetic patient managed perioperatively?

Type 2 insulin-requiring diabetic patients are generally given half their usual dose of long-acting insulin on the morning of the surgery. Their blood glucose is then monitored frequently via finger sticks. Infusions or subcutaneous injections of insulin and glucose are adjusted accordingly.

In general, how should the patient whose diabetes is controlled on oral hypoglycemics be managed for surgery?

Patients should have their oral agent discontinued 1 day before surgery; those on metformin 1 to 2 days before; and those on chlorpropamide 2 to 3 days before. Patients often require no exogenous glucose or insulin, but these may be used if necessary. Serum glucose should be monitored in anticipation of such a possibility.

How is the patient with diet-controlled diabetes managed for surgery?

Diet-controlled diabetic patients can often undergo surgery without any glucose or insulin. Intravenous fluids should lack dextrose, and the patient's blood glucose level should be monitored throughout the procedure. Insulin and glucose should be administered if needed.

What is a reasonable target range for blood sugars in diabetic patients undergoing surgery?

Generally, <140 mg/dL is considered an acceptable range.

In patients whose blood sugar is difficult to maintain, is it better to be on the high side or the low side of the acceptable range?

It is better to have blood sugars run somewhat high than to risk insulin shock. However, it should also be kept in mind that higher blood sugars predispose to worse outcomes owing to infections and wound healing.

Why is the diabetic patient at increased risk of infection?

Small-vessel disease results in tissue ischemia. Also, hyperglycemia impairs phagocytosis, and gastroparesis increases the risk of aspiration pneumonia.

Does the presence of palpable peripheral pulses rule out the presence of tissue ischemia in diabetic patients?

No. The pathology in diabetic circulation is microvascular in nature.

What are the factors that play a role in determining postoperative complications in diabetic patients?

Important elements in the history include duration of disease, current medications, current diet, typical blood sugar levels, and preexisting complications such as retinopathy, nephropathy, and neuropathy. Also, a history of angina, previous MI, claudication, activity limitation, and other major cardiac risk factors (e.g., family history, smoking, hypertension, and hyperlipidemia). The type of surgery planned and type of anesthesia are also factors.

What should be observed on physical examination of a diabetic patient?

Vital signs, heart and lung examination findings, and condition of extremities. Degree of hygiene, any ulcers, evidence of poor perfusion (e.g., decreased hair growth and decreased pulses), and neurologic findings should be noted.

Why is peripheral neuropathy an important perioperative finding?

Patients with peripheral neuropathy are much more prone to extremity complications, with their attendant morbidity and mortality.

What laboratory evaluations are needed for diabetic patients preoperatively?

Blood glucose level, HbA1C, electrolytes (especially sodium and potassium), BUN, creatinine, and urinalysis. Thyroid studies may be indicated if history and physical examination suggest any abnormality.

Is chronic renal insufficiency a contraindication to surgery?

No, but it indicates a need for meticulous attention to volume and electrolyte status perioperatively.

Why might a diabetic patient be instructed to fast for a full 12 hours before surgery?

Diabetic gastroparesis predisposes the patient to aspiration during surgery.

POSTOPERATIVE FEVER

What are the common causes of postoperative fever?	The **5 W's** of postoperative fever are as follows: **W**ind (atelectasis) **W**ater (urinary tract infection) **W**ound (wound infection) **W**alking (DVT) **W**onder drugs (drug reaction)
Which of the five W's is the most common cause of fever?	Atelectasis.
What is the treatment of atelectasis?	Treatment involves incentive spirometry, chest physical therapy, and ambulation.
Should antibiotics be given to patients with postoperative fever?	Antibiotics should be avoided until a source of infection is diagnosed by repeated careful, comprehensive history and physical examinations. Surgical wounds should be carefully evaluated for evidence of infection. Urinalysis and culture as well as culture of blood and all invasive catheters should be carried out.

MISCELLANEOUS MNEMONICS

What is the mnemonic for altered mental status?	**TIPS AEIOU:** **T**rauma and **T**emperature **I**nfection **P**sychiatric disorder or **P**oison **S**epsis, **S**troke, **S**eizure, or **S**pace-occupying lesion **A**lcohol intoxication or withdrawal **E**lectrolyte imbalance **I**nsulin (hyperglycemia or hypoglycemia) **O**verdose or O_2 deficit **U**remia

What is the mnemonic for acidosis without anion gap?	**HEART CCU:**
	Hyperaldosteronism
	Expansion (volume)
	Acid loading
	Renal tubular acidosis
	Turds (diarrhea, pancreatitis)
	Chronic pyelonephritis
	Carbonic anhydrase inhibitors
	Ureterojejunostomy
How do the glucocorticoids compare in potency with respect to hydrocortisone?	**D**on't **S**top **P**rednisone **H**astily:
	Dexamethasone (25 times more potent)
	Solumedrol (5 times more potent)
	Prednisone (4 times more potent)
	Hydrocortisone

ALTERNATIVE MEDICATIONS AND SURGERY

How often do patients use alternative (neutraceutical) medications?	Approximately 30% to 50% of patients use neutraceuticals.
What percent of patients admit to using neutraceuticals?	Approximately 10%
Why should the following herbal medications be discontinued before surgery?	
Echinacea	Associated with liver dysfunction in patients with preexisting liver disease
Ephedra	Associated with hyperpyrexia, hypertension, and coma (when used with monoamine oxidase inhibitors); MI, cerebrovascular accident, cardiovascular collapse (the latter caused by catechol depletion)
Garlic	Associated with bleeding as a result of inhibition of platelet function

Gingko	Potential to increase bleeding
Ginseng	Associated with bleeding as a result of inhibition of platelet function
Kava	May produce prolonged sedation (interaction with anesthetics)
St. John's wort	May increase metabolism of several medications like warfarin, cyclosporine, calcium channel blockers, selective serotonin reuptake inhibitors, midazolam, and nonsteroidal anti-inflammatory drugs
Valerian	Benzodiazepine-like withdrawal after abrupt discontinuation

TRIALS

Goldman L, Caldera DL, Nussbaum SR. Multifactorial index of cardiac risk in noncardiac surgical procedures. *N Engl J Med* 1977;297:845–580.
   A classic perioperative screening tool.
L'Italien GJ, Paul SD, Hendel RC, et al. Development and validation of a Bayesian model for perioperative cardiac risk assessment in a cohort of 1081 vascular surgical candidates. *J Am Coll Cardiol* 1996;27:779–786.
   A perioperative screening tool.
Lee TH, Marcantonio ER, Mangione CM, et al. Derivation and prospective validation of a simple index for prediction of cardiac risk of major noncardiac surgery. *Circulation* 1999;100:1043–1049.
   The Cardiac Risk Index scale.
Lindenauer PK, Pekow P, Wang K, et al. Perioperative beta-blocker therapy and mortality after major noncardiac surgery. *N Engl J Med* 2005;353:349–361.
   An adaptation of the Lee Cardiac Risk Index.
Hertzer NR, Beven EG, Young JR, et al. Coronary artery disease in peripheral vascular patients. A classification of 1000 coronary angiograms and results of surgical management. *Ann Surg* 1984;199:223–233.
   An observational study looking at the incidence of CAD in patients undergoing vascular surgery at the Cleveland Clinic.
Eagle KA, Berger PB, Calkins H, et al. ACC/AHA guideline update for perioperative cardiovascular evaluation for noncardiac surgery—executive summary: a report of the American College of Cardiology/American Heart Association Task Force on Practice Guidelines

(Committee to Update the 1996 Guidelines on Perioperative Cardiovascular Evaluation for Noncardiac Surgery). *J Am Coll Cardiol* 2002;39:542–553.

> The statement of the American College of Cardiology and the American Heart Association on preoperative care.

Landesberg G, Shatz V, Akopnik I, et al. Association of cardiac troponin, CK-MB, and postoperative myocardial ischemia with long-term survival after major vascular surgery. *J Am Coll Cardiol* 2003;42:1547–1554.

> At 5 years patients who suffered a perioperative MI and had a troponin I >3.1 (troponin T >0.2) had a survival rate of only 35% compared with patients with a troponin I of <0.06 (troponin T of <0.03) with a survival of >80%.

McFalls EO, Ward HB, Moritz TE, et al. Coronary-artery revascularization before elective major vascular surgery. *N Engl J Med* 2004;351:2795–2804.

> Survival in 510 patients randomized to revascularization or not. A total of 5859 patients screened at 18 VAs for an expanding AAA, or PAD of the legs. Patients were excluded for emergency surgery, severe comorbids, or prior revascularization without evidence of recurrent ischemia, or LMCA >50%, EF <20% and severe AS. Patients had cath and eligible if >70% stenosis and suitable for revascularization; 240 had revasc: CABG 41% (99) and PTCI 141 (59%) but only 225 had the planned vascular procedure (10 died after CABG or PTCI). This study was underpowered and applicability is limited.

Harvey S, Harrison DA, Singer M, et al. Assessment of the clinical effectiveness of pulmonary artery catheters in management of patients in intensive care (PAC-Man): a randomised controlled trial. *Lancet* 2005;366:472–477.

> The routine use of a PA catheter in medical and surgical patients does not lower the risk of events.

Index

Note: Page numbers followed by a *t* indicate tables.

3-Hydroxy-3-methylglutaryl Coenzyme A
(HMG-CoA), 33
5-acetylsalicylic Acid derivatives, 203–204
5FU, 450
5FU-based Therapy, 448
10s, Rule of, 141

A

AAA. *See* Abdominal aortic aneurysm
(AAA)
Abciximab, 71, 72
ABCs (Airway, Breathing, Circulation),
590
Abdominal aortic aneurysm (AAA), 32,
107
Abdominal-jugular reflux, 41, 42
ABPA. *See* Allergic bronchopulmonary
aspergillosis (ABPA)
Abscesses, 538
brain, 651–652
epidural, 324
Absolute reticulocyte count, 263
Abuse, drugs of, 615–620
Acalculous cholecystitis, 224
Acanthocyte, 262
Acanthosis nigricans, 560–561
ACE. *See* Angiotensin-converting enzyme
(ACE)
ACEI. *See* Angiotensin-converting
enzyme inhibitor (ACEI)
ACEIS, 403
Acetaminophen, 596–598
Acetaminophen hepatotoxicity, 238–239
Acid generation, acid load or, 340
Acid load or acid generation, 340
Acid-base disorders, 340–347
Acid-base disorders, mixed, 346
Acidosis
increased anion gap not associated with
metabolic, 342
metabolic, 341, 354
respiratory, 346

Acne, 555–556
Acquired immunodeficiency syndrome
(AIDS), 329–331, 492
Acquired NDI, causes of, 351
Acrochordon, 575
Acromegaly, symptoms associated with,
128
ACTH. *See* Adrenocorticotropic hormone
(ACTH)
Actinic keratosis, 575–576
Activated charcoal, 593, 594
Acute adrenal insufficiency, 122
Acute and chronic cholecystitis, 223–225
Acute and chronic pericarditis, 102–103
Acute asthma
cromolyn and, 467–468
exacerbation, 672
and initiating noninvasive and invasive
ventilatory support, 468
Acute coronary syndromes
biomarkers in, 69–71
treatment of, 71–74
Acute dystonic reaction, 714–715
Acute esophageal varices, 178
Acute gouty arthritis, 515
Acute hepatitis, 225
Acute HSP, 469
Acute interstitial nephritis (AIN),
366–367
Acute kidney injury (AKI), 364–365
atheroembolic, 370
pigment-induced, 368–369
in setting of cancer, 372–373
Acute lead poisoning, 607
Acute leukemia, 431–432
Acute liver failure (ALF), 240–241
Acute lymphoid leukemia (ALL), 432
Acute mania, 688
Acute meningitis, 322–323
Acute mercury inhalation, symptoms of,
607
Acute myeloid leukemia (AML), 432–433